MW01026262

The Body and Physical Difference

THE BODY, IN THEORY   Histories of Cultural Materialism

The Body and Physical Difference

DISCOURSES OF DISABILITY

David T. Mitchell and Sharon L. Snyder, Editors

Foreword by James I. Porter

Ann Arbor

The University of Michigan Press

Copyright © by the University of Michigan 1997
All rights reserved
Published in the United States of America by
The University of Michigan Press
Manufactured in the United States of America
⊗ Printed on acid-free paper

2004   2003   2002   2001   4   3   2

No part of this publication may be reproduced,
stored in a retrieval system, or transmitted in
any form or by any means, electronic, mechanical,
or otherwise, without the written permission
of the publisher.

*A CIP catalog record for this book is available
from the British Library.*

Library of Congress Cataloging-in-Publication Data

The body and physical difference : discourses of disability / David T.
   Mitchell and Sharon L. Snyder, editors.
       p.   cm. — (The body, in theory: Histories of Cultural Materialism)
   Includes bibliographical references.
   ISBN 0-472-09659-1 (hardcover : acid-free paper). — ISBN
0-472-06659-5 (pbk. : acid-free paper)
   1. Sociology of disability.   2. Humanities—Social aspects—
Methodology.   I. Mitchell, David T., 1962–   .   II. Snyder, Sharon
L., 1963–   .   III. Series: Body, in theory.
HV1568.B63   1997
362.4—dc21   97-20579
                                                              CIP

To Arnold Coran for making ends meet

Acknowledgments

When we first saw an announcement for a conference on "Discourses of Disability in the Humanities" posted on a university bulletin board, we were taken with the idea that our private theoretical musings on disability could be shared at a public event—in a familiar intellectual arena no less. Nandita Bantra and Pierre Etienne-Cudmore organized the conference that was held in Mayaguez, Puerto Rico, in 1992. This event not only provided the impetus for our first writing on representations of disability but also introduced us to several colleagues and (later) friends working in disability studies. Particularly we thank Marcy Epstein and Susan Crutchfield for acting as our tour guides and for their enthusiasm and commitment to the theorizing of disability in the humanities.

Harlan Hahn's work on disability paradigms, as well as his friendship, is much appreciated. Paul Longmore served as our intellectual guru and kept us on track by reading and commenting on an early draft of the introduction. Simi Linton has provided support and encouragement for our work at all stages. Many thanks to Rosemarie Garland Thomson, who has acted as our sounding board every step of the way. She not only put us in contact with several of the volume's essays and potential contributors but also made helpful suggestions on the manuscript. In addition, Rosemarie also participated in the successful establishment of the Modern Language Association Committee on Disability Issues in the Profession. Part of the mission of this committee entails the forwarding and recognition of disability studies. All of its other initial members, Lois Bragg, Brenda Brueggeman, Lennard Davis, Georgina Kleege, Nancy Mairs, and Ellen Stekert, have not only helped to keep the "studies" aspect of this committee's charge a central matter, but have offered collegial support at every turn.

We are grateful for Phyllis Franklin's unflagging committment to this committee. Raymond Ventre let us talk with him about our academic projects, and many thanks to Dean Marsden and Leonard Heldreth for their support and encouragement. Jim Livingston advised us on Shakespearean drama. Thomas Hyslop was unremittingly generous in providing computer counseling. Mary Letts and Rose Rosina have provided administrative support for many aspects of this and other projects. Likewise, staff at the Lydia Olson Library, including Jacquelyn Greising, Kathleen Kroll, Darlene Pierce, Richard Tremblay, and Ernie Young, were incredibly helpful and enabled us to acclimate to the challenge of research work in the "virtual library" of the Upper Peninsula.

Members of the Pediatric Surgery Unit at Mott Children's Hospital at the University of Michigan Medical Center provided both technologically brilliant care for our daughter and just cause for completing this volume. Our thanks to Arnold G. Coran M.D., Professor of Surgery, Head of Section of Pediatric Surgery, and Surgeon-in-Chief of Mott Children's Hospital, Dr. Linda Liu; Dr. Charles Cox; Dr. Donald Liu; Jennifer Chamberlain RN, MS; Marilyn Weimar RN, BSN; Laurie Wild RN, PNP; and Colleen Rauch. Jan Leonard and Debbie Davis at Holden Neonatal not only gave us hope but good advice (several times over).

We recollect, with gratitude, the many people at the University of Michigan who fostered our growth as scholars: Michael Awkward, Lillian Back, Ross Chambers, June Howard, Ira Konigsberg, John Kucich, Jim Porter, Alan Wald, and Susan White. Many thanks to our editor, LeAnn Fields, for nurturing this manuscript and for her friendship.

Horace H. Rackham School of Graduate Studies provided travel funds, as did the English department at Northern Michigan University. A Northern Michigan University Faculty Development Grant supported David Mitchell's work on this project in its early stages.

We are fortunate to have a supportive and caring family. Earl, Geraldine, Marianna, Estel, William, Shirley, Charlie, Laura, "Tight," Michael, and Sharon consoled us through graduate school and beyond. Thanks also to Dale and Kathy (and not only for upholding the integrity of the profession that this volume critiques). Nothing would be worth it without the pleasure that Cameron and Emma Jane bring to our life outside the academy.

Finally, Gary Treumer, Scott Timmerman, and Karen Lillie—our home nursing team in the wilderness—braved record Upper Peninsula snowfalls last winter to help us care for our daughter. It takes a plow to raise a child!

Grateful acknowledgment is made to the following authors, publishers, and journals for permission to reprint previously published material.

"In Search of Al Schmid: War Hero, Blinded Veteran, Everyman." Originally appeared in *Journal of American Studies* 29 (1995): 1–32. Copyright © 1995 Cambridge University Press. Reprinted with the permission of Cambridge University Press.

"Disabled Women as Powerful Women in Petry, Morrison, and Lorde: Revising Black Female Subjectivity." From *Extraordinary Bodies* by Rosemarie Thomson. Copyright © 1996 by Columbia University Press. Reprinted with permission of the publisher.

"Feminotopias: The Pleasures of 'Deformity' in the Mid Eighteenth-Century England." Originally appeared in Felicity A. Nussbaum's *Torid Zones: Maternity, Sexuality, and Empire in Eighteenth Century Narratives* pp. 135, 149–162. Copyright © 1995. The Johns Hopkins University Press.

"Defining the Defective: Eugenics, Aesthetics, and Mass Culture in Early-Twentieth-Century America" from *The Black Stork: Eugenics and the Death of "Defective" Babies in American Medicine and Motion Pictures Since 1915*, by Martin S. Pernick (New York: Oxford University Press, 1996). Copyright © 1996 Oxford University Press.

"Nude Venuses, Medusa's Body, and Phantom Limbs: Disability and Visuality," originally appeared as "Visualizing the Disabled Body" from *Enforcing Normalcy* by Lennard Davis is reproduced by kind permission of the publishers, Verso.

Every effort has been made to trace the ownership of all copyrighted material in this book and to obtain permission for its use.

Contents

PART 2 ▶ A History of Representations

Foreword
James I. Porter

How does one write the disabled body?

Current theories of the body are at a loss to say.

Viewed in itself (an essentializing perspective—but that is part of the point), a disabled body seems somehow *too much* a body, *too real*, too corporeal: it is a body that, so to speak, stands in its own way. From another angle, which is no less reductive, a disabled body appears to lack something essential, something that would make it identifiable and something to identify with; it seems *too little* a body: a body that is deficiently itself, not quite a body in the full sense of the word, *not real enough*.

There is something wrong with these two perceptions, but what is it? The answer has to do with the view of the body they presuppose: the body in itself, which is in fact a product of something else, namely the way in which the body is constructed in our culture today. Averted and silenced, the disabled body presents a threat to the very idea of the body, the body in its pure, empty form. It is this idea that informs the prevailing normativities of the body. And it informs current theoretical views of the body as well.

Either too real or not real enough, the disabled body appears the way it does on these views and in our culture because it disturbs our deepest fascinations with the body, our fantasies of the body. The fashionable exoticism of the body (the mutilated body, the obscene body, the body in pleasure or pain) does not threaten the idea of the body but only enhances it. However, the intrusion of a disabled body into these fantasies is disquieting in the extreme. In the presence of disability, the readily represented and fantasized body—the conventional object of body theory—stands in an awkward way. It seems strangely unreal by comparison.

One can take this comparison further. The implicit essentialism of so many theories of the body, a fact that is elicited in their (non)encounter with disablement, is a defense against the realities of bodies. The mere concept of the body shields theory from its objects; it protects us from confronting the body in any other way than as a fascination.

To recognize that the overwhelming corporealness, or lack thereof, that a disabled body projects is in some sense phantasmatic is not to diminish in any way the reality of disability. It is to locate the source of disability's stigmatization and avoidance. This act of avoidance is more commonplace than we may like to think. To the naked eye, fragments of bodies, widely fetishized in glamorous ads or wrapped in the aura of museums, are literal signs of disablement. In the cultivated imagination, they are ideals of bodily perfection. How culturally shaped is our perception of the body? And how much disavowal or psychic investment must go into the making of that perception? A point that surfaces repeatedly and strikingly in *The Body and Physical Difference: Discourses of Disability* is that disability is as much a symptom of historical and cultural contingencies as it is a physical and psychological reality.

Needless to say, cultural perceptions are not always so innocuous. The slide from denegation to negation and finally destruction, all premised on isolating the pure form of the body, or the pure form of its impurity, is a path that is all too easily taken. Witness, for example, the disastrous effects of the label "degeneracy" under the Nazi regime. The purity of a concept is its danger.

How does one write the disabled body, its history, its cultural forms, and its problematic repression? However one does, the aim must not be to "conquer" disability with comprehension or to drown it out with discourse—least of all through an all too familiar kind of academic industry. Instead, body theory must begin by naming its own incomprehension in the face of disability in all its forms.

The lesson of *The Body and Physical Difference* is clear: writing the disabled body will mean that our most basic conceptions of the body will need to be rewritten. Body theory will itself have to acknowledge its inadequate recognition of disability to date. Like the normative ideologies of the body to which they often stand opposed, theoretical discourses of the body already contain within themselves a series of unacknowledged and/or disavowed assumptions and theories about disability. Bringing these out for inspection is one way that body theory can begin to learn something from disability studies and can intervene in them in turn.

Their collaboration already looks promising.

Introduction ▶ Disability Studies and the Double Bind of Representation

David T. Mitchell and Sharon L. Snyder

> I want to speak to the despisers of the body. I would not
> have them learn and teach differently, but merely say
> farewell to their own bodies—and thus become silent.
> —Friedrich Nietzsche, *Thus Spoke Zarathustra*[1]

Defining Disability

This volume introduces questions on the representation of disability to critical discourses in the humanities such as the body, cultural studies, minority studies, history, and aesthetics.[2] Historically, disability has been the province of numerous professional and academic disciplines that concentrate upon the management, repair, and maintenance of physical and cognitive incapacity. Medicine, rehabilitation, special education, sociology, psychology, and a panoply of sub-specialties have all established their scientific and social credentials (as well as their very professional legitimacy) through the "humane" study and provision of services to disabled populations that are at the outermost margins of social interest and cultural value. In fact, the value of these "healing professions" has been largely secured by their willingness to attend to populations seen as inherently lacking and unproductive within the social circuit. We rarely consider that the continual circulation of professionally sponsored stories about disabled people's limitations, dependencies, and abnormalities proves necessary to the continuing existence of these professional fields of study.[3] Disability has spawned and bolstered an array of professional and academic fields by symbolizing the purest example of a "special needs" community.

The predominance of disability in the biological, social, and cognitive sciences parallels an equally ominous silence within the humanities. Perhaps because disabilities are exclusively narrated as debilitating phenomena in need of medical intervention and correction, the humanities have not privileged disability as a foundational category of social experience or symbolic investment. In fact, while literary and cultural studies have resurrected social identities such as gender, sexuality, class, and race from their attendant obscurity and neglect in the social and hard sciences, disability has suffered a distinctly different disciplinary fate.[4] In spite of the historical reliance upon images of disability in artistic discourses and critical practices (as the essays in this volume demonstrate), our professional vocabularies and methodologies eschew analyses that allow readers to attend to the meanings of disability's omnipresent utility.[5] What is certain in this contradictory treatment of disability in the sciences and the humanities is that in either case the disabled experience is never imagined to offer its own unique and valuable perspective.[6]

Our notion in this volume of the pervasive absence of a disability perspective is twofold. First, we want to demonstrate that rarely do scholarly discussions of the body in the sciences or the humanities anticipate that people with disabilities are part of their readership. Thus, the idea of disabled populations, patients, or individuals is usually introduced as if they represent a separate entity outside of the written and research context of the work itself. This is still the case even in recent work on disability. For example, in a 1995 essay collection entitled *Disability and Culture,* the editors include work by only one author out of nearly forty contributors who identifies himself as having a disability. This problem is indicative of writing mobilized from a service-oriented perspective on behalf of people with disabilities rather than research and writing that self-consciously issues from a community of scholars with disabilities. Second, while this collection does not seek to promote scholarship on disability written only by those with disabilities, the paucity in the field of academics and researchers with disabilities points to the invisibility of disabled academics in general. As with other marginalized constituencies such as women, ethnic, and racial scholars, the study of disability will help to clear a path for a more inclusive representation of this population in the profession. A visible increase in the numbers of scholars with disabilities would radically affect the ways in which we imagine this constituency's relationship within and to social institutions.

In this volume we use the term *disability* to designate cognitive and physical conditions that deviate from normative ideas of mental ability and physiological function. Borrowing from the legislative definition of disability that was outlined in section 504 of the Rehabilitation Act of 1973 (29 USC 794), the Americans with Disabilities Act recognizes three distinct facets of disability: (1) the impairment of a major life function, (2) an official diagnostic record that identifies a history of an individual's impairment; and (3) a trait or characteristic that results in the stigmatization of the individual as limited or incapacitated.[7] Such an expansive definition identifies the terms *disability* and *disabled* as denoting more than a medical condition or an essentialized "deformity" or difference. Unlike the terms *handicapped* and *crippled,* which suggest inherent biological limitations and individual abnormalities, this collection employs a definition of disability that denotes the social, historical, political, and mythological coordinates that define disabled people as excessive to traditional social circuits of interaction and as the *objects* of institutionalized discourses. The term does not seek to diminish or deny the variables and limitations that comprise the physical lives of disabled people, but rather to forward a notion of physicality that is cross-sectioned with and informed by narratives of malignancy, excessive dependency, and the parasitism of a special needs community. *Disability* provides a definition of a limited physical body that is not simultaneously assumed to be extraneous to definitions of citizenry and humanity. Approaching questions of disability in this manner allows scholars to consider the social, artistic, and political uses that disability has served. The study of disability in the humanities simultaneously delineates a unique subjectivity of disability and identifies the social phantasms projected upon the disabled subject in history.

The medical philosopher Georges Canguilhem has pointed out that "[l]ife rises to the consciousness and science of itself only through maladaption, failure and pain," thus placing disability, illness, and the aging process all along a continuum of normative physiology rather than labeling them as abnormal pathological states of being.[8] Yet, while categories such as illness and aging also come replete with associations of physical debility and social suspicions of diminished productivity, disability bears the onus of a permanent biological condition such as race and gender from which the individual cannot extricate him- or herself. People with disabilities, as Robert Murphy explains, suffer "a contamination of identity," for their conditions are understood to be embedded in the very fabric of their physical and moral personhood.[9] This socially defined experience of organismic contamination situates the disabled person as one who harbors more than just a physical/cognitive limitation or difference: disability infuses every aspect of his or her social being. This equation of physical disability with social identity creates a tautological link between biology and self (imagined or real) that cannot be unmoored—the physical world provides the material evidence of an inner life (corrupt or virtuous) that is secured by the mark of visible difference. Disabled people, by definition, do not enjoy the biological luxury of recovery that informs the more transient experiences of illness, disease, or disorder. As Julia Epstein points out: "whatever their cause, diseases remain *processes* that follow a *course* . . . [whereas] disability is the absence of ability."[10]

Since diseases "follow a *course*" and therefore prove familiar and domesticated by virtue of a belief in their determinate status (i.e., the ability to confidently narrate their future), disability might be characterized as that which exceeds a culture's predictive capacities and effective interventions. Since effective predictions and interventions change over history, bodily differences classified as nonnormative, monstrous, or disabling also shift from one epoch to another. Yet the particular and peculiar nature of disability is this definitive unpredictability within social narratives. Disability defies correction and tends to operate according to its own idiosyncratic rules. In fact, this resistance to cure or successful rehabilitation determines disability's unnatural status in medical and social discourse: people with disabilities are said to be fated or unsalvageable and, thus, somehow stubbornly inhuman. They constitute a population in possession of differences that will not respond to treatment, and the resulting *stigma*—to use Erving Goffman's term[11]—consequently situates the disabled person within the social space of difference that forever alienates the "afflicted" from the normative conventions of everyday social and scientific interaction.

> [A]n individual who might have been received easily in ordinary social inter-course possesses a trait that can obtrude itself upon attention and turn those of us whom he meets away from him, breaking the claim that his other attributes have on us. He possesses a stigma, an undesired differentness from what we had anticipated.[12]

This "undesired differentness" hypermarks the chance encounters of daily life with the discomfort of a stigma that becomes the subject (stated or not) of the social exchange itself. Goffman analyzes how the insinuation of one's disability into social interactions demonstrates that physical difference structures and pervades all aspects (linguistic, bodily, personal) of one's relational identity. As Goffman points out, the violation of expectations here hinges upon an unnatural claim made by the disability upon the attentions of the participants. There seems to be no getting away from it, and the consequences are such that it must serve as the topic of every exchange with affected individuals or cause a break in the claims that the individual's other characteristics attempt to make. The ill or the aged participate in a natural cycle of biological processes and breakdowns, but people with disabilities possess a biology that does not conform to even the most radical operations of normalization.

The Minoritization of Disability

Despite the renewed visibility of a vigilant civil rights activism that led to the passage of the Americans with Disabilities Act in 1990, disabled identities pose significant difficulties for inclusion alongside other minority and identity models. This is despite the fact that 69.1 percent of disabled individuals in the United States live below the poverty line,[13] and thus by extension disabled populations exist on the outermost margins of social access to all influential cultural institutions. Recent figures of the World Health Organization identify disabled people as comprising 6 or 7 percent of any given population and indicate that there are about 240 million disabled people globally.[14] Such figures define a population that represents one of the largest minority groups in the world. Although cultures radically vary in their treatment and definition of this value-laden constituency, the editors of *Disability and Culture* (the work containing the previously mentioned figures) make it clear that in the majority of cultures physical difference is understood in terms of physical incapacity, special needs accommodations, and statistical deviance.[15]

Consequently, while disability, at first glance, would seem to share with other socially stigmatized identities visible physical characteristics that link external or perceptible differences to internal deficits, critical parallels with other minoritized identities have been slow in coming.[16] Whereas feminist and racial discourses in the humanities have produced a significant corpus of work that exposes race, gender, sexuality, and nationality as physical markers that have accumulated historical and symbolic associations of limitation and deviance, disability has rarely been included in catalogs of marginalized social groupings. Indeed, the push to expose physical difference as an ideological phantasm has, ironically, resulted in the further reification of disability as the term absented from our social models. While physical aberrancy is often recognized as constructed and historically variable it is rarely remarked upon as its own delegitimized or politically fraught identity.

This omission spans a range of academic discourses on the "body" extending from philosophy to film studies. In the past two years alone we have seen a veritable explosion of works that foreground terms such as *the body, the corporeal,* and *the grotesque* as the material of their scholarly investigations.[17] Selected titles that emphasize these terms include the following: *American Anatomies: Theorizing Race and Gender,*[18] *Bodies That Matter: On the Discursive Limits of "Sex,"*[19] *Body Criticism,*[20] *Deviant Bodies: Critical Perspectives on Difference in Science and Popular Culture,*[21] *The Female Grotesque: Risk, Excess, and Modernity,*[22] *Thinking Bodies,*[23] *Troubled Bodies: Critical Perspectives on Postmodernism, Medical Ethics, and the Body,*[24] and *Volatile Bodies: Towards a Corporeal Feminism.*[25] The current popularity of the body in critical discourse seeks to incorporate issues of race, gender, sexuality, and class while simultaneously neglecting disability. These studies share a penchant for detecting social differences as they are emblematized in corporeal aberrancies. Within this common critical methodology physical difference exemplifies the evidence of social deviance even as the constructed nature of *physicality itself* fades from view.

Among a multitude of examples, Judith Halberstam's study of the racial and sexual codings of gothic fiction, *Skin Shows: Gothic Horror and the Technology of Monsters,* provides us with a case in point.

Within the nineteenth-century Gothic, authors mixed and matched a wide variety of signifiers of difference to fabricate the deviant body. Dracula, Jekyll/Hyde, and even Frankenstein's monster before them are lumpen bodies, bodies pieced together out of the fabric of race, class, gender, and sexuality.[26]

The preceding quotation crystallizes the strategic move endemic to much of our current critical commentary.[27] The location of monstrosity with visible bodily deformation demonstrates that monsters themselves host an array of disabilities that hypermark them as social abominations.[28] Yet, when we turn our critical attention to the rationale undergirding this superfluous bodily distortion, inevitably disability metamorphoses into the signifier of "race, class, gender, and sexuality." While this important critical elision is not intended to deny that "lumpen bodies" are racialized, sexed, and/or classed, their identification quickly usurps and outdistances the physical characteristics that signaled an ideologically constructed body in the first place.

Such an observation marks the representational double bind of disability. While disabled populations are firmly entrenched on the outer margins of social power and cultural value, the disabled body also serves as the raw material out of which other socially disempowered communities make themselves visible. While deformities of the surface signal an ideologically inflected body, disability is rarely coupled with the othering terms of this critical chain of identities. In fact, once the bodily surface is exposed as the phantasmatic facade that disguises the workings of patriarchal, racist, heterosexist, and upper class norms, the monstrous body itself is quickly forgotten. This jettisoning of the monstrous body allows critics to point out that physical difference is a constructed phenomenon. Any attempt to distance disenfranchised communities from the fantasy of deformity further entrenches the disabled as the "real" abnormality from which all other nonnormative groups must be distanced.[29] Within these theories the disabled body represents both a projection of dominant ideology and the source of a verifiable malignancy that must be refuted.

These scenarios point to a veritable panic in our current critical discussion of the meaning of monstrosity and physical (or cognitive) aberrancy. Not only has disability been used as a sign that links politics to aesthetics in criticism, it has held down the terms of a critique of a uniquely modern social disorder. The influential postmodern philosopher, Paul Virilio, in concert with other commentators who bemoan the vagaries and insubstantialities of the age of hypertext, designates disabled constituencies as the common denominator of a contemporary penchant for self-willed immobility and technological dependency. In the opening essay of the collection *Re-Thinking Technologies*, Virilio quotes Francois Mitterand's peroration at an international colloquium on the handicapped: "Cities will have to be adapted to their citizens, and not the other way around. We must open the city to handicapped citizens. I demand that a global politics for the handicapped become a strong axis of social Europe."[30] Virilio includes Mitterand's articulation of the politicized nature of architecture and city planning in order to demonstrate how demands for accessible environments threaten to make special needs citizens of us all. His commentary upon the demand to adapt cities appropriates Mitterand's point as symptomatic of a dangerous postmodern mind-set.

> If every one of us is obviously in agreement that the handicapped person has to live as others do and therefore *with others,* it is no less revealing to note the similarities that now exist between the reduced mobility of the equipped invalid and the growing inertia of the over-equipped, "valid" human population.[31]

Even though Virilio begins his remark with a nod toward liberal inclusivity, disabled populations become the exemplary consumers of a world characterized by the alienating distance of telecommunications that keep citizens at home and out of the loop of a more genuine and robust social interaction. Virilio's comparison of the "reduced mobility of the equipped invalid" with the "growing inertia of the over-equipped, 'valid' human population," though deliberately scandalous, nonetheless betrays key precepts of an ableist philosophy. His admonition to audiences about the dangerous lure hidden in technological prostheses results in a stereotypical equation of disabled populations, technological fetishism, and welfare state dependency.[32]

One has to appreciate Virilio's flamboyance; he exposes the extent to which postmodern liberation politics are premised upon disability panic. This logic reifies a normative lifestyle of the able bodied at the same time that it turns an "invalid" population into paradigmatic consumers of technology and accessibility. Clearly, a primary objective of an international disability rights movement—to expose the ableist ideology that underpins architecture and city planning—has put disability rights advocates at odds with cultural critics such as Virilio, who would invoke memories of nonartificial neighborhoods and terrorize audiences with comparisons between the involuntary "heavy metal" body of an "invalid" and the compensations afforded by high-tech prosthetic luxuries. In contrast, the disability community has been founded upon the understanding that ability serves public policy and philosophy alike as a historically and culturally variable term. It is through their common association with incapacity and aberrancy that people with enormously varied bodily experiences and capacities come to share a political and communal identity. Disability acts as a loose rubric and as an amalgam of dissimilar physical and cognitive traits that often have little in common other than the social stigma of limitation, deviance, and inability.

Virilio's staging of the problem enables us to contemplate the extent to which a disabled citizenry is central to social theory and postmodern philosophy. Over the past twenty years, even as disability rights advocacy has become more prominent, cultural critics have worked to demonstrate how the definitions of human "wholeness" and "integrity" are shifted by technological innovations. In this way, and in a more benign and sweeping fashion, disability underwrites the cultural studies of technology *writ large*. Unlike Virilio, essayists on postmodern science and culture such as N. Katherine Hayles, Avital Ronell, and Donna Haraway deploy disabled bodies as proof of our fascination with "cyborglike" prosthetic enhancement.[33] The apparatus of disability shows up in numerous postmodern catalogs without comment on the conflictual relationship of disabled people to the equipment that theoretically affords them access to able-bodied populations, architectural structures, and cultural commodities. Nor is there any serious effort to specify the nature of this usage within disabled communities themselves.[34] As N. Katherine Hayles comments:

> Already about 10% of the U.S. population are cyborgs in the technical sense, including people with electronic pacemakers, prosthetic limbs, hearing aids, drug implants, and artificial joints. V[irtual] R[eality] would substantially increase this percentage. If the extent to which one has become a cyborg is measured in terms of impact on psychic/sensory organization rather than difficulty detaching parts, VR users . . . are more thoroughly cyborgs than people with pacemakers.[35]

Such a comparison inverts Virilio's alarmist message by competitively squaring off the prosthetic agility and technological dependencies of disabled people against virtual reality buffs. In doing so, Hayles levels the cyborgian playing field in order to establish a more inclusive definition of the "prosthetically altered" body. While one may debate whether or not "difficulty [in] detaching parts" adequately describes the psychic/sensory impact of living one's life on a respirator, with an artificial limb, or in a wheelchair, Hayles forgoes a discussion of disabled people's more obvious status as "cyborgs" in order to privilege the *chosen* prosthetic identification of computer hackers and video junkies. Between Virilio and Hayles we have come full circle, from a discussion of the dangers of technological fetishism to an embrace of the titillating sensations of artificial augmentation. Yet, rarely do critics venture toward an elucidation of the experience of the population that underwrites either critical system.

All of these examples speak to the glaring omission of a disability studies perspective. Indeed, if one of the most common experiences of disabled people is that they are made to feel alone in their attempts to procure environmental access or to challenge the pathological narratives of their bodies presented in medicine and by the culture at large, disability scholars have experienced their own disciplinary and professional segregation and isolation. In response, this volume brings together essays by scholars seeking to understand the nature of such a critical and cultural elision by privileging disability as their own methodological objective. In the past few years we have witnessed the publication of works that either approach the question of disability from a humanities perspective or self-consciously announce themselves as proffering a disability studies perspective: Lennard Davis's *Enforcing Normalcy: Disability, Deafness, and the Body*,[36] Arthur Frank's *The Wounded Storyteller: Body, Illness, and Ethics*,[37] Diane Price Herndl's *Invalid Women: Figuring Feminine Illness in American Fiction and Culture, 1840–1940*,[38] David Hevey's *The Creatures That Time Forgot: Photography and Disability Image*,[39] Martin Norden's *The Cinema of Isolation: A History of Disability in the Movies*,[40] Rosemarie Garland Thomson's *Extraordinary Bodies: Figuring Physical Disability in American Culture and Literature*,[41] and David Wills's *Prosthesis*.[42] The publication of these texts establishes that the study of disability helps to explain the complex contours of able-bodied persons' mythologies about disability and also provides a field of inquiry within which to imagine a more humane constellation of stories about physical and cognitive difference.

The Private Subject of Disability

The discourse of disability has been largely defined by the genre of autobiography. Guided by the assumption that people with disabilities need to write their own stories in order to counteract the dehumanizing effects of societal representations and attitudes, these personal narratives usually offer the narrator as a disputatious figure critiquing the less than humane responses of a flat, often hostile, and uniformly able-ist culture. Such an impulse has inevitably invested its literary capital in personal narrative models that project the disabled subject as a lone figure against the uncomprehending universe of social discrimination and institutional disenfranchisement. As we follow the first person narrator through vignettes that illustrate the daily round of humiliations and insensitivities that comprise the lives of disabled people, the reader grows increasingly aware that inaccessibility involves more than the provision of ramps, curb cuts, and accessible public toilets (although the lack of these structural features literally prevents people with disabilities from engaging in meaningful participation in communities and institutions). The autobiographical narrator also provides a glimpse at a unique subjectivity that evolves out of the experience of disability as a physical, cognitive, and social phenomenon.

In one of the best known essays among disability studies scholars in the humanities, "On Being a Cripple," Nancy Mairs formulates some of the curious paradoxes of physical incapacitation and being. For Mairs, disease and disorder serve up frustrating personal scenarios that must be creatively negotiated, and her inclination is to approach the question of life as a "cripple" from a private point of view that foregrounds the "hassles" of "being crippled." Such a scrutiny of attitudes that comprise the interior life of the autobiographical subject of disability (she has multiple sclerosis) serves to direct attention to her own "peculiar history" of responses to physical "limitation."[43]

Because Mairs focuses upon the personal travails and negotiations that define living with a disability, the essay's perspective strategically shifts attention away from institutional pathology and social attitudes toward the individual's experience of disability. Hence, while Mairs goes on to assess the "discomforts" of parents, doctors, colleagues, and children, her analysis remains cloistered in the "less comfortable" arena of personal depression, "self loathing," and debilitating paranoia. Mairs describes the private coordinates of bodily experience as a sporadic and unpredictable biological march into future deterioration. The value and appeal of her work hinge upon its no-nonsense approach to the traumas and ironies of a life that remains ambiguously tethered to the daily experience of pain and bodily breakdown. Her narrative style offers a shockingly intimate portrait of a disabled woman who unveils her most private thoughts and scathing self-critiques as a way of using disability to burrow down into the psychic and physical depths of human affairs.

Mairs's approach dovetails with many contemporary attempts by autobiographers of disability to expand the array of options from which to imagine the lives of people with disabilities. The genre of "life stories" that has come to be synonymous with the literature of disability serves as an important gateway into the interior conflicts and psychology of disability. Such first person narratives provide readers with an alternative perspective on what it means to live with a disability in a culture obsessed with forging equations between physical ability, beauty, and productivity. Autobiographical narratives demand that the disabled subject develop a voice that privileges the agency of a bona fide perspective of disability. Given the presupposition that the "able-bodied" could never adequately dramatize the encounters between disability, personal experience, and "unaware" social policies, what motivates these stories is the pressing need for true-life verification that disability provides a specific and distinct perspective of its own.

The autobiographical narrative of disability tools disability as a private and "minority" concern, one that requires the attention of the culture because the social arena has proven inadequate to the task of responding—both legislatively and morally—to a population located on the fringes of institutional access. Nonetheless, first person narratives of disability have historically fed a public appetite for confessional writing that promises the revelation of personal catastrophe as the evidence of a more truthful access to secreted lives. The confessional mode places physical and cognitive limitation and difference on display to be consumed, and the mainstream parading of personal misfortune inevitably assures the reader/viewer of his or her comparative good fortunes or assuages a shared societal sense of guilt and insensitivity. Disability falls readily into conventional scenarios of triumph over tragedy or stories of saintly suffering where the afflicted fades away (physically and intellectually) into private martyrdom. As Lennard Davis points out, "by narrativizing an impairment, one tends to sentimentalize it, and link it to the bourgeois sensibility of individualism and the drama of an individual story."[44] The personal narrative expands the boundaries of our understanding of disability on an individual level, but its attendant social and political contexts tend to be overshadowed by the emotions of pity and/or sympathy evoked by the reader's identification with the narrator's personal plight. Consequently, first person narratives cannot singularly provide the interpretive paradigms needed to revise cultural understandings of disability.

While wide-ranging social critiques of disability are often downplayed or ignored in the public reception of autobiography, such recent histories of disability activism as those documented in Lennard Davis's *Enforcing Normalcy*,[45] David Hevey's *The Creatures Time Forgot: Photography and Disability Imagery*,[46] and Joseph P. Shapiro's *No Pity: People with Disabilities Forging a New Civil Rights Movement*[47] contextualize disability as a socially constructed identity. The main thrust of these political treatises has been to reject the trite sentiments of mainstream representations of disabilities as "pitiful," "leprous," or "catastrophic" individual conditions. Critiques of social responses to disability have extended to such institutional fixtures as Jerry Lewis's MDA telethon, the human genome project, Social Security regulations, welfare laws, mainstream movies, television "disease-of-the-week" portrayals, art photography, federal funding for the nursing home industry, and the "right-to-die" movement. These philosophical explorations endeavor to place the neglected moral, legislative, and social issues of disability at the center of an evolving national agenda.

While the reasons for the historical omission of disabled communities from prevailing social agendas have been construed from many vantage points and attributed to many causes, disabled writers and scholars of disability have consistently agreed upon one point: the neglect of people with disabilities has resulted in their preeminent social invisibility. For instance, two groundbreaking anthologies published in the 1980s—Alan Gartner and Tom Joe's collection, *Images of the Disabled/Disabling Images* and Michelle Fine and Adrienne Asch's volume, *Women with Disabilities: Essays in Psychology, Culture, and Politics*[48]—argue in their introductions that disabled people can be most accurately defined as an ignored population in academic and public discourses of identity, civil rights, and representation. As with most minority populations who have sought to break down the barriers of racial, class, and gendered discrimination, disability studies scholars define their political program as an effort to redress the social "voicelessness" and institutional neglect of disabled people. This absence of models for comprehending the lives of people with disabilities has led to the articulation of two parallel problems: (1) disabled people have been portrayed inadequately in mainstream media presentations and have suffered from their historical invisibility in other representational arenas; and (2) in the wake of the passage of the 1990 Americans with Disabilities Act the new visibility of disabled constituencies has produced the need for cultural institutions to locate alternative vocabularies for responding to this population.

While critiques of stereotypes have comprised a significant portion of the literature and criticism of disability thus far, these studies often overlook narrative as a privileged space for contemplating disability as an individual *and* social phenomenon. *The Body and Physical Difference: Discourses of Disability* outlines the coordinates of a disability studies approach in the humanities by interrogating a pervasive cultural and artistic dependency upon disability. All the essays in this volume have taken as a guiding principle that a disability studies approach to representations of disability will yield more than symptomatic, flat characterizations of disabled people. Analyses of disability in art, popular media, and history have much to teach us about the role of disability in culture than the assumption that lives defined as disabling (and hence unlivable or unworthy) go unrepresented and un(der)appreciated by audiences and cultures. This research inquires into the impact of representational discourses such as literature, film, television, and photography upon social perceptions of disability and the subjectivities of the disabled alike.

Characterizing Disability Studies

In part, investigating the impact of representational discourses upon perceptions of both disabilities and disabled communities involves the scrutiny of character types developed through the differentiating function of physical and psychological difference. Disability studies grapples with the metaphorical and symbolic values that disability has represented. Other than in autobiography, disability seldom has been explored as a condition or experience in its own right; instead disability's psychological and bodily variations have been used to metaphorize nearly every social conflict outside of its own ignoble predicament in culture. Consequently, the essays in this volume seek to forward an understanding of the discourses of disability in ways that are not strictly connected to elucidating the experience of disability itself. Each essay in this collection seeks to explore the historical, social, political, and metaphorical contours of disability in order to discern the manner and method of the category's symbolic deployment in art.

Of the collections currently available in disability studies, only Marsha Saxton and Florence Howe's edited volume, *With Wings: An Anthology of Literature by and about Women with Disabilities,* describes the significance of literature to questions of disability and representation. Saxton and Howe explain literature's applicability to questions of disability and disabled populations with a humanistic formula.

Literature is an important and effective tool for education and social change. Literature illuminates the details of daily living, the tiniest aspects of life experience, and at the same time the deepest meanings of this experience. Literature may point out social ills, while offering new possibilities; it communicates pain and transcends it. Literature speaks powerfully and profoundly, as well as subtly, delicately.[49]

Saxton and Howe provide a brief outline of a more positivistic program located in the promise of literature's commitment to the detailing of lives and experiences that artistic portraits often provide. The passage points to the authority that readers attribute to literary endeavor as a social instrument of change, for personal pain can sometimes prove a catalyst for the correction of social injustice. At the same time, the passage sidesteps the ways in which even the most revered literary texts embody the prejudices and debilitating attitudes of their own historical moments of production. This double-edged formulation makes literature both a utilitarian tool of transformation and a medium for further stigmatizing disability in the imaginations of its audience.

This volume seeks to demonstrate that disabled bodies and lives have historically served as the crutch upon which artistic discourses and cultural narratives have leaned to ensure the novelty of their subject matter. While these essays share a respect for art's often profound abilities to weave the intricate web of public lives and private negotiations of disability, each openly scrutinizes literature's often hazardous complicity in the "ideology of the physical." The ideology of the physical constructs an imagined bridge between bodily differences and individual abilities. Historically, the physical surface has existed as a medium that exposes the more abstract and intangible landscapes of psychology, morality, and spirituality. We use the terms *physical* and *bodily* here to designate any discernible characteristic designated by a culture as definitively abnormal and tending toward the pathological. Thus, the ideology of the physical trades upon perceptions of functional disabilities such as missing or "stunted" appendages, mobility impairments, blindness, and deafness, as well as cosmetic distortions such as cleft palates, facial tics, or the presence of an extra finger or toe. Yet, physical or bodily differences also include "nonmaterial" traits that mark one as disabled, such as the sound of a voice filtered through an electronic vocal cord stimulator or the cognitive impairments associated with the speech and thought patterns of people with traumatic head injuries or the "mentally defective." The bridge constructed by the ideology of the physical seeks to lure the reader/viewer into the mystery of whether discernible defects reveal the presence of an equally defective moral and civil character.

The most frequently cited literary example of this phenomenon occurs in Shakespeare's *Richard III*. Shakespeare's play mercilessly trades for its dramatic interest upon the villainous behavior of the hunchbacked Duke of Gloucester in his "unnatural" ascent to the throne. From the outset Richard's treachery appears to issue from the severity of his physical deformities. The protagonist, himself, openly conspires with the audience in the ascription of his villainy to his misshapen figure.

> [B]ut I, that am not shaped for sportive tricks,
> Nor made to court an amorous looking glass;
> I that am rudely stamped and want love's majesty
> . . . .
> And therefore, since I cannot prove a lover
> . . . .
> I am determined to prove a villain.[50]

Throughout the play, Richard soliloquizes upon the relationship between his illegitimate usurpation of the throne and his multiple physical deformities that mark him as "so lamely and unfashionable that dogs bark at me as I halt by them."[51] His assassinations of friends, family members, and children display a vicious and essentialized brutality, while also garnering significance and dramatic interest for the political issue Richard makes of his own deformity. His motives issue from his exclusion, as a disabled man, from the "idle pleasures" of England in peacetime, but while he claims vengeance upon the world, witches, and "dissembling Nature" that brought him into the world "before [his] time" and "scarce half made up" (calling upon the sixteenth-century belief that maternal misdeeds bring about "defects" in their offspring),[52] he faults those who would point out his moral defects, claiming that they discriminate against a "misshapen" man.

Richard's character openly engages the audience in a performance of the multiple and contradictory significations of a disabled body. His figure evidences all of the following attributes over the course of the play: a social burden; metaphysical sign of divine disfavor; evidence of the machinations of a divine plan in history; that a disabled child is retribution for parental weakness; that a disabled subject follows a deterministic trajectory in life; he is the bearer of an entrenched identity (pathetic or vengeful); he is the literal embodiment of the evidence of the fall of man; he personifies the fiendish specter of war; he is singular and exceptional rather than common and ordinary; he can be viewed as the most interior to a social order (the most human in suffering) or the most exiled (lacking in natural human affections); his physical excesses provide a ready source material for caricature. Finally, a scapegoat patterning to the play reiterates exile as a culturally sanctioned historical solution to the social disruption that disabled people are perceived to present. Shakespeare solidifies an array of perverse motivations while ventriloquizing these associations through Richard's perspective and thus, lends them the cast of factuality by placing them in the mouth of a disabled character. Overall, *Richard III* offers a cautionary tale in the formula of a double negative: do not distrust a natural correspondence between physical "imperfections" and villainy.[53]

Indeed, historical repetition has so naturalized the *ideology of the physical* that it has become a generic convention: even if it does not bear the markings of factuality and truth, it yields the pleasure of universal recognition. Al Pacino's recent restaging of the play as a documentary film, *Looking for Richard,* sets into motion (once again) the search for the meaning of the mystery that Richard's character embodies.[54] The generational imperative to "pursue" the essence of such an elusive figuration brings Pacino back full circle to what every generation of critics before has already discovered: disablity *is* motivation embodied. This tautological equation becomes the artistic holy grail itself; what begins as the most alien and inexplicable of life forms yields what is most commonplace and familiar. Generations of artists and critics willingly set out on this ritualized artistic travel narrative in search of the assurance that the mystery can be resolved, and in so doing we confirm that disability's physical and psychological *disorder* can be recontained and domesticated from the safe distance of art's voyeuristic gaze.

Representational media secure our attention as readers and viewers in the double bind of our fascination/repulsion with physical difference. This titillating oscillation between binary sentiments develops out of the voyeuristic promise upon which poetry, plays, fiction, and films trade. Physical and cognitive differences mark lives as inscrutable and mysterious, and thus we approach these artistically embellished differences with a distanced curiosity that simulates intimacy while staving off the risk of an encounter. We experience disability through an anticipation of our desire to "know" the secret labyrinths of difference, without significantly challenging our investment in the construction of difference itself. Whether the narrative in question cements the link between disability and moral corruption or severs the association between difference and impurity, we find ourselves fascinated with the exploration of their potential alliance and repulsed by the possibility, fulfilled or not. Once narrative mobilizes the question of disability's ambiguous relationship to morality a duality is established, and the point is not whether the connection is forged or broken but rather that the two perpetually coexist and define each other. Readers' experience of the dual pleasures of fascination and repulsion also evolve out of an ability to leave the site of a fiction with our own membership in normalcy further consolidated and assured.

Consequently, the productive relationship between narrative discourses in the humanities and disability often proves to be a precarious one. As Dierdre Lynch explains in her study of eighteenth-century portraiture and caricature, the line between mimetic art and cartoonish satire is a fine one that disabled characters always threaten to collapse: "quantity undermines the positive claims of singularity by threatening inflation: more description and more detail may well define but they eventually disfigure. Added strokes, intended to flesh out a character, turn a portrait into a worthless lampoon or, worse, into something monstrous and unnameable."[55] Is Shakespeare's portrait of Richard III a historical portrait or a regal caricature because of the prominence given to his disabilities? While the introduction to the aforementioned *With Wings* volume proffers a glimpse into the promise that literature affords, art's relationship to social and political change refuses any purely positivist program. Scholars working in disability studies survey and analyze the range of uses for disability in narrative, provide methods for assessing the potential of these representational devices, and trouble our own predispositions to secure a privileged space for artistic vision.

The arguments offered in the essays that follow all scrutinize disability's link to the *modus operandi* of genre in order to comprehend the means by which disabled figures provide a creative license to the process of character definition itself. Many of the essays that follow work toward definitions of the common disabled types that populate and help to define generic formulas. For example, Felicity Nussbaum interprets Sarah Scott's eighteenth-century novel, *Millenium Hall,* as offering a glimpse of a homosocial utopian women's community founded, in part, upon the social inclusion of women with disabilities. David Yuan's essay identifies narratives of the unsightly Civil War amputee who offends civil society's protocols for acceptable presentation. Cindy LaCom explores the centrality of the bedridden female protagonist of Victorian fiction as both a monstrous, asexual creation and as a new alternative for representing female sexuality and power. Jan Gordon evolves a theory of the gout-ridden patriarchy in order to symbolize crises within the patrilineal lines of the fin de siècle British upper class. David Gerber examines the divergent institutions and ideologies at work in the narration of blinded World War II veteran, Al Schmid. Paul Longmore identifies the story of the innocent victim of biological tragedy as a product of the U.S. telethon industry's manipulation of a middle class ethos of civic duty and moral obligation. Caroline Molina analyzes Jane Campion's use of her mute female protagonist in *The Piano* to represent women's voicelessness within patriarchy. Finally, Rosemarie Garland Thomson explores the ways in which twentieth-century African American women writers have used disabled female characters to symbolize the violence of racism and alternative values of bodily difference. Such a catalog reveals the pervasive presence of disability in film and literature by documenting an expansive array of disabled prototypes who populate our imaginative worlds.

Taking the primacy of disability in the discourses of the humanities as a starting point for the rationale and necessity of disability studies in the humanities, one comes immediately upon the paradox of disability's definitive invisibility in the cultural imaginary. Disability has been formulated as an inherently marginalized (and therefore "invisible") community within even the most "liberal" discussions concerning questions of representational politics, human rights, and institutional access. Yet, a survey of discourses in the humanities would demonstrate that disability has served not only as a category of artistic and social fascination but as one of the instrumental devices of narrative production.

Paul Longmore's foundational essay, "Screening Stereotypes: Images of Disabled People in Television and Motion Pictures," begins with a provocative question that clearly formulates this curious paradox: "Why do television and film so frequently screen disabled characters for us to see, and why do we usually screen them out of our consciousness even as we absorb them?"[56] For Longmore, this question can be partially answered by an analysis of the ways in which visual media pursue a quick fix to the distressing moral and social issues involved in the representation of disability. Longmore and other disability scholars demonstrate that popular media narrate disability as an isolated phenomenon that is largely a matter of individual fortitude, will power, and perseverance, rather than delving into questions of social accommodation. According to Longmore, the visual media have traditionally used disability as a sop to our beleaguered cultural consciences by assuring the viewer that the problem is a largely isolated affair that needs to be treated one disorder at a time.

Here we come to the crux of the problem that Longmore introduces: narratives of disability have relied upon the production of physical and psychological difference in every historical epoch, yet this dependency has rarely led to a widespread understanding of disability as a communal identity. The consequences of the paradoxical relationship between a desire to parade disability on the screen and the simultaneous assurance to audiences that these isolated situations are being taken care of situates visual media in a unique position with respect to our understanding of disability. Disability acts as a shorthand method of securing emotional responses from audiences because pathos, pity, and abhorrence have proved to be an integral part of the historical baggage of our understandings of disability. Repetitive associations between these more superficial emotive responses and the differences of physical and cognitive anomalies segregate disabled individuals as the exotic specimens of our most pervasive cultural narratives. The narrative theories of Susan Stewart explain that this contradictory process results in the invention of an "overheated social organism" that functions as an "outlet or exit" for continuously constructing fictional notions of normalcy and social acceptability.[57] In Stewart's words, "[t]he idiosyncratic [those populations that stand in for our notions of aberrancy and impropriety] occupies a space-time, more often than not, of the private room in the public square."[58] Disability studies seeks to understand the ways in which we produce the "private room" of disability in our most public discourses. This paradoxical representational process demonstrates the complexity of delineating disability as a symbolic space.

Such a history of metaphorical opportunism sits at the heart of the profound ambivalence that disabled populations inevitably feel when faced with the question of disability as a tool of artistic production. Literature, film, television, folklore, history, and philosophy (the primary discursive vectors in the humanities) straddle a critical divide that is not necessarily rehabilitative; instead they act as the textual space where physical limitations can be reworked as strengths, aberrancies can be deployed as compelling idiosyncracies, and villainous characters can be made comprehensible through psychic, sensory, and physical distortions. If disability has been summoned within the humanities to serve as a symbol of social conflict disability studies scrutinizes the nature and rationale of its symbolic manipulation within these discourses.

Studies of Disability in the Humanities

When one endeavors to locate vocabularies and disciplines about disability the options prove limited. For instance, medical interpretations of disability posit physical condition as a factual catalog of symptoms and diagnostic limitations that bind disability to a purely deterministic biological condition. One prominent historian of medicine and medical narratives, Ivan Illich, has characterized this objectifying process as the "degradation of intimate and meaning-endowing human experiences by transforming them into mere technical events."[59] The taxonomic impulse of empirical discourses in the biological and social sciences proves only to literalize and obscure the intangibles of individual variation. To limit humanity to the factual record of a deterministic biological catalog ultimately proves as devastating as any tradition of metaphorical application and appropriation of disability.

While medicine certainly provides an empirical antithesis to the more ephemeral products of art, the historical and mythic meanings embedded in the scientific terminology of empiricism that constructs physical and cognitive disability usually lie unanalyzed and, therefore, uncomprehended. A host of studies conducted by historians of medical science in the humanities, such as Sander Gilman, Ruth Bleir, Emily Martin, Paula Treichler, and others, have proved invaluable to an increasing suspicion and critical scrutiny of medicalized discourses.[60] The professional desire to prove scientifically the biological bases of pathology has historically reflected an elusive attempt to solidify cultural definitions of normalcy and superiority. Disability studies in the humanities must inevitably attend to the permutations of medical language as one crucial key to the social reception and construction of physical deviation.

This important avenue of critique in disability studies has its methodological roots in the work of Michel Foucault. Rather than accede to the authority of professional diagnosis, Foucault interrogates disciplinary investments in the will to diagnose as an effect of the pleasure-knowledge dyad.

Perhaps this production of truth, . . . multiplied, intensified, and even created its own intrinsic pleasures. We have at least invented a different kind of pleasure, the pleasure of knowing that truth, of discovering and exposing it, the fascination of seeing it and telling it, of captivating and capturing others by it, of confiding it in secret, of luring it out in the open—the specific pleasure of the true discourse on pleasure.[61]

Although Foucault's territory in this excerpt is the domain of the nineteenth-century prototype of contemporary sexologists, his exposé proves instructive for disability studies and the critique of diagnostic discourses. Rather than refuting the diagnosis itself—and thus in turn calling attention to the enunciation of its titillating bodily contours and physical prognoses—Foucault turns the medicalized gaze back upon itself. In doing so, he exposes a pleasure at the heart of professional activity that results in the will to produce a pathological subject of diagnosis.

Disability studies inevitably emphasizes a similar methodological objective. The essays in this collection attempt to return the products of a medicalized gaze—in history, science, art, and electronic media—back upon the source. Disability studies does not refuse or repress the uncertainties and limitations of biological conditions, but rather it exposes the pleasurable investments undergirding discourses that reproduce, expand, and tediously detail taxonomic catalogs of disability's pathological trajectories. What is the professional titillation that accompanies the exotic land of dysfunction and biological breakdown? How is the attempt to contain and control the chaotic text of disability integral to modern science's ability to manufacture itself as normalizing and authoritative? How have disabled populations been used to solidify and secure definitions of the altruistic service and moral commitments of diagnostic disciplines? Following some of the key tenets of Foucaultian theory, disability studies scholars endeavor to analyze the self-serving values and advantages of disability's circulation within all disciplines and cultural discourses. Collectively, scholars of disability seek to understand the various motivations, pleasures, and professional interests that are at stake in the historical construction of disability.

In part, as many of the essays in this collection demonstrate, the pursuit of alternatives to pathological models of disability is a historical project. All of the essayists in *The Body and Physical Difference* seek to unearth and understand the varied attitudes that have characterized disability across history and cultures. Since we arrive in our own historical moment replete with an awareness of disability's malignant repertoire, one is tempted to assume that disability has always played host to a similar array of deforming and malignant associations. Yet, while this has been the case during many historical periods (particularly near the end of centuries when millennial scenarios of future utopias and cultural collapse loom large),[62] one cannot generalize about the social meanings of disability across historical epochs or cultures. For instance, Martha L. Edwards's essay, "Constructions of Physical Disability in the Ancient Greek World: The Community Concept," analyzes the ways in which the Greek aesthetic of ideal bodily forms did not automatically lead to the parallel stigmatization of disability as a corruption of that utopic and artistic impulse. Using a methodology that she terms a "community model of disability" that defines physicality as a culturally constructed phenomenon, Edwards argues that the category of disability was largely an absent term in Greek vocabularies. This absence for Edwards suggests that having a disability did not result in one's ostracism from significant cultural activities. Felicity Nussbaum's reading of Sarah Scott's novel, *Millenium Hall,* identifies a narrative of an eighteenth-century utopian women's community that privileges physical "monstrosity" as one criterion of membership. Capitalizing upon disabled women's expulsion from heterosexual and patriarchal rituals of courtship, maternity, and domesticity, Scott presents an alternative female society that functions "as a harmonious community of reason, reflection, and freedom to speak that is unattainable outside of its confines." These alternative historical moments identified by Edwards and Nussbaum proffer a glimpse into the historical variables of disability's representation.

In discussions of the ways in which disability has been historically represented in literature and history, disability studies scholars have also begun to identify a working catalog of disability's cultural meanings. Such a catalog reflects ableist projections onto disability, and consequently, a compilation of these restrictive narrative possibilities reveals the method by which disability has been colonized in rhetoric and metaphor. Martin S. Pernick's essay, "Defining the Defective: Eugenics, Aesthetics, and Mass Culture in Early Twentieth-Century America," explores the enactment of physical violence upon babies designated as malformed and unfit to carry on viable lives. Through a discussion of the film, *The Black Stork,* that fictionalized the "heroic" program of euthanasia against disabled infants pursued by Chicago surgeon Harry Haiselden, Pernick argues that an aesthetics of normalcy inevitably rationalizes extraordinary campaigns of professionally sanctioned genocide against disabled populations. This further demonstrates the idea of "the disabled" or "nonviable" itself to be reliant upon historically variable values—as opposed to medical—precepts.

For Lennard Davis this connection between physical aesthetics and disability is demonstrated as fictional by the art history critic who imaginatively "re-members" the fragmented statue of the Venus de Milo into an object of aesthetic pleasure and illusory wholeness. Using Lacan and Freud, Davis demonstrates that the psyche continuously attempts to re-member its own conception of the body as whole and nonfragmented even though this ideal of wholeness is necessarily false. Elizabeth C. Hamilton's essay, "From Social Welfare to Civil Rights: The Representation of Disability in Twentieth-Century German Literature," explores the relationship between representations of disability and genocidal histories in twentieth-century Germany. Using as a starting point the Nazi death camps that killed between 100,000 and 125,000 German citizens with disabilities during World War II, Hamilton analyzes how postwar social policies and literature ironically perpetuate the devaluation of disabled communities. Hamilton's essay concludes with a consideration of novelist Gunter Grass's symbolic treatment of disability as an allegory of a disabling German nationalism and concludes with a consideration of disabled German autobiographers such as Andrea Buch and Sigride Arnade who challenge this ambivalent representational heritage. For Hamilton, first person narrations of disability provide important counterpoints to the symbolic impulses of fiction that, in metaphorizing disability, overlook the individual and political struggles of disabled populations. In each of these cases, disability studies scholars endeavor to reflect the pathological impositions and moral investments in disability back upon cultural ideologies of able bodiedness.

The most common methodological approach to the question of disability in the humanities is the analysis of cognitive and physical differences that symbolize other social conditions. Stigmatized social positions founded upon gender, class, nationality, and race have often relied upon disability to visually underscore the devaluation of marginal communities. The essayists in this volume demonstrate that while disability is often used as the physical evidence of "damaged" populations, it also serves storytellers for its transgressive and subversive potential. For instance, narrative explorations of feminine subjugation within patriarchy often find a metaphorical alliance in the female protagonist's disabling condition. Cindy LaCom's essay, " 'It Is More Than Lame': Female Disability, Sexuality, and the Maternal in the Nineteenth-Century Novel," examines the pervasive use of the female invalid to comment upon Victorian ideas of sexuality, domesticity, and feminine authority. Analyzing the works of canonical authors such as Anthony Trollope, as well as lesser known women writers such as Charlotte Yonge, LaCom argues that disability was closely connected with metaphors of seduction and desire throughout the nineteenth century. While the melodramatic prototype of the female invalid most often represented the asexual monster of patriarchal imaginations, she also represented the alternative power of a repressed feminine sexuality. In Caroline Molina's analysis of Jane Campion's contemporary feminist allegory, The Piano, Ada's muteness provides the symbolic material of "the universal problematic of linguistic interpretation, of speaking and understanding the 'Other.' " By using both Ada's self-willed silence and her later mutilation at the hands of her husband as a symbol of the historical voicelessness of women, Molina demonstrates that the film "aesthetisizes and eroticizes the disabled woman in unprecedented ways." Such a strategy places Campion's use of her mute heroine as an important innovation in the female romance genre.

While disability in narratives of gender serves as a useful metaphor for feminine alterity, stories that privilege class concerns tend to position disability as a synecdoche for the collapse of aristocracies or the amelioration of middle class anxieties. In "The 'Talking Cure' (Again): Gossip and the Paralyzed Patriarchy," Jan Gordon argues that British literature has traditionally portrayed disability within the aristocracy as a defect of the head and heart. Such an emphasis upon disability as a dis-ease of the psychological realm provides literature with a textual syndrome that can be successfully "treated" and often cured with the salve of conversation. Within this tradition that includes classical British works such as *Lady Chatterley's Lover, Middlemarch, The Expedition of Humphry Clinker, Bleak House,* and *Waverley,* supposedly class-bound disorders such as gout, impotence, and paralysis have exemplified the collapse of aristocratic lines and the lethality of pure bloodlines. Paul K. Longmore also examines class and disability in his essay, "Conspicuous Contribution and American Cultural Dilemmas: Telethon Rituals of Cleansing and Renewal." Longmore documents a history of the U.S. telethon industry in terms of its appeals to middle class notions of civic and moral duty. The promotion of charity networks such as the Muscular Dystrophy Association, Easter Seals, and the United Cerebral Palsy Association in the name of "catastrophic" biological disorders seeks to assuage a perennially beleaguered sense of economic greed and abundance. Such suspicions of capitalist corruption present a portrait of a historical U.S. conflict wherein material acquisition must be offset by ritualized acts of "conspicuous charitable contribution." In the midst of this moral and economic exchange the disabled child as tragic innocent is transformed into the recipient of American beneficence.

Rosemarie Garland Thomson's essay, "Disabled Women as Powerful Women in Petry, Morrison, and Lorde: Revising Black Female Subjectivity," demonstrates a historical alliance between disability and racialized femininity. Using the work of Ann Petry, Toni Morrison, and Audre Lorde, Thomson examines the ways in which the dual marginalization of being black and female conspires to undermine African American women's sense of autonomy and self-worth. An analysis of disabled black women characters reveals that traditionally stigmatized markers such as race, gender, and disability are transformed into a powerful elaboration of a transgressive social identity. Rather than succumbing to the denigrating projections of an able-ist and racist culture, these writers all describe the "aberrantly embodied" black woman as one who "both embodies and transcends her subjugated identities by claiming corporeal difference as exceptionality rather than inferiority." Thomson demonstrates that this relationship between race and disability will be a fertile area of analysis for disability studies.

In addition to these metaphorical alliances with gender, class, and race, disability can also serve to symbolize and expose the workings of nationalist ideologies. Because cultures often base their sense of morality upon the "humane" treatment of disabled citizenries, national identity—particularly during wartime—is often closely tied to attitudes about war wounds that result in physical infirmity and bodily loss. In "Disfigurement and Reconstruction in Oliver Wendell Holmes's 'The Human Wheel, Its Spokes and Felloes'" David D. Yuan argues that the development of a modernized prosthetics industry in the postbellum United States was explicitly linked to the Republic's hopes for a reintegrated nation. The invention of the Palmer leg signaled the possibility of a modern prosthesis that could make the "unsightliness" of Civil War amputees less obtrusive to the class protocols and fragile sensibilities of the Victorian era. In doing so, Yuan explores the ways in which the war amputee threatened a traditional myth of American innocence that was artificially restored by the sleight of hand that prosthetics promises. David A. Gerber's essay, "In Search of Al Schmid: War Hero, Blinded Veteran, Everyman," details the ways in which a veteran's blinding acts as the symbolic material for patriotic resuscitation. Moving between the politicized agendas of the marines, the U.S. government, "communist" Hollywood, and the Blind Veterans Association, Gerber documents the ways in which Al Schmid's blindness was mobilized to serve various national ideologies. Like Yuan, Gerber contemplates the ways in which narratives of disability prove integral to quintessentially American mythologies of masculinity, racial supremacy, and manifest destiny. Both essays provide a pivotal understanding of the centrality of disability to definitions of nation, nationalism, and national identity. In addition, Gerber documents the ways in which disabled individuals' lives are both subjected to and exceed the limits of the state institutions that ensnare them.

Implicitly, all the essays in the volume explore how disabled subjectivities are constituted in a struggle with the able-bodied public's projections and investments in maintaining disability as alterity. Finally, disability studies methodologies also involve the identification of artistic models that provide dimension to our ideas of disabled subjectivities. Such projects privilege works that delineate the unique and even perverse psychic lives of people with disabilities as they refract and reflect the myriad ideologies that compose the conflictual subject of disability. Maria Frawley looks at Harriet Martineau's delineation of a subjectivity of the invalid in her essay, "'A Prisoner to the Couch': Harriet Martineau, Invalidism, and Self-Representation." Frawley argues that Martineau, in order to critique the objectifying principles of medicine, inverts the socially isolated space of the "sickroom" into its own philosophical vantage point. By unseating conventional associations of physical ability with insight and interpretive control, Frawley argues that Martineau invites readers to see the world through the eyes of the "invalid" rather than adopting the traditionally medicalized gaze that turns the bedridden into an object of investigation and horror. The result is Martineau's development of an alternative ideology of "healthy illness" that threatens to "unravel traditional binary pairings such as those of sickness and health, mind and body, and reason and emotion." In "'Making up the Stories as We Go

Along': Men, Women, and Narratives of Disability," Madonne Miner analyzes the influence of gender upon the narrative structure of contemporary stories of "physical catastrophe." In order to demonstrate the ways gender expectations influence the narration of disability narratives, Miner contrasts Andre Dubus's sense of the irretrievable loss of masculine agency with Nancy Mairs's creation of a newfound sexual identity that evades more traditional sexual objectifications of women's bodies. Miner's work foregrounds the multiple social identities that necessarily inform any theorization of a disabled subjectivity. These affiliations, as Elizabeth Hamilton's research into disability autobiography also demonstrates, often override the disabled subject's sense of sharing a common experience with other disabled people. By researching disability as narrative, Miner and Frawley both examine how disabled subjectivities must be understood as multiply inflected across gender, class, and racial lines.

Collectively these essays afford a more expansive and complex understanding of the cultural and artistic tropes and types that have come to dominate our ideas of disability as a social narrative. Each essay highlights the socially freighted meanings, mythologies, and stereotypes that have accrued around disabled persons and communities. Through careful interrogations of the historical nature of definitions such as limitation, incapacity, monstrosity, physicality, humanity, and being itself, disability studies scholars seek to expose the symbolic investments that produce and reproduce disabled communities as inherently inferior and parasitic. In the face of pervasive ableist ideologies, the theorization of disability as a socially constructed category will prove integral to our understanding of the body and bodily limitation.

NOTES

1. Friedrich Nietzsche, *Thus Spoke Zarathustra*, trans. Walter Kaufmann (1954; reprint, New York: Penguin Books, 1978), 34.

2. *Disability studies* is a relatively recent rubric that seeks to group research that focuses upon the historical, political, social, and professional meanings ascribed to disability and disabled populations. As this introduction will go on to demonstrate, the study of disability has been largely relegated to the empirical sciences that seek to categorize and catalog disorders and impairments in order to further consolidate definitions of normative physiology. Disability studies takes the medicalized model of disability as its primary object of critique. In this volume we seek to introduce this critical rubric into the humanities by collecting essays that comment upon the centrality of disability in history, literature, film, and the arts.

3. This particular critique of disability as central to the rationale and justification for the necessity of numerous professions comes by way of Michel Foucault. For Foucault, the very viability of professions is secretly maintained by the ceaseless production of aberrancy that in turn provides a perennial object of investigation in need of treatment. In *The*

History of Sexuality: An Introduction (1978; reprint, New York: Random House, 1990), for instance, Foucault designates the disciplinary exposé of sexual abnormality and deviance as an addictive professional pleasure that both ensures the longevity of the profession itself and assures the insertion of patients within a determinant catalog of perversions. Disability studies critiques a similar history of professional parasitism. Disabled communities traditionally have been defined through scientific narratives about aberrancies and physiological dysfunctions that in turn further sustain the need for the professional discourses that define them.

4. All of the previously mentioned social identities have developed critiques of empirical objectivity through the humanities. By arguing that heterosexist, racist, masculinist, and class-bound ideologies undergird our notions of normative cultural ideals, criticism in the humanities has effectively politicized our understanding of the inherently biased nature of all information while arguing that professional neutrality represses structuring social differences. In this way disability has taken a decidedly different direction from other identity discourses due to its omnipresence in the empirical sciences, and yet it still suffers from the lack of a voice within those very disciplines.

5. One recent foray into the prevalence of disability imagery is Martin Norden's *The Cinema of Isolation: A History of Disability in the Movies* (New Brunswick, NJ: Rutgers University Press, 1994). Norden chronicles the use of disability from the earliest moments of silent film to the recent fascination with disability stories in the 1980s. Norden hypothesizes that disability has been characterized most typically as an experience of isolation where the disabled character is depicted as existing outside of all social and communal circuits.

6. Although there is much debate within the disability community over appropriate terminology, we use the following designations interchangeably throughout our introduction: "disabled people," "disabled populations," "people with disabilities," "disabled constituencies," and so forth. While many have argued that using disability as a modifying adjective (as in "disabled people") dangerously usurps the personhood of the specified individual or population, our position is that disability acts as a structuring feature through which one is interpellated into an identity (whether that identity is chosen or not). See, for instance, the comments of Harlan Hahn (professor of political science) and Mary Duffy (visual and performance artist) on this question in the documentary *Vital Signs: Crip Culture Talks Back,* dir. Sharon Snyder and David Mitchell, 48 min., Brace Yourselves Productions, 1996, videocassette.

7. This paraphrase of the definition of disability comes from M. Golden, L. Kilb, and A. Mayerson, *Explanation of the Contents of the Americans with Disabilities Act of 1990* (Berkeley, CA: Disability Rights Education and Defense Fund, circa 1991).

8. Georges Canguilhem, *The Normal and the Pathological* (New York: Zone Books, 1991), 209.

9. Robert Murphy, "Encounters: The Body Silent in America," in *Disability and Culture,* ed. Benedicte Ingstad and Susan Reynolds Whyte (Berkeley, CA: University of California Press, 1995), 140–58.

10. Julia Epstein, *Altered Conditions: Disease, Medicine, and Storytelling* (New York: Routledge, 1995), 11.

11. Erving Goffman, *Stigma: Notes on the Management of Spoiled Identity* (Englewood Cliffs, NJ: Prentice Hall, 1963).

12. Ibid., 5.

13. Susan Reynolds Whyte and Benedicte Ingstad, "Disability and Culture: An Overview," in *Disability and Culture,* ed. Benedicte Ingstad and Susan Reynolds Whyte (Berkeley, CA: University of California Press, 1995), 3–32.

14. Ibid.

15. Even in the editors' examples of cultures that more naturally include people with disabilities, such integration occurs only on the heels of an exceptional story that attempts to linguistically accommodate a group that exists outside of a normative definition of physicality. Their examples of more positive understandings of disability include the disabled child who is "a gift from God" or the heightened capacities of one sensory organ that develops to help overcome the absence or limitations of another. These mythologies of "exceptional" inclusion have long been the target of disability scholars seeking to debunk malignant *and* romanticized narratives ascribed to people with disabilities.

16. Even in the Reynolds and Whyte introduction with its emphasis upon cultural variability in the international approach to disability there is a nagging criterion of humanity that people with disabilities must struggle to achieve in most cultures. See their discussion of "personhood" and "humanity" in Barbados, North America, and European countries on pages 10–12.

17. Current theories of the body share a penchant for unveiling a mapping of gendered, racialized, classed, and sexed coordinates onto bodies. Efforts to be inclusive of the range of ideological meanings ascribed to bodies inevitably reveal important limitations when it comes to disability. The very proliferation of politicized identities that attach to our notion of the body as a construct reveals a neglect of disabled bodies as a crucial nexus of physical experience. For instance, Elizabeth Grosz explains it in this way: "The specificity of bodies must be understood in their historical rather than simply their biological concreteness. Indeed, there is no body as such: there are only *bodies*—male or female, black, brown, white, large or small—and the gradations in between." *Volatile Bodies: Toward a Corporeal Feminism* (Bloomington, IN: Indiana University Press, 1994), 19. In *The Female Grotesque: Risk, Excess and Modernity* (New York: Routledge, 1994), Mary Russo articulates a connection between feminine bodies and images of degraded materiality: "The word [grotesque] itself, as almost every writer on the topic feels obliged to mention sooner or later, evokes the cave—the grotto-esque. Low, hidden, earthly, dark, material, imminent, visceral. As bodily metaphor, the grotesque cave tends to look like (and in the most gross metaphorical sense be identified with) the cavernous anatomical female body" (1). In Robyn Wiegman's introduction to her collection *American Anatomies: Theorizing Race and Gender* (Durham, NC: Duke University Press, 1995) , she says that "[i]n this sense, the economies of visibility that produce the network of meanings attached to bodies (their specific race, gender, ethnic, sexual and national demarcations) are more than political in hierarchical practices: they are indelibly subjective ones as well" (4). Even in books on the body and medicine, as in Paul Komesaroff's "Introduction: Postmodern Medical Ethics," in *Troubled Bodies: Critical Perspectives on Postmodernism, Medical Ethics, and the Body,* ed. Paul A. Komesaroff (Durham, NC: Duke University Press, 1995), we witness the same tendency to ascribe a limited series of social meanings to corporeal states: "As it is

lived, the body is marked, inscribed, and made meaningful in relation to the culturally specific forms of intersubjectivity and language. The identity it acquires in this process is a gendered one, inscribed on the biological raw materials" (15). All of these outgrowths of our current ideas regarding the absolute constructed nature of the body can be related to Jean-Luc Nancy's influential proposition that the body lacks any tangible essence in his essay "Corpus," in *Re-Thinking Technologies,* ed. Verena Andermatt Conley (Minneapolis, MN: University of Minnesota Press, 1993): "There is no whole, no totality of the body—but its absolute separation and sharing out. There is no such thing as *the* body. There is no body" (31).

18. Robyn Wiegman, ed., *American Anatomies: Theorizing Race and Gender* (Durham, NC: Duke University Press, 1995).

19. Judith Butler, *Bodies That Matter: On the Discursive Limits of "Sex"* (New York: Routledge, 1993).

20. Susan Stafford, *Body Criticism: Imaging the Unseen in Enlightenment Art and Medicine* (New York: Zone Books, 1993).

21. Jennifer Terry and Jacqueline Urla, eds., *Deviant Bodies: Critical Perspectives on Difference in Science and Popular Culture* (Bloomington, IN, and Indianapolis, IN: Indiana University Press, 1995).

22. Mary Russo, *The Female Grotesque: Risk, Excess, and Modernity* (New York: Routledge, 1994).

23. Juliet Flower MacCannell and Laura Zakarin, eds., *Thinking Bodies* (Stanford, CA: Stanford University Press, 1994).

24. Paul A. Komesaroff, ed., *Troubled Bodies: Critical Perspectives on Postmodernism, Medical Ethics, and the Body* (Durham, NC: Duke University Press, 1995).

25. Elizabeth Grosz, *Volatile Bodies: Towards a Corporeal Feminism* (Bloomington, IN: Indiana University Press, 1994).

26. Judith Halberstam, *Skin Shows: Gothic Horror and the Technology of Monsters* (Durham, NC: Duke University Press, 1995), 3.

27. One of the defining difficulties for disability studies scholars is going to be a grappling with ideas and experiences of physicality in a historical moment of constructivism. Influential philosophers such as Judith Butler and Sander Gilman have argued in tandem that physical deformities ascribed to gay or Jewish populations are nothing more than phantasmatic projections of normative cultural narratives. In doing so, both Gilman and Butler demonstrate that physicality is a fiction embodied by a normative frenzy to make unacceptable cultures visible and, therefore, recognizably deviant. Yet, undergirding their rhetoric of constructed deviancy is that they strategically distance their interest in "abject communities" from the tangible evidence of physical aberrancy. Subsequently, disabled communities that are defined by virtue of the presence of physical differences will be hard pressed to utilize the same rhetorical tactic.

28. Both David Hevey in *The Creatures Time Forgot: Photography and Disability Imagery* (New York: Routledge, 1992) and Lennard Davis in *Enforcing Normalcy: Disability, Deafness, and the Body* (London: Verso Press, 1995) point to the ironic fact that Frankenstein is constituted as a monster through a variety of disabilities yet we have no critical tradition that attends to this fact.

29. In "The Third Interval: A Critical Transition," in *Re-Thinking Technologies,* ed.

Verena Andermatt Conley (Minneapolis, MN: University of Minnesota Press, 1993), Paul Virilio points out that the demands of the disabled community that threaten to pull us all into an artificial world of social (non)interaction can be understood as a crisis of the human versus nonhuman binary that informs much of the criticism of technology. David Wills's *Prosthesis* (Stanford, CA: Stanford University Press, 1995) points out that the alignment of disability with fears of the inhuman highlights a perennial conflict that informs the utilization of language itself. Since language is always burdened with the task of passing off an artificial re-presentation of events as natural and "in process," the act of speaking or writing is one best characterized by the idea of prosthesis (the substitution of the artificial for the natural): "In this way the wooden leg represents the duality of every prosthesis, its search for a way between emulating the human and superceding the human . . . But what are demonstrated in the leg's simultaneous advances towards the human and the nonhuman are two competing conceptions of mechanical operations, one based on analogy with the human model and that opts for the difference of the digital, a digital reduced, however, to a binary. But they are also two competing models of the human, of difference, of conceptualization itself. For they continue to compete throughout the development of high technology into the domain of the robotic operations and into the question of artificial intelligence, and it is hard to know where the force of analogy has ever abandoned the field in favor of something that might be called the purely mechanical, or the electronic" (27). The critical formulation that would expose Virilio's philosophy as an artificial construct here is that Wills perceives a historical continuity that persists into the electronic age. Since Virilio sees disabled people as "robotic" in their technologized existences and thus more closely aligned with the "nonhuman," they serve as emblematic of this postmodern terror.

30. Paul Virilio, "The Third Interval: A Critical Transition," in *Re-Thinking Technologies,* ed. Verena Andermatt Conley (Minneapolis, MN: University of Minnesota Press, 1993), 11.

31. Ibid., 11–12.

32. One irony of such an association of disabled people with technological prosthesis is that nearly 70 percent of the disabled population lives below the poverty line. Consequently, disabled people are often prevented from gaining access to necessary equipment that can facilitate their access to able-bodied cultures and institutions. This fact alone demonstrates the depths of insensitivity that inform the politicized use of disability employed by Virilio and other philosophers of technology.

33. Though we go on to explore N. Katherine Hayles's use of disabled populations, Avital Ronell's *The Telephone Book* (Lincoln, NE: University of Nebraska Press, 1991) and Donna Haraway's *Simians, Cyborgs, and Women* (New York: Routledge, 1991) both use disability as a means by which to establish the arrival of a modern era founded upon technological prosthesis. Ronell develops her theories around readings of Alexander Graham Bell's invention of the telephone to communicate with his deaf wife. In doing so, she theorizes that the nineteenth-century freak show serves as the repressed term in scientific and medical discourses that would seek to ameliorate suffering, isolation, and monstrosity by containing physical and cognitive difference within the diagnostic categories of empiricism.

Donna Haraway's "A Manifesto for Cyborgs," in *Simians, Cyborgs, and Women* (New York: Routledge, 1991) provides another example of disability's unremarked-upon centrality to definitions of contemporary culture. Haraway valorizes "monsters" and other "boundary creatures" as exemplary of high-tech subjectivities that undermine old world dualisms but footnotes the disabled in order to demonstrate some patriarchal ironies of high-tech culture: military tech "tames" technological research by advertising its applica-tion for disabled users. Her point is that disabled people are supplemented with technology only in order to *re-humanize* patriarchal culture. Haraway then delights in the postmodern point that a "perverse" aspect of technology involves its way of "[m]aking the always context-relative social definitions of 'ableness' particularly clear, and military high-tech has a way of making human beings disabled by definition, a perverse aspect of much auto-mated battlefield and Star Wars R & D" (248). In this way, disabled people exemplify, in a footnote, the self-evident cyborgs of modernity—transhuman subjects who rework the nature/culture divide.

34. Note the difference between these representations of disability and the recent work of journalist John Hockenberry. In *Moving Violations* (New York: Harper and Row, 1994), Hockenberry analyzes his relationship as a disabled person to his journalistic sub-jects. Such a relationship is a complex one for it involves a negotiation of his disability from a variety of perspectives. For instance, in one of the opening chapters, "Walking with the Kurds," Hockenberry discusses his trek on horseback across the mountains separating Iraq and Turkey. In such a landscape his wheelchair is of no use to him, yet riding horseback allows him a sense of mobility that he rarely experiences back in the States. Also, Hocken-berry speculates throughout the work about the ways in which his disability often allows him a form of intimacy with his subjects that nondisabled journalists do not necessarily enjoy. Such an irony exposes one way in which disability can prove to be an advantage as well as an obstacle in the pursuit of professional objectives.

35. N. Katherine Hayles, "The Seductions of Cyberspace," in *Re-Thinking Tech-nologies,* ed. Verena Andermatt Conley (Minneapolis, MN: University of Minnesota Press, 1993), 178.

36. Lennard Davis, *Enforcing Normalcy: Disability, Deafness, and the Body* (London: Verso Press, 1995).

37. Arthur Frank, *The Wounded Storyteller: Body, Illness, and Ethics* (Chicago, IL: University of Chicago Press, 1995).

38. Diane Price Herndl, *Invalid Women: Figuring Feminine Illness in American Fiction and Culture, 1840–1940* (Chapel Hill, NC: University of North Carolina Press, 1993).

39. David Hevey, *The Creatures Time Forgot: Photography and Disability Imagery* (New York: Routledge, 1992).

40. Martin Norden, *The Cinema of Isolation: A History of Physical Disability in the Movies* (New Brunswick, NJ: Rutgers University Press, 1994).

41. Rosemarie Garland Thomson, *Extraordinary Bodies: Figuring Physical Disability in American Culture and Literature* (New York: Columbia University Press, 1997).

42. David Wills, *Prosthesis* (Stanford, CA: Stanford University Press, 1995).

43. Nancy Mairs, *Plaintext: Deciphering a Woman's Life* (New York: Perennial Li-brary, 1987), 16.

44. Lennard Davis, *Enforcing Normalcy: Disability, Deafness, and the Body* (London: Verso Press, 1995), 3–4.

45. Ibid.

46. While David Hevey's book, *The Creatures Time Forgot: Photography and Disability Imagery* (New York: Routledge, 1992), is not exclusively devoted to a history of disability activism, chapters 4 and 6 attend specifically to the struggle of politicized disabled constituencies. Underpinning the entire book is an argument about a historical movement to bring a disability perspective into circulation in various social arenas.

47. Joseph P. Shapiro, *No Pity: People with Disabilities Forging a New Civil Rights Movement* (New York: Times Books, 1993).

48. The majority of studies on disability outside of medical discourses begin by re-iterating that people with disabilities can best be described as suffering from cultural invisibility. Michelle Fine and Adrienne Asch begin their introduction to *Women with Disabilities* (Philadelphia, PA: Temple University Press, 1988) by stating: "Despite the prevalence of disability in this society, disabled persons tend to be invisible" (1). In *Images of the Disabled/Disabling Images* (New York: Prager Publishers, 1987), Alan Gartner and Tom Joe make a parallel point about the relative absence of images of disability in main-stream media: "They [the image makers] include literature and the movies; telethons with their infantilized portrayal of the disabled, and the news presentations; the print media, which like the TV news, rarely include the disabled and then most often as a human interest feature—not news" (3). This volume (and disability studies in general) adopts a position more akin to that made by David Hevey in *The Creatures Time Forgot: Photography and Disability Imagery* (New York: Routledge, 1992): "Disabled people have had more images launched in their name than Helen ever had ships" (7).

49. Marsha Saxton and Florence Howe, *With Wings: An Anthology of Literature by and about Women with Disabilities* (New York: Feminist Press, 1987), xiii–xiv.

50. William Shakespeare, *Richard III* (New York: Bantam Books, 1988), 5–6.

51. Ibid., 5.

52. Marie-Helene Huet has most recently traced out the historical lineage of the rela-tionship between women's maternal imaginations and monstrous offspring in *Monstrous Imagination* (Cambridge, MA: Harvard University Press, 1993).

53. The play's enduring reputation as Shakespearean drama with mass appeal has also mitigated against its cultural value amongst commentators and critics. Many trace out the egregiousness of Shakespeare's reiteration of a Tudor myth of Gloucester's deformity—one that was culled from Sir Thomas More's account, kept alive by Hollinshed, and is traceable to an orignary source in Bishop Ely who, historians suggest, *invented* the deformity of the king as a stratagem for deriding the wholesale malignity of the previous regime. Members of the Richard III society point to Richard's hump, withered arm, and limp as indicative of Shakespeare's distortion of historical reality: "In reality, Richard was quite normal looking . . . [he] was known as an accomplished solider. He would not have been able to fight on horseback with heavy armor and weapons if he were Shakespeare's hunchback with a withered arm" (Richard III Society Web-Page http://www.webcom.com/ blanchrd/ index.html). These efforts at rescuing the historical Richard from the slander of physical deformity were begun as early as the mid-eighteenth century by Horace Walpole. The restoration of Richard's physical form in an effort at historical accuracy, however, leaves intact a more resonant equation at the root of cultural mythologies of disability—that between external shape and internal disposition.

54. *Looking for Richard,* 35 mm, 112 min., Fox Searchlight Pictures, 1996.

55. Dierdre Lynch's arguments are carefully summarized by Veronica Kelly and Dorothea E. Von Mucke in their collection, *Body and Text in the Eighteenth Century* (Stanford, CA: Stanford University Press, 1994), 15.

56. Paul Longmore, "Screening Stereotypes: Images of Disabled People in Television and Motion Pictures," in *Social Policy* (summer 1985): 31–38.

57. Susan Stewart, "On Ghosts and Prime Numbers," in *Textual Analysis: Some Readers Reading*, ed. Mary Ann Caws (New York: Modern Language Association of America, 1986), 307.

58. Ibid., 307.

59. Paul A. Komesaroff, "Introduction: Postmodern Medical Ethics," in *Troubled Bodies: Critical Perspectives on Postmodernism, Medical Ethics, and the Body*, ed. Paul A. Komesaroff (Durham, NC: Duke University Press, 1995), 2.

60. The work of these four scholars has proven integral to our understanding of medicine as a culturally and ideologically inflected institution. In *Difference and Pathology* (Ithaca, New York: Cornell University Press, 1985), *The Jew's Body* (New York: Routledge, 1991) and *Picturing Health and Illness* (Baltimore, MD: Johns Hopkins University Press, 1995), Sander Gilman analyzes the pathological societal investments in the construction of the Jew that were forwarded by medicine in the nineteenth and early twentieth centuries. Ruth Bleier's *Science and Gender: A Critique of Biology and Its Themes on Women* (New York: Pergamon Press, 1984) and Emily Martin's *The Women in the Body: A Cultural Analysis of Reproduction* (Boston, MA: Beacon Press, 1987) discuss the masculinist biases that inform medical discourses on gender. Paula Treichler discusses the patriarchal narratives at work in biological constructions of femininity.

61. Michel Foucault, *The History of Sexuality*, vol. 1, *An Introduction* (New York: Vintage Books, 1980), 71.

62. One of the most sweeping analyses of the genocidal tendencies of cultures nearing the millennium is Richard Powers's *Operation Wandering Soul* (New York: William Morrow and Company, 1993). Powers uses disabled children in a Los Angeles children's ward as the springboard into his history of myths that turn upon the apocalyptic sacrifice of "innocent" and "flawed" populations.

PART 1 ▶ Representations in History

Constructions of Physical Disability in the Ancient Greek World ▶ The Community Concept
Martha L. Edwards

As scholars begin to compose an account of physical disability in the ancient world,[1] it is crucial to avoid imposing twentieth-century assumptions about physical disability onto other cultures. Two models have emerged from the field of disability studies that serve as core organizational principles. The medical model describes modern assumptions about people with physical impairments in the developed world; the community model offers an alternative perspective that can be applied to an investigation of physical impairment in ancient—or any—society.[2]

Two interrelated assumptions, both of which distort interpretation of the ancient material, comprise the medical model. First, the medical model assumes that disability is a medical condition that is inherent in the individual and that the disabled person's functional ability deviates from that of the normal human body. People with physical disabilities are commonly seen as dependent on others for practical and financial help. By extension, disabled people are often seen as heroic when they participate in ordinary activities such as sports or careers. Second, by the assumptions of the medical model, if one displays any of a number of physical conditions, one is automatically "disabled," and one's life is defined by membership in this deviant class. From the perspective of the medical model, the inability to walk, for example, is a condition that condemns one to a life of economic and physical dependence.

The community model presents physical disability as a cultural construct in which "physical disability" has no inherent meaning but is defined by any given community's understanding of people's roles. The degree to which one is able to fulfill the tasks of membership in the community determines the degree of one's physical ability or disability. The community model is much more applicable to the ancient world than the medical model. The Greeks had no fixed definition of physical disability. This is not to suggest that there was no such concept as physical disability in the ancient Greek world; rather, the meaning of physical disability depended on the community's understanding of people's roles—what they were supposed to do. In other words, the criteria of physical disability rested not on one's ability to function as an individual but on one's functional ability within the community. The definition of ability and disability, then, shifted according to one's socially prescribed role.

35

The Greek material that mentions or depicts physical disability comes from a wide variety of sources, and mention is rarely explicit. The evidence for physical disability is scattered, scant, and often contradictory.[3] Because of the nature of the evidence, this essay is painted with extremely broad strokes, including in "the ancient Greek world" all areas with predominantly Greek culture from the eighth century B.C. through the Hellenistic period. There were differences, surely, between the experiences of a wealthy Athenian man who had cerebral palsy and the lame daughter of a poor island family. Yet even such a huge distinction is lost, to say nothing of subtle differences.

One of the contributing factors to this state of the evidence is that the Greeks had not reached the level of abstraction in perceiving a category of physical disability in which people were a priori banned from carrying out certain roles and expected to fulfill others.[4] In fact, the Greeks may not have known what to make of this discussion of physical disability. Permanent physical disability was not part of the realm of Hippocratic medicine,[5] and partly as a result of this, the Greek vocabulary for physical disability appears vague, at best, to the modern eye. Most of the terms are generic, even interchangeable, taking on specific meaning only in the individual contexts in which they were used.[6] The modern term *disabled,* which has so many social and political connotations, is at first glance close in meaning to the Greek term *unable (adunatos).* In fact, the two terms differ significantly, and it is crucial to recognize the differences between them. In order to avoid confusion between the modern and ancient terms, I will henceforth avoid the modern term *disabled* in favor of the older terms *handicapped* and *impaired.*

The Greeks saw the human body as a whole; we in the developed world see it as the sum of its parts. Furthermore, we are accustomed to medical categorizations of physical conditions. Inherent in a modern term such as *cerebral palsy* or *muscular dystrophy,* for example, is the etiology, range of symptoms, prognosis, and so on. In the ancient world, the term *maimed (pêros)* or *formlessness (amorphia)* also implied a set of conditions, so that a Greek would form a mental picture of a maimed or formless person. The difference, though, is that the image intended by any given term varied from usage to usage, informed by the context and by the reading or performance.[7] Without the context, the specifics of the Greek terms are usually lost, to say nothing of subtle shifts in meaning between audiences and over time. It is also important to note that no Greek term refers exclusively to physical impairment.[8]

Physical impairment was a common phenomenon. This is no surprise, since vaccines and antibiotics were lacking in the ancient world. Still, a brief summary of the many physical variations is a counterweight to the persistent neoclassical image of the Greek human body, as reflected for example in David's *Death of Socrates,* in which the mathematically perfect classical representation of the human body is depicted on canvas. Congenital handicaps resulted from heredity, the circumstances of gestation, and the conditions of birth. Even those born without handicaps could acquire them from a variety of circumstances. Permanent physical impairment could result from injured, diseased, and lost limbs; from diseases such as arthritis; and from several other conditions such as multiple sclerosis. In addition, other diseases, some epidemic, caused permanent physical handicaps.

While information is sparse about the consequences of physical impairment, we can see, in broad outline, some of the social consequences of physical impairment. I will discuss economic and military consequences, then practical aspects of mobility, and finally, the aesthetic implications.

Economic Consequences of Physical Impairment

A key source of information about the economic aspects of physical handicaps is the defense speech "On the Refusal of a Pension" (Lysias 24) that the orator Lysias composed for an anonymous client, probably in the last years of the fifth century B.C. As a persuasive speech, it is bound to contain some exaggeration; nevertheless, the speech does highlight the differences between the Greek term *unable* and the modern term *disabled,* and it does show us some basic economic attitudes toward handicapped people.

The defendant had been classed among the unable *(tôn adunatôn),* and had been receiving a pension. This pension is outlined briefly by Aristotle (*Athenian Constitution* 49.4), who tells us that the Athenian Boule, the council of citizens, annually inspects the men who are classed as unable *(adunatous).* People in this class, who have very little wealth and who are physically maimed so as to be unable to work, receive a small grant for food. The defendant is now accused of being able-bodied, thus ineligible for the grant. Specifically, he is charged with mounting and riding horses, carrying on a trade, and associating with wealthy friends. (4–5)

The defendant has a physical handicap.[9] Well into his speech (12), Lysias mentions the "two sticks" on which the defendant relies to walk and which, of course, the jurors would have seen all along. This man obviously had a significant mobility impairment, which may have consisted of anything from gnarled legs to missing legs—we are not told. Yet his defense could not consist of simply appearing before the Boule and displaying his condition.

Physical impairment alone, in any degree, did not earn one a place among the "unable." Although it would have been obvious to every council member that this man had a great deal of difficulty walking, Lysias has his client present a triple misfortune: a father who left him nothing; a mother whom he had to support until recently; and an absence of children to take care of him (5–6). Compounded with this, he is now growing older and weaker (7). These factors, not just the physical impairment, are important in deciding whether this man should be counted as able or not able to make a living.

There were consequences associated with belonging to the class of people unable to fend for themselves. Lysias's speech suggests that people who received the dole were not eligible to serve as *archon* (official in important state office) (13). It is important to note, though, that he does not suggest that people with physical impairments were ineligible to serve as *archon*. He only suggests that people—with or without physical impairments—who were unable to support themselves were ineligible to serve as *archon*. It could be that people with physical impairments so severe as to prevent them from doing any sort of work were more likely to be categorized officially as "unable." Some handicapped people, no doubt, begged for their living. There are important differences between modern and ancient notions of begging. Modern thought distinguishes between legitimate, handicapped beggars and impostors who mimic a missing leg or a limp. This distinction rests on the assumption that a physical handicap in itself signifies helplessness and merits alms, a notion that was foreign to the Greeks.[10]

A physical impairment in itself did not constitute a need for money.[11] Lysias's speech demonstrates that one could be "unable in body" yet not in need of a pension. This is, after all, what the accuser is charging, and the charge is serious enough to merit a hearing before the Boule. Xenophon (*Cavalry Commander* 9.5–6) provides another example of physically handicapped people who did not need financial help when he suggests that the money for cavalry should come from, among other parties, wealthy men who are "unable *(adunatôn)* in body."

A physically handicapped person earning a living would not have been a remarkable sight; thus the phenomenon appears in the surviving material infrequently and incidentally. We usually learn about people's physical handicaps because permanent physical characteristics were personal, individual attributes that among other things established people's identity.[12] A permanent physical handicap was an efficient means of identification. A private letter from the fourth century A.D., for example, identifies a certain Isaac as "the mutilated one."[13]

We see people with physical handicaps involved in a wide range of economic activities. Alciphron depicts a tailor who limped;[14] a fragment of Aristophanes's comedy may refer to a lame peddler;[15] and a first-century A.D. contract for a division of property included a lame slave.[16] A Hippocratic author (*On Joints* 12) mentions that people who have congenitally withered arms, though unable to raise their elbows, can still use tools such as saws, picks, or spades. Metalworkers and miners were especially vulnerable to physical impairment[17] and, having acquired a physical impairment, would have no reason to stop working or change trades if they were capable of carrying on their livelihoods. The connection between artisans and physical impairment is reflected both in Amazon lore[18] and in the figure of the divine smith Hephaestus, the Crook-Foot god.[19] Men with physical handicaps were not thought incapable of farming the land, the occupation of the bulk of the Greek population.[20] The phenomenon of handicapped men farming the land appears between the lines in the tale of the apocryphal horde of old Greek men upon whom Alexander the Great chances.[21] The men were pitiable because of their spectacular mutilations and because of the humiliating circumstances of their mutilations: all their extremities except those necessary to their various crafts had been amputated by their Persian captors.[22] Rather than returning to their various native cities, the men decided to live out their lives as a group, farming, or at least managing, the land that Alexander assigned them.[23]

Physical Impairment and Military Service

The ultimate measure of a Greek man's worth and stance in his community was his capacity to participate in the military. Notoriously, in World War II, flat feet were enough to keep men from seeing active duty, but this was not the case in the Greek world. Among the Greek military forces of the *Iliad,* for example, Thersites's physical characteristics that identified him as a buffoon—he was "bandy legged"; he limped; and his back was humped (2.216–19)—did not bar him from war. The *Iliad* is a fantastic tale rather than a historical one; nevertheless, the details and background of fantasy are based in reality.[24] Thersites is one of several examples in Greek lore of a soldier with a variation of gait. Hephaestus is also portrayed going to battle, limping.[25] Plutarch (*Moralia* 234e) tells the story of a limping Spartan who explains that a limp does not prevent participation in battle: one needs to hold his ground in battle, he says, not run away.[26] These anecdotes may tell us more about Plutarch's view of Spartan valor in bygone days than they do about the real experience of lame soldiers. Nevertheless, we can see, in broad outline, that one could both limp and take an active part on the battlefield,[27] as the career of the Spartan king Agesilaus demonstrates.[28] Plutarch (*Agesilaus* 1) tells us that King Agesilaus was trained as an ordinary Spartan citizen-soldier because his older brother Agis was expected to take the throne,[29] which suggests that a limp was not considered a deterrent to enduring the rigors of the Spartan military education. The seventh-century B.C. Spartan poet and general Tyrtaeus was also lame, at least in later tradition (*Suidae Lexicon,* s.v. *Turtaios*).

Alexander's father, Philip II, himself was, by Demosthenes's account (*On the Crown* 67), quite physically handicapped. We learn that he had lost an eye, fractured his collar bone, and mutilated his hand and leg and was prepared to sacrifice every part of his body to battle. We do not know if Demosthenes is portraying Philip's characteristics accurately or if he is exaggerating, but in either case, his rhetoric suggests a perception that the physical signs of a man's willingness to sacrifice his body and keep fighting made him a dangerous foe.[30] We can trace this theme—that the signs of endurance of bodily hardship were the signs of a good soldier—over several centuries. The eighth-century Homeric warrior Diomedes, injured in the shoulder with an arrow, is made even more ferocious by his wound when he returns to the ranks (*Iliad* 5.134–43). The seventh-century Archilochus (frag. 114 West), in visualizing his bowlegged general, is not, of course, applauding the state of being bowlegged itself but is illustrating someone who, through action and experience, is tough. This theme appears again in the second century A.D. in Plutarch's tale (*Pelopidas* 1.1–2) of a good soldier with poor health and a ruined body who, when he was cured, became a bad soldier, no longer holding life cheap. This theme suggests that a man who had become permanently impaired as the result of a war injury may have been perceived as a tough and experienced soldier, with the full capacity to continue to serve in active battle.

Of course, these accounts are idealized, exaggerated situations. In everyday life, there must have been a limit to the degree of bodily hardship that would make one appear to be a good soldier. A limp in battle is one thing; an inability to walk at all is another. Still, we see such physically incapacitated men who could not take part in active battle playing other roles in the military. "No wounded man can fight," Nestor says bluntly to Agamemnon (*Iliad* 14.63). The wounded Homeric heroes, unable to fight, go to the field and organize the weapons, exhort the soldiers, and advise.[31] A later and more dramatic example of a physically handicapped person serving in the role of advisor is provided by Plutarch's account (*Pericles* 27.3–4) of Artemon, who designed siege engines. Artemon was lame enough that he needed to be carried to all of his projects. Because of this he was nicknamed Periphoretus, or "Carried-Around."[32] Artemon, though not on the front lines, accompanied Pericles on all his military campaigns. Similarly, Aratus, the third-century general of the Achaean confederacy, was carried in a litter on his campaigns after he put his leg out of joint (Plutarch *Aratus* 33.4; 34.4).

The preceding examples include handicapped men of extraordinary talent. Not every man who could not walk was an engineering genius or a brilliant strategist. That ordinary men with physical handicaps also played a military role can be inferred, though not proved, by examining the term *useless (achreios)* in its military context. The term *useless* was used to refer to the class of men who were noncombatants. For example, Thucydides (2.6.4) writes that, at Plataea, the Athenians took away the young, the old, and the "useless."[33] *Useless (achreios)* is not a subtle term. It refers to old, worn-out things.[34] Even this class of so-called useless men, which might have included men with significant physical impairments, sometimes played a military role. Thucydides (1.93.6) reports that

Themistocles wanted to guard the Piraeus walls with the useless men *(tôn achreistatôn)*. The tradition of noncombatants guarding the city's walls is long: in the *Iliad* (8.517–19), Hector calls for the young men and the gray-haired men to bivouac all around the walls; this was such an emblem of war that Achilles's shield showed a scene of a city that had left its walls defended by the wives, children, and old men (*Iliad* 18.514–15).[35] While we never hear directly that handicapped men took part in guarding walls, garrison duty was indeed an appropriate military task for men who could not take part in active battle.[36] In fact, so many men of military age were physically incapable of active fighting in the field that there may have been an official class of men at Athens designated for garrison duty. Even the "useless," a category that could reasonably include those with significant physical handicaps, had some opportunity to be of service in the military.

Physical Care for Handicapped People

From the Homeric writings on, war injuries were noted as causes of permanent physical handicaps. Even if people who had been made physically handicapped in battle were maintained by the state at Athens, as Plutarch (*Solon* 31) suggests, the maintenance was a small monetary amount, and no provision for physical care was made.[37] Physical care for an ordinary handicapped person was a family matter.[38] We can only guess at the range of conditions that must have existed for physically handicapped people who required care, for we do not have any direct information. The surviving literature shows us only the extremes of solicitousness and neglect and only the case of old or ill people, not permanently physically handicapped people. On one hand, Cleobis and Biton were so dutiful that they yoked a cart to themselves in order to transport their old mother (Herodotus 1.31). In contrast, we see in a third-century B.C. petition (*Sel. Pap.* 2.268) a man who complains that although he is stricken with bodily infirmity and failing eyesight, his daughter won't care for him in his old age. We also get a glimpse of at least one person's attitude toward caring for a family member—again, not a physically handicapped family member but rather an old and sick one—in a speech of Isocrates. Isocrates (*Aegineticus* 24–29) has helped his client argue for the right to the inheritance of his father by describing the drudgery of caring for him when he lay bedridden for six months.[39] In any case, independence is a modern notion; "interdependence" better describes the ancient relationship of an individual within the family and community.[40]

Mobility

Mobility is another practical matter of daily life for a handicapped person. People who had difficulty walking probably used staffs or canes. As Plutarch (*Moralia*

922b) puts it, the lame man makes no progress without his stick.[41] Indeed, the staff was an emblem of the unsteady feet of the old, part of Odysseus's disguise as a hobbling beggar (*Odyssey* 17.203, 336–38).[42] In addition to crutches or staffs, apparently there were other aids for people who had difficulty walking.[43] Perhaps this equipment included the corrective boots and shoes mentioned incidentally in the Hippocratic Corpus (*On Joints* 62). Plutarch (*Moralia* 18d) may have such a boot in mind in his story of Damonidas the music master, who prayed, when he lost his boots, specially made for his lame feet, that they would fit their finder.[44]

Prosthetic devices do not appear at all in the Hippocratic Corpus. The scraps of evidence that survive indicate that prosthetic aids were individually crafted items.[45] Herodotus (9.37) tells us that Hegesistratus, the diviner on the staff of the Persian general Mardonius, forced to cut off his own foot in order to escape from a Spartan prison, fashioned his own prosthetic foot out of wood.[46] An archaeological example confirms that wooden prosthetic devices existed in the ancient world: an artificial leg of wood, covered with bronze sheathing, was found on a skeleton from Capua, from about 300 B.C.[47]

People who were missing limbs or who had other severe mobility impairments probably got around as best they could, using crutches if necessary. There is absolutely no evidence for the wheelchair in the ancient Greek world, nor is there evidence for small carts on which people could propel themselves. A Hippocratic writer (*On Joints* 52) describes young children with dislocated limbs who "crawl about *(eileontai)* on the sound leg,"[48] supporting themselves with the hand on the sound side on the ground, and indicates that some adults crawl around as well. For distances, the ancient equivalent of a wheelchair was probably the donkey, such as Hephaestus rides,[49] and this transportation perhaps produced the mildly obscene expression, "the lame man rides best."[50]

People who could not walk, temporarily or permanently, could be transported in carts, presumably, though we only see people who were able to walk carried in carts, such as the oxcart in which Cleobis and Biton transported their mother (Herodotus 1.31). Teiresias and Cadmus, too, discuss whether or not to ride in carriages to the mountain (Euripides *Bacchae* 191). Litters were also available for transporting the sick and the injured, as well as people permanently unable to walk.[51] Artemon, the lame siege engine designer, was carried in a litter (Plutarch *Pericles* 27.3–4).

Aesthetic Considerations

Given the Greek philosophical ideal of symmetry and balance, it is not surprising that physical handicaps usually had negative aesthetic consequences.[52] Thersites's physical characteristics, for example, are as unappealing as Achilles's are appealing; his lameness is one of the characteristics that comprises the portrait of this most ugly man.[53] Still, the aesthetic consequences of physical impairment were, like the economic, military, and practical consequences, relative to the context. Recognizing an individual's physical impairment as ugly, funny, or both is quite different from the institutionalized horror of physical impairment that is so lavishly reflected in the media today.

Plato (*Hippias Minor* 374c) has Socrates call limping a faultiness and ungracefulness of the feet. This perception of limping as an ungraceful unevenness, an uneven meter, allows Aristophanes (*Frogs* 845–46) to call Euripides "Cripple-maker."[54] Actual limping, too, is portrayed as a cosmetic defect. Diogenes Laertius (*Pittacus* 1.81) writes that the sixth-century poet Alcaeus mocked his political opponent Pittacus with various epithets, such as "Potbelly" and "Broom-foot," "because he had flat feet and dragged them in walking." Plutarch (*Moralia* 621e–f) lumps together bald, lame, and lisping guests in one aesthetic category in his etiquette tip to refrain from requesting bald men to comb their hair or lame guests to dance on a greased wineskin.[55]

In contrast to the ideals of symmetry expressed in classical depictions of the human body, actual human bodies varied enormously.[56] Even if classical statuary represented the human body in mathematical perfection,[57] a cosmetic defect could be overlooked, even admired, in a real human being. Plato himself, so concerned with symmetry in physical appearance, concedes that any physical characteristic, such as a tilted nose, can be taken as a sign of good in the object of one's desire.[58] While some divergence was acceptable and even pleasing, we see a boundary between a simple cosmetic trait and ugliness. Aristotle, in his metaphor for the state (*Politics* 1309b), for example, writes that a nose that is hooked or snub can still be pretty but, when taken farther in the direction of excess, it loses its symmetry and doesn't end up looking like a nose at all. Aristotle's viewpoint is, of course, the aristocratic voice: "We do not think a man happy of very ugly appearance or low birth."[59] Among other subtleties that are lost to us, the boundary between cosmetic trait and ugliness must have shifted according to gender, between classes, and over time.

Conclusions

In summary, the consequences of physical handicaps varied according to the context and to the individual. Without a codified notion of "able bodied" on one hand and "disabled" on the other, people were not automatically assigned to one category or the other on the basis of medical diagnosis or appearance. While we can piece together a few aspects of some physically handicapped people's daily lives, it is impossible to draw conclusions about the circumstances of people with physical handicaps as a distinct group.

No one set of attitudes toward people with disabilities is apparent because the notion of physical disability as an abstraction was foreign to the Greeks. The Greeks did not recognize a dichotomy of ability or disability. Rather, we see a range of conditions to which the human body was always susceptible. The state of Greek medicine is one of the contributing factors to this lack of a rigid notion of physical disability. The conditions that we in the modern world would call physical disability were not in the domain of the Hippocratic practitioners. The medical model did not exist in Greece. We see very few instances in which people with physical handicaps were banned a priori from certain roles. Men who could not walk at all were unable to participate in the front lines of battle, but this was not a codified restriction. Only a modern perspective would see this practical circumstance as a restriction related to disability.[60]

Overall, we see people with a wide variety of physical handicaps participating in a wide variety of social, economic, and military roles. People with even the most severe handicaps were integrated into communities that accommodated all ranges of ability. We have seen, for example, that there were military roles for men who could not walk at all. The integration of people with severe physical handicaps into their communities was not an early form of charity. Rather, the Greeks did not waste manpower.

One of the reasons that it is difficult to find information about people with disabilities in Greek society is that they were integral to the society. There is no indication that people with physical handicaps in the ancient Greek world identified themselves or were identified as a distinct minority group, as is the case today. At some point, people with physical handicaps became a distinct group, the object of pity and fear, deserving charity and scorn. While much of modern, western culture rests on the institutions of ancient Greece, this set of attitudes toward people with disabilities does not have Greek origins.

NOTES

This essay is based on the first two chapters of my doctoral thesis, "Physical Disability in the Ancient Greek World." I thank Natalie Alexander, David Christiansen, and Janet Davis for their many suggestions. Other chapters of the dissertation examine the consequences of impairments of hearing, speech, and sight; this essay deals exclusively with bodily disabilities.

1. See, for example, Eleftheria Bernidaki-Aldous, *Blindness in a Culture of Light, Especially in the Case of* Oedipus at Colonus *of Sophocles* (New York: P. Lang, 1990). Veronique Dasen couched her iconographic study of dwarfs, *Dwarfs in Ancient Egypt and Greece* (Oxford: Clarendon Press, 1993), in terms of "physical minorities" (but see Nicholas Vlahogiannis, *Medical History* 39 [1995]: 119–20, for an assessment of the success of her approach). Michael Garmaise has recently completed a doctoral dissertation, "Studies in the Iconography of Dwarfs," McMaster University, 1996 [unseen]; also see Robert

Garland's study of disability in Greece and Rome, *The Eye of the Beholder: Deformity and Disability in the Graeco-Roman World* (Ithaca, NY: Cornell University Press, 1995). See also Nicholas Vlahogiannis, *Images of Disability in Antiquity* (forthcoming).

2. Several disability studies models are summarized by Beth Haller, "Rethinking Models of Media Representation of Disability," *Disability Studies Quarterly* 15 (1995): 29–30.

3. Literary material from the Homeric writings through the corpus of Galen has been relevant. I have used some later literary material, such as the commentary of the Byzantine writer Johannes Tzetzes and the tenth-century encyclopedic collection, the *Suidae Lexicon*. I have also used papyrological material up to the sixth century A.D. This material is late in date and from Egypt, not Greece, and it is not always clear whether any given piece reflects Hellenistic or imperial culture. Nevertheless, the material is written in Greek and therefore has, at least, linguistic continuity. Although the Christian Gospels are also recorded in Greek, I omit them from my investigation because they reflect hellenized Jewish attitudes more than Greek or even Graeco-Roman attitudes. Scholarship on disability in the Hebrew and Christian Scriptures has been carried out as a separate undertaking; for work with the Hebrew Scriptures, see for example, David Stewart, "Semantic Development of Disability Terminology" (Berkeley, University of California at Berkeley, 1995). I am grateful to Mr. Stewart for providing me with a copy of this essay and for discussing with me his ongoing work with disability terminology.

4. Marion Hathway, *The Young Cripple and His Job,* Social Service Monograph 4 (Chicago, IL: University of Chicago Press, 1928), 66, provides a blatant example of the level of abstraction in which a physically disabled person is banned from her societal role solely on the basis of physical disability: a 1928 social worker reports the case of Elizabeth Morris, "a woman who walks with the aid of one crutch and limps only slightly," yet who was ineligible to be a school clerk solely because of her physical handicap. In the present quarter of the century, assumptions about physically disabled people are more subtly expressed. Joseph Shapiro, *No Pity: People with Disabilities Forging a New Civil Rights Movement* (New York: Random House, 1993), 16, observes the flip side of the poster child, the "supercrip," whose ordinary feats are admired out of proportion.

5. Heinrich von Staden, "Incurability and Hopelessness: The *Hippocratic Corpus,*" in *La maladie et les maladies dans la Collection hippocratique*, ed. P. Potter, G. Maloney, and J. Desautels (City of Québec: Les Éditions du Sphinx, 1990), 110–11.

6. Edwin Rosner, "Terminologische Hinweise auf die Herkunft der frühen griechischen Medizin," in *Medizingeschichte in unserer Zeit*, ed. H. Eulner et al. (Stuttgart: Ferdinand Enke, 1971), 1–22, catalogs early Greek medical terms and finds (15–16) a preponderance of terms for visible physical characteristics such as rashes and deformities, especially of the trunk and limbs, for which he finds thirty-two terms. Included in these thirty-two terms, one should note, is everything from the broadest of terms, *maimed (pêros),* to the fairly specific term *lame in the leg (chôlos).* Mirko Grmek, *Diseases in the Ancient Greek World,* trans. M. Muellner (Baltimore, MD: Johns Hopkins University Press, 1989), 18, argues that the variety of terms suggests a "refined differentiation," but the variety of terms could just as well suggest a lack of codification.

7. We have only the written terms, for the most part. Alan Boegehold, "Some Modern Gestures in Ancient Greek Literature," *Transactions of the Greek Humanistic Society* 1

(forthcoming), urges scholars to remember that Greek text was meant to be read aloud complete with wordplay and gesture.

8. Theophrastus *On the Causes of Plants* 3.5.1, for example, uses "maimed" to refer to parts of plants of inferior quality.

9. When he refers to his bodily condition, he never calls himself "unable" *(adunatos)*. He refers vaguely to "the afflictions of the body" (3) and to the misfortune that makes it difficult for him to make long journeys (10).

10. Arthur Hands, *Charities and Social Aid in Greece and Rome* (London: Thames and Hudson, 1968), 77–78. Garland, *Eye of the Beholder,* notes (37) that the defendant of Lysias 24 does not appeal to pity, even though an appeal to pity was a conventional, even formulaic, part of such speeches.

11. As Henri-Jacques Stiker, *Corps infirmes et sociétés* (Paris: Aubier Montage, 1982), 59, points out.

12. In mythology, we see the grand revelation of Odysseus's scarred foot, *Odyssey* 19.298; 21.221. Odysseus's limp was earlier, 17.203, 336–38, a reverse identification—that is, a disguise. Perhaps the most dramatic revelation is that of Oedipus's pierced ankles, in Sophocles *Oedipus the King* 1034. Maybe in mockery of these dramatic moments, Aristophanes *Acharnians* 418–29 uses a series of physical clues that lead to Telephus's identity. In other comedy, we see ordinary people identified by a variety of permanent physical characteristics, including physical handicaps; for example, Eupolis "Golden Race" frag. 298 *Poetae Comici Graeci* identifies spectators as blind, hunchbacked, red-headed, and so on. Herodotus 4.161 distinguishes the younger from the elder Battus by writing that the younger was "lame and not stable on his feet."

13. *P.Oxy.* 46.3314.23. Several other papyri show physical handicaps as efficient iden-tification, such as a real estate transaction from 101 B.C., *Sel. Pap.* 1.29, which identifies the owner of a house by the scar on his cheek and the limp in his right foot.

14. *Letters of Farmers* 24.1.

15. Aristophanes "Anagyrus" frag. 57 *Poetae Comici Graeci.*

16. *P.Tebt.* 2.323–25.

17. Alison Burford, *Craftsmen in Greek and Roman Society,* Aspects of Greek and Roman Life (Ithaca, NY: Cornell University Press, 1972), 72.

18. A Hippocratic writer, *On Joints* 53, relates the tale that the Amazons dislocate their sons' joints at the hip and knees and use them as artisans in leather and copper.

19. This epithet is seen in *Iliad* 8.371; 20.270; 21.331. The significance of Hephaestus's impairment is discussed more thoroughly in "On Misinterpreting Hephaistos the Crook-Foot God," a paper that Tamara M. Green and I presented at the meeting of the Society for Disability Studies, 14 June 1996, Washington, DC.

20. Alison Burford, *Land and Labor in the Greek World* (Baltimore, MD: Johns Hopkins University Press, 1993), 1.

21. Diodorus 17.69.2–9; Curtius Rufus 5.5.5–24; Justin 11.14.11–12.

22. The authors who describe this scene lived in periods in which amputation was known. Amputation had probably been practiced by the Alexandrians.

23. Diodorus 17.69.8; Curtius Rufus 5.5.5–24; Justin 11.14.11–12. Whether we are supposed to picture the men as wealthy landowners, peasant farmers, or something in between is unclear. Burford, *Land and Labor,* 182–222, discusses the wide range of people

who would work the land, from the landowner himself to the seasonally employed, landless thete. At any rate, even extreme physical mutilation did not automatically mean that a man was incapable of carrying on this typical occupation, whether by his own labor or by hired labor.

24. Although it is not the main point of his essay, W. G. Thalmann, "Thersites: Comedy, Scapegoats, and Heroic Ideology in the Iliad," *Transactions of the American Philological Association* 118 (1988): 1, points out that Thersites portrays a common soldier rather than one of the military leaders.

25. "and yet his shrunken legs moved lightly beneath him." *Iliad* 20.36–37.

26. Plutarch was fond of this story and repeats it seemingly every chance he gets: in another version, a lame Spartan soldier is limping off to war, enquiring after a horse. Agesilaus sees him and tells him that the army has need of those who stand and fight, not those who run away. *Moralia* 210f. Closely following this tale, we read of Androcleidas, who has a crippled leg and is being questioned about his military competence. He replies that he does not have to run away but rather to stand and fight. *Moralia* 217c. And in yet another version, a lame Spartan is limping off to war, but no one is laughing this time: he is accompanied by his mother. She admonishes him, laconically, to remember his valor with every step. *Moralia* 241e. This version is repeated when Philip, injured in the thigh and troubled by his lameness, is urged by Alexander to go forth and to remember his valor with every step. *Moralia* 331b.

27. Victor Hanson, *The Western Way of War: Infantry Battle in Classical Greece* (New York: Alfred Knopf, 1989), 95, points out that in hoplite battle neither speed nor agility was necessary but that the crucial quality was determination to stand one's ground, keeping the line intact.

28. Plutarch enjoyed the tale that the Delphic oracle's warning against a "lame kingship" manifested ironically in the lame Agesilaus. The "lame kingship" is mentioned by Xenophon *Hellenica* 3.3.3; Plutarch *Moralia* 399b–c; *Lysander* 22.5; *Agesilaus* 3.4–5 and 30.1; and *Comparison between Agesilaus and Pompey* 2.2.1. Another lame king is seen in Herodotus 4.161, where Battus, the great-great-grandson of Battus, the founder of Cyrene, is described as lame and weak in the foot.

29. In addition, Alexander the Great's leg was "shattered beneath his knee" according to Plutarch *Alexander* 45, though we are not told if the injury was temporary or permanent. It seems that one had to be quite extremely mutilated not to fight. When the otherwise unknown Aristogeiton wanted to get out of military service, Plutarch *Phocion* 10.1–2 tells us, he appeared with both legs bandaged, using a staff. Also, it is interesting that in Diodorus' account of the Amazons, 2.45.1–3, the women had to maim not just one but all four limbs of the male offspring to incapacitate them for the demands of war.

30. Whether Demosthenes portrayed Philip's physical characteristics accurately or not, Plutarch *Moralia* 739b shows that Philip II was remembered as having a lame leg.

31. Onosander 1.9–10; *Iliad* 14.128–32; 14.370–87; 19.47–73. On the value of the experience of those too old to fight: Lysias *Funeral Oration* 50–51; Demosthenes *Third Olynthiac* 34–35.

32. Here—*Pericles* 27.3–4—Plutarch relates Heracleides of Pontus's version of the origin of the nickname: Artemon was weak and panicky and was carried around so as to escape injury. Fritz Wehrli, *Der Schule des Aristoteles 7: Herakleides Pontikos* (Basel:

Benno Schwabe, 1953), 80–81, explains that underlying this (frag. 60) is Heracleides's familiarity with the carried-around Artemon, the debaucher of Anacreon's poetry, frag. 27 *Poetae Melici Graeci.*

33. Also Thucydides 2.78.3: the Plataeans send away their wives, children, old, and most of the useless men. The Amazons maimed their sons, Diodorus 2.45.3 explains, so that they would be useless *(achrêstous)* in battle.

34. For example, *Supplementum Epigraphicum Graecum* 38.1210 lists a temple inventory from Miletus from the end of the second century B.C., in which several linen garments are "useless" *(achreiai),* worn-out items.

35. Other, later examples of the phenomenon include Herodotus 4.135: Darius abandons his men who were worn out by leaving them at camp on the pretext that they will guard it; whether or not this describes actual Persian practice, Herodotus's Greek audience would understand that soldiers could be tricked that way. Diodorus 15.65.2 tells us that the Spartans left their women, children, and old men in the city to guard Sparta against Epaminondas; and a few chapters later, 15.83.3, writes that King Agesilaus instructed the oldest children and the aged to station themselves on the roofs to defend themselves against the enemy.

36. It is no surprise to find an account of the watchmen of Oxyrhynchus, *P.Oxy.* 1.43.verso.5.6, in which a watchman posted on a certain street is identified as a "cripple."

37. As we have seen, this maintenance for handicapped war veterans that Plutarch mentions probably represents the origins of the classical Athenian pension for those unable to fend for themselves. P. J. Rhodes, *A Commentary on the Aristotelian* Athenaion Politeia (Oxford: Clarendon Press, 1981), 570, assembles the evidence for the amount of the dole and points out that the pension was barely sufficient, less than what an unskilled laborer would earn; see also Garland, *Eye of the Beholder,* 36. Garland goes on to suggest that relatives had equal responsibility for the well-being of those unable to take care of themselves.

38. Garland, *Eye of the Beholder,* 30, points out that while the very rich might employ a staff of slaves, this would be the exception. Hands, *Charities and Social Aid,* 17–18, discusses the difference between charities as institutions that exist in their own right and the charity of the classical city-state, which had no legal personality and which was a matter of individual arrangements.

39. Isocrates *Aegineticus* 28. This is testimony that Isocrates hopes will win his client's case and so is probably exaggerated, but exaggeration is often the nature of complaint.

40. As Margaret Louck, "Cultivating the Body: Anthropology and Epistemologies of Bodily Practice and Knowledge," *Annual Review of Anthropology* 22 (1993): 138, points out.

41. Just as fire makes no progress without wood: this is Plutarch's explanation for the lame Hephaestus's association with fire. This is repeated in Porphyry frag. 8.10, J. Bidez, *Vie de Porphye le philosophe néo-platonicien* (Hildesheim: George Olds, 1964). We see an example in Emma Edelstein and Ludwig Edelstein, *Asclepius: A Collection and Interpretation of the Testimonies,* vol. 1 (Baltimore, MD: Johns Hopkins University Press, 1945), 233, of the lame man with his stick on a stele from the fourth century B.C. at Epidaurus.

42. Other examples of the staff as an emblem of weak old age include, for example, Aristophanes *Acharnians* 680–83; *Clouds* 540–41; Cratinus "The Laws" frag. 133 *Poetae*

Comici Graeci; and Plutarch's account of Solon, *Solon* 29.5, in which we see that when Solon returns to Athens, he has become old: he carries a staff.

43. Aristotle *Eudemian Ethics* 8.3.1248b compares the invalid who does not profit from the diet of a healthy man and a weak or maimed man who does not profit from the equipment of a healthy man.

44. Athenaeus 8.338a tells a nearly identical story.

45. Lawrence Bliquez, "Classical Prosthetics," *Archaeology* 36 (1983): 29, suggests that if craftsmen, not physicians, created artificial parts, this would explain their absence in medical writings.

46. Plutarch *Moralia* 479b repeats the story of this Hegesistratus. Lucian *The Ignorant Book-Collector* 6 tells the tale of a man who, having lost his feet to frostbite, strapped on wooden feet and hobbled with the help of servants. Pliny *Natural History* 7.28.104–5 relates the story of the Roman general Sergius, who, having lost his right hand, has a very unlikely prosthetic hand made of iron. It is difficult to believe that any prosthetic device would have been helpful—that is, practical as well as cosmetic. Even today, with advanced understanding of preprosthetic preparation and a wide array of prosthetic choices, such as cataloged by Carol Stube Hammersley, "Prosthetic Prescription," in *Lower Extremity Amputation,* 2d ed., ed. L. Karacoloff, C. Hammersley, and F. Schneider (Gaithersburg, MD: Aspen, 1992), 59–65, Yeongchi Wu and Preston Flanigan, "Rehabilitation of the Lower Extremity Amputee," *Gangrene and Severe Ischemia of the Lower Extremities,* ed. J. Bergan and J. T. Yao (New York: Grune and Stratton, 1978), 437, report that 66 percent of people with above-knee amputations who are given prostheses discard them within six months. They theorize that it is the far greater energy expenditure that it takes to walk with a prosthesis that leads most people to discard the device.

47. Reported by Lawrence Bliquez, "Classical Prosthetics," *Archaeology* 36 (1983), who (29) writes that it is not clear how functional the leg would have been: its owner may have walked with a cane or crutch.

48. The same verb is used by Sophocles *Antigone* 340, where the chorus describes the ever-circling motions of the plough in the field.

49. Axel Seeberg, "Hephaistos Rides Again," *Journal of Hellenic Studies* 85 (1965): 103–4, catalogs the four Corinthian vase paintings that depict the Return of Hephaistos; he is seated on a mule in all cases.

50. Mimnermus frag. 23 West; Athenaeus 13.568e. Jeffrey Henderson, *The Maculate Muse: Obscene Language in Attic Comedy* (New York: Oxford University Press, 1991), 154, 157, catalogs the verb "to ride" *(oifein)* as a Doric word meaning "to mount," used only of human beings and used as a euphemistic—not coarse—term for sexual congress in comedy.

51. People unable to walk were carried into the Asclepiadic temple at Epidaurus on litters; see E. Edelstein and L. Edelstein, *Asclepius,* 236. Injured people could expect to be carried except perhaps in Sparta, at least according to Plutarch *Moralia* 241e, who tells us that a young man came back from war wounded, crawling on all fours rather than walking, and humiliated by it. His mother, of course, admonished him to rejoice in his valor.

52. As Robert Garland discusses in "The Mockery of the Deformed and Disabled in Graeco-Roman Culture," *Laughter down the Centuries,* vol. 1, ed. S. Jäkel and A. Timonen (Turku, Finland: Turun Yliopisto, 1994), 71–84.

53. *Iliad* 2.216–19. Thalmann, "Thersites," 1, points out that Thersites is the antithesis of the Homeric hero.

54. Also, *Acharnians* 410: "not for nothing do you make lame heroes." It is more likely that Aristophanes was taking a jab at Euripides's style than making a reference to Euripidean characters. While it is Euripides's most artful plays, probably, that survive, not all of his verse was graceful, as Gilbert Norwood, *Essays on Euripidean Drama* (Berkeley, CA: University of California Press, 1954), 41, points out.

55. Sven-Tage Teodorsson, *A Commentary on Plutarch's Table Talks,* Studia Graeca et Latina Gothoburgensia 51 (Göteborg: Acta Universitatus Gothoburgensis, 1989), 105–6, explains that dancing—or, more specifically, hopping and balancing—on a greased wineskin was an entertainment practiced at the Rural Dionysia. In the same passage, *Moralia* 621e–f, Plutarch tells the tale of Agamestor the academician who, when challenged at a drinking party to balance himself on his withered leg, retaliated by challenging all of the other guests to put a foot in a jug.

56. Harlan Hahn, "Disability and Classical Aesthetic Canons" (Los Angeles, University of Southern California, 1993), 20, points out that the classical sculptors, in using a mathematical ratio to express absolute beauty, set a standard of evaluation of physical beauty to which "generations of Westerners have remained steadfastly wedded." It is important to avoid projecting twentieth-century interpretations of classical statuary onto fifth-century Greeks. Mathematical measurements of conformation to an ideal were probably not applied, as they are to a fanatical degree in the twentieth century, to the actual human body.

57. Robert Charles,"Etude anthropologique des nécropoles d'Argos," *Bulletin de correspondance hellénique* 82 (1958), 275, argues that the Greek artists modeled the human form purely on mathematical canons, producing images that did not resemble their own ethnic type.

58. *Republic* 5.19.474d–e. Along these lines, Plutarch *Moralia* 821f claims that the Persians, because Cyrus was hooknosed, consider hooknosed men attractive.

59. *Nichomachean Ethics* 1099a–1099b. As another example of Aristotle's aristocratic bias, he tells us, *Eudemian Ethics* 1219b, that even the imaginations of the virtuous are better than the base, as long as they're not perverted by disease or deformity.

60. Claire H. Liachowitz, *Disability as a Social Construct: Legislative Roots* (Philadelphia, PA: University of Pennsylvania Press, 1988), 19–44, clearly demonstrates that expectations shape reality in an analysis of eighteenth- and twentieth-century military pension legislation. Among other results, these laws "construct disability by promoting particular expectations among the ablebodied segment of the population" (19).

Nude Venuses, Medusa's Body, and Phantom Limbs ► Disability and Visuality
Lennard J. Davis

> A human being who is first of all an invalid is *all* body,
> therein lies his inhumanity and his debasement. In most
> cases he is little better than a carcass.
> —Thomas Mann, *The Magic Mountain*

> the female is as it were a deformed male.
> —Aristotle, *Generation of Animals*

> When I begin to wish I were crippled—even though I am
> perfectly healthy—or rather that I would have been better
> off crippled, that is the first step towards *butoh*.
> —Tatsumi Hijikata, cofounder of the Japanese
> performance art/dance form *butoh*.

She has no arms or hands, although the stump of her upper right arm extends just to her breast. Her left foot has been severed and her face badly scarred, with her nose torn at the tip and her lower lip gouged out. Fortunately, her facial mutilations have been treated and are barely visible, except for minor scarring visible only up close. The big toe of her right foot has been cut off, and her torso is also covered with scars, a particularly large one between her shoulder blades, one that covers her shoulder, and one covering the tip of her breast where her left nipple was torn out.

Yet, she is considered one of the most beautiful female figures in the world. When the romantic poet Heinrich Heine saw her he called her "Notre-Dame de la Beauté."

He was referring to the Venus de Milo.

Consider, too, Pam Herbert, a quadriplegic with muscular dystrophy, writing her memoir by pressing her tongue on a computer keyboard, who describes herself at twenty-eight years old: "I weigh about 130 pounds; I'm about four feet tall. It's pretty hard to get an accurate measurement on me because both of my knees are permanently bent and my spine is curved, so 4' is an estimate. I wear size two tennis shoes and strong glasses; my hair is dishwater blonde and shoulder length."[1] In this memoir, she describes her wedding night.

> We got to the room and Mark laid me down on the bed because I was so tired from sitting all day. Anyway, I hadn't gone to the bathroom all day so Mark had to catheterize me. I had been having trouble going to the bathroom for many years, so it was nothing new to Mark, he had done it lots of times before. It was time for the biggest moment of my life, making love. Of course, I was a little nervous and scared. Mark was very gentle with me. He started undressing me and kissing me. We tried making love in the normal fashion with Mark on top and me on the bottom. Well, that position didn't work at all, so then we tried laying on our sides coming in from behind. That was a little better. Anyway, we went to sleep that night a little discouraged because we didn't have a very good lovemaking session. You would have thought that it would be great, but sometimes things don't always go the way we want them to. We didn't get the hang of making love for about two months. It hurt for a long time.[2]

I take the liberty of bringing these two women's bodies together. Both are disabled. The statue is considered the ideal of Western beauty and eroticism, although her image is armless and disfigured. The living woman might be considered by many normal people to be physically repulsive and certainly without erotic allure. The question I wish to ask is, why does the impairment of the Venus de Milo in no way prevent "normal" people from considering her beautiful, while Pam Herbert's disability becomes the focal point for horror and pity?

In asking this question, I am really raising a complex issue. On a social level, the question has to do with how people with disabilities are seen and why, by and large, they are deeroticized. If disability is a cultural phenomenon rooted in the senses, one needs to inquire how a disability occupies a field of vision, of touch, of hearing; and how that disruption or distress in the sensory field translates into psychodynamic representations? This is more a question about the nature of the subject than about the qualities of the object; more about the observer than the observed. The "problem" of the disabled has been put at the feet of people with disabilities for too long.

Normalcy, rather than being a degree zero of existence, is more accurately a location of biopower. The "normal" person (clinging to that title) has a network of traditional ableist assumptions and supporters that empowers the gaze and interaction. The person with disabilities, until fairly recently, had only his or her own individual force or will. Classically, the encounter has been, and remains, an uneven one. Anne Finger describes vividly that encounter between abled and disabled in strikingly visual terms. Finger relates an imagined meeting between Rosa Luxemburg and Antonio Gramsci, each of whom was a person with disabilities, although Rosa is given the temporary power of the abled gaze.

We can measure Rosa's startled reaction as she glimpses him, the misshapen dwarf, limping towards her in a second-hand black suit so worn that the cuffs are frayed and the fabric is turning green with age, her eye immediately drawn to this disruption in the visual field; the unconscious flinch; the realization that she is staring at him, and the too-rapid turning away of the head. And then, the moment after, the consciousness that the quick aversion of the gaze was as much of an insult as the stare, so she turns her head back but tries to make her focus general, not a sharp gape. Comrade Rosa, would you have felt a slight flicker of embarrassment? shame? revulsion? dread? of a feeling that can have no name?[3]

In this encounter, what is suppressed, at least in this moment, is the fact that Rosa Luxemburg herself is physically impaired, walking with a limp her whole life. The contention then moves from the cultural norm to the deviation; the subject gazing places herself in the empowered position of the norm, even if that position is not warranted.

Disability, in this and other encounters, is a disruption in the visual, auditory, or perceptual field as it relates to the power of the gaze. As such, the disruption, the rebellion of the visual, must be regulated, rationalized, contained. Why the modern binary—normal/abnormal—must be maintained is a complex question. But we can begin by accounting for the desire to split bodies into two immutable categories—whole and incomplete, abled and disabled, normal and abnormal, functional and dysfunctional.

In the most general sense, cultures perform an act of splitting (*Spaltung*, to use Freud's term). These violent cleavages of consciousness are as primitive as our thought processes can be. The young infant splits the good parent from the bad parent—although the parent is the same entity. When the child is satisfied by the parent, then the parent is the good parent; when the child is inevitably not satisfied, then the parent is bad. As a child grows out of the earliest phases of infancy, she learns to combine those split images into a single parent who is sometimes good and sometimes not. The residue of *Spaltung* remains in our inner life, personal and collective, to produce monsters and evil stepmothers as well as noble princes and fairy godmothers.

In this same primitive vein, culture tends to split bodies into good and bad parts. There are cultural norms considered good and others considered bad. Everyone is familiar with the "bad" body—too short or too tall, too fat or too thin, not masculine or feminine enough, not enough or too much hair on the head or other parts of the body, penis or breasts too small or (excepting the penis) too big. Further, each individual assigns good and bad labels to body parts—good: hair, face, lips, eyes, hands; bad: sexual organs, excretory organs, underarms.

This psychological dimension may partly explain why it becomes imperative for society at large to engage in *Spaltung*. The division neatly seals off the frightening writing on the wall that reminds the hallucinated whole being that its wholeness is in fact a hallucination, a developmental fiction. The primitive reaction creates the absolute categories of abled and disabled, with the concomitant defenses against the repressed fragmented body.

But a psychological explanation alone is finally insufficient. Historical specificity makes us understand that disability is a social process with an origin. So, why certain disabilities are labeled negatively while others have a less negative connotation is a question tied to complex social forces. It is fair to say, in general, that disabilities would be most dysfunctional in postindustrial countries where the ability to perambulate or manipulate is so concretely tied to productivity, which in itself is tied to production. The body of the average worker, as we have seen, becomes the new measure of man and woman. Michael Oliver, citing Ryan and Thomas, notes:

> With the rise of the factory . . . [during industrialization], many more disabled people were excluded from the production process for "The speed of factory work, the enforced discipline, the time-keeping and production norms—all these were a highly unfavourable change from the slower, more self-determined and flexible methods of work into which many handicapped people had been integrated."[4]

This aspect of production and standardization of the human body has had a profound impact on how we split up bodies.

We tend to group impairments into either the category of disabling (bad) or just limiting (good). For example, wearing a hearing aid is seen as much more disabling than wearing glasses, although both serve to amplify a deficient sense. But loss of hearing is associated with aging in a way that nearsightedness is not. Breast removal is seen as an impairment of femininity and sexuality, whereas the removal of a foreskin is not seen as a diminution of masculinity. The coding of body parts and their selective function or dysfunction is part of a much larger system of signs and meanings in society and is constructed as such.

"Splitting" may help us understand one way in which disability is seen as part of a system in which value is attributed to body parts. The disabling of the body part or function is then part of a removal of value. The gradations of value are socially determined, but what is striking is the way that rather than being incremental or graduated, the assignment of the term *disabled* and the consequent devaluation are total. That is, the idea of disabled seems to be an absolute rather than a gradient concept. One is either disabled or not. Value is tied to the ability to earn money. If one's body is productive, it is not disabled. People with disabilities continue to earn less than "normal" people, and, even after the passage of the Americans with Disabilities Act, 69 percent of people with disabilities were unemployed.[5] Women and men with disabilities are seen as less attractive and less able to marry and be involved in domestic production.

The ideology of standards of the body goes back to preindustrial origins. Myths of beauty and ugliness have laid the foundations for normalcy. In particular, the Venus myth is one that is dialectically linked to another. The story of the embodiment of beauty and desire is tied to the story of the embodiment of ugliness and repulsiveness. So the appropriate mythological character to compare the armless Venus with is Medusa.[6] Medusa was once a beautiful sea goddess, but, because she lay with Poseidon at one of Athena's temples, she was turned by Athena into a winged monster with glaring eyes, huge teeth, protruding tongue, brazen claws, and writhing snakes for hair. Her appearance, so hideous, had the power to turn people into stone. Athena eventually completed her revenge by having Perseus kill Medusa. He found Medusa by stealing the one eye and one tooth shared by the Graiae and withholding these items until the Graiae agreed to help him. Perseus killed Medusa by decapitating her while looking into his brightly polished shield, which neutralized the power of her appearance, and then he put her head into a magic wallet that shielded onlookers from its effects. When Athena received the booty, she used Medusa's head and skin to fashion her own shield.

In the Venus tradition, Medusa is a poignant double. She is the necessary counter in the dialectic of beauty and ugliness, desire and repulsion, wholeness and fragmentation. Medusa is the disabled woman to Venus's perfect body. The story is a kind of allegory of a "normal" person's intersection with the disabled body. This intersection is marked by the power of the visual. The "normal" person sees the disabled person and is turned to stone, in some sense, by the visual interaction. In this moment, the normal person suddenly feels self-conscious, rigid, unable to look but equally drawn to look. The visual field becomes problematic, dangerous, treacherous. The disability becomes a power derived from its otherness, its monstrosity, in the eyes of the "normal" person. Thus, the disability must be decapitated and then contained in a variety of "magic wallets." Rationality, for which Athena stands, is one of the devices for containing, controlling, and reforming the disabled body so that it no longer has the power to terrorize. And the issue of mutilation comes up as well because the disabled body is always the reminder of the body about to come apart at the seams. It provides a vision of, a caution about, the body as a construct held together willfully, always threatening to become its individual parts—cells, organs, limbs, perceptions—like the fragmentary shared eye and tooth that Perseus steals from the Graiae.

In order to understand better how normalcy is bred into ways of viewing the body, it might be productive to think about the body as it appears in art, photography, and the other visual media. There has been a powerful tradition of representing the body in Western art in a way that has served to solidify, rather early on in history, a preferred mode of envisioning the body. This tradition, identified by Kenneth Clark, has been most clearly articulated in "the nude." The nude, as Clark makes clear, is not a literal depiction of the human body but rather a set of conventions about the body: "the nude is not the subject of art, but a form of art."[7] Or, as he says, the nude is "the body re-formed" (3). If that is the case, then the nude is really part of the development of a set of idealized conventions about the way the body is supposed to look.

While some nudes may be male, when people talk about "the nude" they most often mean the female nude. As in so many other areas, the female has been the focus of men's attention, obsession, and control. Lynda Nead, in a feminist correction of Clark, points out that "more than any other subject, the female nude connotes 'Art'."[8] And in that tradition, the Venus becomes the vortex for thinking about the female body. The Venus is, rather than a subject, a masculine way of fashioning the female body or remaking it into a conceptual whole.

I emphasize the word *whole,* because the irony of the Venus tradition is that there are virtually no intact Venuses from antiquity. Indeed, one of the reasons for the popularity of the Venus de Milo was that from the time it was discovered in 1820 and until 1893 when Furtwangler's scholarship revealed otherwise, the statue was, according to Clark, "believed to be an original of the fifth century and the only free-standing figure of a woman that had come down from the great period with the advantage of a head" (89).

The mutilation of the statues is made more ironic by the fact that their headless and armless state is usually overlooked by art historians—barely referred to at all by Clark, for example, in the entirety of his book. The art historian does not *see* the absence and so fills the absence with a presence. This compensation leads us to understand that in the discourse of the nude one is dealing not simply with art history but with the reception of disability, the way that the "normal" observer compensates for or defends against the presence of difference. This is a way of seeing not often discussed in art criticism. Of course, one can consider that art historians are really just making the best of a bad situation: that the statues they wish to observe have been destroyed over time. But if one wishes to make more of this state of affairs, it is possible to say a number of things.

First of all, the headlessness and armlessness of Venuses link them, although subtly, with the Medusa tradition. Many of these Venuses have in effect been decapitated. There seems to be a reciprocal relationship between the decapitations of Medusa in myth and of Venus in reality. It seems that the Venus is really only made possible in coordination with the Medusa—that Aphrodite can romp because Medusa can kill. So it is a fitting dialectic that Medusa's beheading is contained within every broken Venus. The speechlessness of the art historian about the mutilation of his objects of beauty and desire is the effect of his metaphoric transformation to stone. This lapsus in speech is really an avoidance, a wish to avoid the castrating, terrifying vision of Medusa—the disabled, the monster, who is also the disabler. In a larger sense, as Nead suggests, all visions of the female nude, particularly in the Venus tradition, are attempts of male artists

and critics to gird themselves against the irrationality and chaos of the body—
particularly the female body.

> It begins to speak of a deep-seated fear and disgust of the female body and of
> femininity within patriarchal culture and of a construction of masculinity
> around the related fear of the contamination and dissolution of the male ego.[9]

In thinking about disability, one can extend this argument and say that the fear of
the unwhole body, of the altered body, is kept at bay by these depictions of whole,
systematized bodies. The unwhole body is the unholy body. Or as Kaja Silverman
points out about images of the body in film, society creates a "protective shield"
that insulates it against the possibility of mutilation, fragmentation, castration.[10]

Indeed, the systematization of the body by artist and critic suggests a linearity,
a regularity, a completeness that belie the fragmentary, explosive way the body is
constitutively experienced. Clark exemplifies this systematic approach in discussing the Esquiline Venus of the fifth century, the first embodiment of these
conventions.

> But she is solidly desirable, compact, proportionate; and, in fact, her propor-
> tions have been calculated on a simple mathematical scale. The unit of mea-
> surement is her head. She is seven heads tall; there is the length of one head
> between her breasts, one from breast to navel, and one from the navel to the
> division of the legs . . . fundamentally this is the architecture of the body that
> will control the observations of classically minded artists till the end of the
> nineteenth century. (75)

The amnesia of art historians upon the subject of mutilation and decapitation
(the Esquiline Venus has no head) is not accidental. The most we get from Clark
in his entire book is one wistful mention of a Greco-Roman depiction of the three
graces as "a relief in the Louvre, headless, alas" (91). The "alas" speaks volumes.
This amnesia, this looking away from incompleteness, an averting of the attention, a sigh, is the tip of a defensive mechanism that allows the art historian still to
see the statue as an object of desire. So the critic's aim is to restore the damage,
bring back the limbs, through an act of imagination. This phenomenon is not
unlike the experience of "phantom limb," the paradoxical effect that amputees
experience of sensing their missing limbs. In the case of the art historian, the
statue is seen as complete with phantom limbs and head. The art historian does
not see the lack, the presence of an impairment, but rather mentally re-forms the
outline of the Venus, so that the historian can return the damaged woman in
stone to a pristine state of wholeness. His is an act of re-formation of the visual
field, a sanitizing of the disruption in perception.

This is the same act of imagination, or one might say control, that bans from the nude the representation of normal biological processes. For example, there are no pregnant Venuses and there are no paintings of Venuses who are menstruating, micturating, defecating—lactating and lacrimating are the only recognized activities of idealized women. There are no old Venuses (with the exception of a Diana by Rembrandt). One might think of a pregnant Venus as a temporarily disabled woman and as such banned from the reconstruction of the body we call "the nude." Clark distinguishes between prehistoric fertility goddesses, like the Willendorf Venus, images of fertility and pregnancy, and the differently ideal Grecian versions, which are never pregnant. As Nead notes, "Clark alludes to this image of the female body [the Willendorf Venus] as undisciplined, out of control; it is excluded from the proper concerns of art in favour of the smooth, uninterrupted line of the Cycladic [Greek] figure."[11] As artists and art historians shun the fluids and changes in shape that detract from the process of forming the regular body, the evidentiary record of mutilated Venuses must be repressed by a similar process.

A cautionary word on the decapitated and armless Venuses. While it is true that male statues are equally truncated, the incompleteness of the female statues suggests another obvious point that has been repressed for so long—violence. Did all these statues lose their arms and heads by sheer accident? Was the structural fragility of head and limbs more likely to deteriorate than the torso? Were there random acts of vandalism? Or was there a particular kind of symbolic brutality committed on these stone women? Did vandals, warriors, and adolescent males amuse themselves by committing focused acts of violence, of sexual bravado and mockery, on these embodiments of desire? An armless woman is a symbol of sexual allure without the ability to resist; a headless nude captures a certain kind of male fantasy of submission without the complication of the individuality and the authority granted by a face, even an idealized one. We do not now and will probably never know what happened to these statues, although the destruction of the Parthenon Marbles has been documented as the act of occupying soldiers. But the point is that the violence against the body, the acts of hacking, mutilation, and so on, has to be put in the same context we have been discussing. An act of violence against a female statue is constitutively different from that against a male statue—and these acts are ones that can be placed in a range of terrorist acts against women during war. Such acts create disabled people, and so in a sense, these Venuses are the disabled women of art. To forget that is again to commit acts of omission of a rather damning nature.

Of course, a statue is not a person. But as representations of women, the Venus statues carry a powerful cultural signification. The reaction to such statues, both by critics and by other viewers, tells much about the way that we consider the body both as a whole and as incomplete. One point to note is that the art historian, like Clark, tends to perform a complex double act. On the one hand, the critic sees the incomplete statue as whole, imagines the phantom limbs to defend against incompleteness, castration, the chaotic or "grotesque body," as Peter Stallybrass and Allon White have, using Bakhtinian terminology, called it.[12] On the other hand (if indeed our standard is *two* hands), the critic and the artist are constantly faced with the fragmentary nature of the body, analyzing parts, facing the gaze of the missing part that must be argued into existence.

The model for the fragmentary nature of the nude is best illustrated by the famous story of Zeuxis, as told by Pliny. When Zeuxis painted his version of Aphrodite, he constructed her from the parts of five beautiful young women of his town of Kroton. His vision of the wholeness of Aphrodite was really an assemblage of unrelated parts. Likewise, the critic in regarding the whole nude must always be speaking of parts: "their torsos have grown so long that the distance from the breasts to the division of the legs is three units instead of two, the pelvis is wide, the thighs are absurdly short."[13] The whole can only be known by the sum of its parts—even when those parts are missing. John Barrel detailed the reactions of eighteenth-century men to the Venus de Medici and noted how they tended to examine every detail of the statue. Edward Wright, for example, tells observers to "strictly examine every part," and a typical account read:

> One might very well insist on the beauty of the breasts . . . They are small, distinct, and delicate to the highest degree; with an idea of softness . . . And yet with all that softness, they have a firmness too . . . From her breasts, her shape begins to diminish gradually down to her waist; . . . Her legs are neat and slender; the small of them is finely rounded; and her feet are little, white, and pretty.[14]

Another carped:

> The head is something too little for the Body, especially for the Hips and Thighs; the Fingers excessively long and taper, and no match for the Knuckles, except for the little Finger of the Right-Hand.[15]

These analyses perform a juggling act between the fragmentation of the body and reuniting it into a hallucinated erotic whole.[16] In imagining the broken statues, the critic must mentally replace the arms and the head and then criticize any other restoration, as does Clark in attacking the reconstruction of the Venus of Arles: "the sculptor Girardon . . . not only added the arms and changed the angle of the head, but smoothed down the whole body, since the King was offended by the sight of ribs and muscles" (87). The point here is that the attempt of the critic to keep the body in some systematic whole is really based on a repression of the fragmentary nature of the body.

One might also want to recall that for the Greeks, these statues, while certainly works of art, were also to be venerated, since they were representations of deities.

For the Greeks, Aphrodite was not a myth; she was a goddess whose domain was desire. It somehow seems appropriate that the ritualistic or reverential attitude toward these statues, pointed out by Walter Benjamin[17]—indeed their very appearance in stone, which Page Dubois sees as a cultic representation of the bones of the female spirits—has been reproduced in the attitude of that most secular of worshippers—the art critic. For the Venus has a double function: she is both a physical and a spiritual incarnation of desire. In that double sense, the critic must emphasize her spiritual existence by going beyond her physical incarnation in fallible stone, and her mutilations, to the essential body, the body of Desire, the body of the Other.

We can put this paradox in Lacanian terms. For Lacan, the most primitive, earliest experience of the body is actually of the fragmented body *(corps morcelé)*. The infant experiences his or her body as separate parts or pieces, as "turbulent movements."[18] For the infant, rather than initially experiencing the body as a whole, the body is an assemblage of arms, legs, surfaces. These representations/images of fragmented body parts Lacan calls *imagos* because they are "constituted for the 'instincts' themselves." (11)

> Among these *imagos* are some that represent the elective vectors of aggressive intentions, which they provide with an efficacity that might be called magical. These are the images of castration, mutilation, dismemberment, dislocation, evisceration, devouring, bursting open of the body, in short, the *imagos* that I have grouped together under the apparently structural term of *imagos of the fragmented body*. (11)

The process that builds a self involves the enforced unifying of these fragments through a hallucination of a whole body, "a Gestalt, that is to say, in an exteriority" (2), as Lacan has pointed out. This movement "extends from a fragmented body-image to a form of its totality . . . and, lastly, to the assumption of the armour of an alienating identity" (4). When the child points to an image in the mirror, at that stage Lacan calls "the mirror phase," the child recognizes (actually misrecognizes) that unified image as his or her self. That identification is really a donning of an identity, an "armor" against the chaotic or fragmentary body.

In this sense, the disabled body is a direct imago of the repressed fragmented body. The disabled body causes a kind of hallucination of the mirror phase gone wrong. The subject looks at the disabled body and has a moment of cognitive dissonance, or should we say a moment of cognitive resonance with the earlier state of fragmentation. Rather than seeing the whole body in the mirror, the subject sees the repressed fragmented body; rather than seeing the object of desire, as controlled by the Other, the subject sees the true self of the fragmented body. For Lacan, because the child first saw its body as a "collection of discrete part-objects, adults can never perceive their bodies in a complete fashion in later life."[19] This repressed truth of self-perception revolves around a prohibited central, specular moment—of seeing the disabled body—in which the "normal" person views the Medusa image, in which the Venus nude cannot be sustained as a viable armor. In Lacanian terms, the *moi* is threatened with a breaking up, literally, of its structure, with a reminder of its incompleteness. The kind of fragmentary images of the body we have are often found in dream work. But in a specular, face-to-face moment, the ego is involved in what J. B. Pontalis calls "death work," which involves the "fundamental process of unbinding [of the ego], of fragmentation, of breaking up, of separation, of bursting."[20] Thus the specular moment between the armored, unified self and its repressed double—the fragmented body—is characterized by a kind of death work, repetition compulsion in which the unified self continuously sees itself undone—castrated, mutilated, perforated, made partial. In this context, it is worth noting that the Venus tradition involves castration at its very origin. Aphrodite is said to have been born from the foam of Uranus's genitals, which Cronus threw into the sea after castrating his father.[21] The dynamic is clear. Male mutilation is mitigated by the creation of the desirable female body. The disabled body is corrected by the wholeness of the constructed body of the nude. But, as has been noted, the emphasis on wholeness never entirely erases the foundation of the Venus tradition in the idea of mutilation, fragmented bodies, decapitation, amputation.

If we follow these terms, then the disabled Venus serves as an unwanted reminder that the "real body," the "normal body," the observer's body, is in fact always already a "fragmented body." The linking together of all the disparate bodily sensations and locations is an act of will, a hallucination that always threatens to fall apart. The mutilated Venus and the disabled person in general, particularly one who is missing limbs or body parts, will become in fantasy a visual echo of the primal fragmented body—a signifier of castration and lack of wholeness. Missing senses, blindness, deafness, aphasia, in that sense, will point to missing bodily parts or functions. The art historian in essence dons or retains the armor of identity, needs the armor as does Perseus, who must see Medusa through the polished shield. The art historian's defense is that mirrorlike shield that conjures wholeness through a misrecognition linking the parts into a whole.

What this analysis tells us is that the "disabled body" belongs to no one, just as the normal body, or even the "phallus," does not belong to anyone. Even a person who is missing a limb or is physically "different" still has to put on, assume, the disabled body and identify with it.[22] The disabled body, far from being the body of some small group of victims, is an entity from the earliest of childhood instincts, a body that is common to all humans, as Lacan would have it. The "normal body" is actually the one that we develop later. It is in effect a Gestalt— and therefore in the realm of what Lacan calls the "imaginary." The realm of the "real" in Lacanian terms is where the fragmented body is found because it is the body that precedes the ruse of identity and wholeness. Artists often paint this vision, and it often appears in dreams "in the form of disjointed limbs, or of those organs represented in exoscopy . . . the very same that the visionary Hieronymus Bosch has fixed for all time" (4).

In understanding this point, we can perhaps see how the issue of disability transcends, by definition, the rather narrow category to which it has been confined. It is in tracing our tactical and self-constructing (deluding) journeys away from that originary self that we come to conceive and construct that phantom goddess of wholeness, normalcy, and unity—the nude. The element of repulsion and fear associated with disability results perhaps from that repression of the primal fragmentariness of the body. As Freud wrote, "the uncanny is in reality nothing new or foreign, but something familiar and old-established in the mind that has been estranged only [in] the process of repression" (*Studies in Parapsychology*, 47).[23] The feelings of repulsion associated with the uncanny, *das Unheimlich*, the unfamiliar, are not unlike the feelings associated with the "normal" visualizing of the disabled. The key to the idea of the uncanny is in its relation to the normal. *Heimlich* is a word associated with the home, familiarity, and the regular, comfortable, predictability of the home. The disabled body is seen as *unheimlich* because it is the familiar become estranged. Freud notes that the terror or repulsion of the uncanny is found precisely in its ambivalent relation to the familiar and yet its deviance from that standard. That the uncanny can be related to disability is made clear when Freud cites specifically "dismembered limbs, a severed head, a hand cut off at the wrist" as *unheimlich* (49). What is uncanny about dismemberment seems to be the familiarity of the body part that is then made *unheimlich* by its severing. As Freud wrote, "the *unheimlich* is what was once *heimisch*, home-like, familiar; the prefix 'un' is the token of repression" (51).

But in this equation, I think Freud is actually missing the earlier repression of the inherently fragmentary nature of the original body imagos. The homeyness of the body, its familiarity as whole, complete, contained, is based on a dynamic act of repression. Freud is assuming that the whole body is an a priori given, as he had done with the concept of the ego. But as Lacan has shown more than adequately, the ego is a multifaceted structure to be understood in its philosophical complexity. Likewise, the ground of the body, its materiality given by Freud, needs a reanalysis. The route of disability studies allows for this revisioning. In this case, the *heimisch* body becomes the *unheimlich* body, and the fragment, the disabled parts, can be seen as the originary, familiar body made unfamiliar by repression. Dominant culture has an investment in seeing the disabled, therefore, as uncanny, as something found outside the home, unfamiliar, while in fact where is the disabled body found if not at home?

The Venus, neatly enclosed in its marmoreal skin, represents an unperforated body, despite the mutilations that have disfigured it. Most of the visual arts eschew disability and disabled images, except perhaps for the romanticized images around madness. A notable exception to this reluctance to think of living Venuses without arms as the equivalent of Medusa is the work of Mary Duffy, a contemporary performance artist without arms. In the first plate of a photographic series entitled *Cutting the Ties That Bind,* we see a standing figure draped entirely in white cloth against a dark background so that the figure beneath the drapery is not visible. In the second plate, the drapery is partially removed so that it covers mainly the thighs and legs, revealing to us a female body, the artist's, without arms. The figure is clearly mean to reproduce the Venus de Milo in the flesh. The third picture in the series shows the figure stepping away from the drapery with a triumphant smile. The work serves to show how the female disabled body can be reappropriated by the artist herself. Duffy writes:

> By confronting people with my naked body, with its softness, its roundness and its threat, I wanted to take control, redress the balance in which media representations of disabled women is usually tragic, always pathetic. I wanted to hold up a mirror to all those people who had stripped me bare previously . . . the general public with naked stares, and more especially the medical profession.[24]

The Medusa gaze is rerouted so that it comes not from the object of horror, the "monstrous" woman, but from the gaze of the "normal" observer. It is the "normal" gaze that is seen as naked, as dangerous. And unlike Perseus slaying Medusa by holding up a mirror, it is now the "object of horror" who holds the mirror up to the "normal" observer.

This reappropriation of the "normal" gaze is further carried out by the British photographer Jo Spence. Recognizing the inherent and unstated pose of normalcy imposed by the camera and by the photographic session, Spence has revisioned her photography to be capable of representing the nude model as a person with disabilities. Her work, detailed in many shows and in her book *Putting Myself in the Picture: A Political, Personal, and Photographic Autobiography,* partly focuses on her mastectomy. Spence links this operative and postoperative process to an understanding and participating gaze that seeks to touch, not recoil from, bodily changes. In addition to the simple fact of the partial mastectomy, Spence also includes in her work photographs and text that question assumptions about age and beauty. Her body is middle-aged, irregular, and defies the canons of ideal feminine beauty. Her work is involved with "explaining my experience as a patient and the contradictions between ways in which the medical profession controls women's bodies and the 'imaginary bodies' we inhabit as women."[25]

The visual arts have done a magnificent job of centralizing normalcy and marginalizing different bodies. Photographer David Hevey has written about the paucity of images of the disabled in photographic anthologies. He concludes that "disabled people are represented but almost exclusively as symbols of 'otherness' placed within equations which take their non-integration as a natural by-product of their impairment."[26] When he looked for any images of disabled people, he found either medical photographs in which the "patients" appear "passive and stiff and 'done to,' the images bear a bizarre resemblance to colonial pictures where 'the blacks' stand frozen and curious, while 'whitey' lounges confident and sure"[27] or images like those of Diane Arbus that show the disabled as "grotesque." However, ungrotesque, routine pictures of disabled people in advertising, "art" photography, films, and so on, are hard to find. With the same regularity that bodies of color were kept out of the mainstream, and even the avant-garde, media in the pre–civil rights years, so too are disabled bodies disqualified from representing universality.

One of the ways that visual images of the disabled have been appropriated into the modernist and postmodernist aesthetic is through the concept of the "grotesque." The word was used by Bakhtin to describe the aesthetic of the Middle Ages that reveled in presenting the body in its nonidealized form. The grotesque, for Bakhtin, was associated with the people, with a culture that periodically turned the established order upside down through the carnival and the carnivalesque. Gigantic features, scatological references, inverse political power were all hallmarks of the grotesque—an aesthetic that ultimately was displaced by humanistic notions of order, regularity, and of course power during the Renaissance.

While the term *grotesque* has had a history of being associated with this counterhegemonic notion of people's aesthetics and the inherent power of the masses, what the term has failed to liberate is the notion of actual bodies as grotesque. There is a thin line between the grotesque and the disabled. Hevey examines, for example, how critics have received Diane Arbus's photographs of the disabled. Susan Sontag writes that Arbus's "work shows people who are pathetic, pitiable, as well as repulsive, but it does not arouse any compassionate feelings." Later she adds, "Do they see themselves, the viewer wonders, like *that?* Do they know how grotesque they are?"[28] The grotesque, in this sense, is seen as a concept without the redeeming sense of class rebellion in Bakhtin's formulation. Here is simply the ugly, what makes us wince, look away, feel pity—more allied with its dictionary definition of "hideous," "monstrous," "deformed," "gnarled." Though artists and writers may use the grotesque, they rarely write about that state from the subject position of the disabled. The grotesque, as with disability in general, is used as a metaphor for otherness, solitude, tragedy, bitterness, alterity. The grotesque is defined in this sense as a disturbance in the normal visual field, not as a set of characteristics through which a fully constituted subject views the world. The problem with terms like *disability* and *the grotesque* is that they disempower the object of observation. The body is seen through a set of cultural default settings arrived at by the wholesale adoption of ableist cultural values.

In no area is this set of cultural values related to the visual more compelling than in film. Film is a medium whose main goal, one might say, is the construction and reconstruction of the body. The abnormal body plays a major role in the defining of the normal body, and so one might assume that film would be concerned with the issue of disability. Martin F. Norden has recently published the most complete account of disability in the film industry to date, *The Cinema of Isolation: A History of Physical Disability in the Movies*. The film industry has been obsessed with the depiction of the disabled body from the earliest silent films. The blind, the deaf, the physically disabled were singled out from the very dawn of cinema. Norden finds movies about disability from as early as 1898, and the earliest one-reeler silent films of the period 1902–9 include such representative titles as *Deaf Mute Girl Reciting "Star Spangled Banner"* (1902), *Deaf Mutes' Ball* (1907), *The Invalid's Adventure* (1907), *The Legless Runner* (1907), *The One-Legged Man* (1908), *The Hunchback Brings Luck* (1908), *The Little Cripple* (1908), *A Blind Woman's Story* (1908), *The Blind Boy* (1908), *The Cripple's Marriage* (1909), *The Electrified Humpback* (1909) to name only a few. Later multi-reeler silent films routinely told the stories of the disabled. D. W. Griffith made a few disability-related films, culminating his efforts in the famous *Orphans of the Storm* (1921), in which two hapless sisters (Lillian and Dorothy Gish), one of whom is blind, try to survive on the streets of Paris. But the noteworthy fact about this film is not merely its disability-related content but that Griffith's version was the *fifth* filmic remake of the 1874 French play *Les Deux Orphelines*. With film only in its infancy, this particular disability story had been told approximately every four years from 1900 through 1921.

The point that Norden's book makes clear is that the cinematic experience, far from including disabilities in an ancilliary way, is powerfully arranged around the management and deployment of disabled and "normal" bodies. Stories of the disabled, stories of people's bodies or minds going wrong, make compelling tales. But more than that, as with any obsession, there has to be an underlying reason that films are drawn obsessively to the topic of disability. In order to understand why filmmakers routinely incorporate disabled bodies into films, it might be relevant to ask what else routinely appears in films. The answer is more than obvious—sex and violence. While it is fashionable for liberals and conservatives to decry the violent content of films, it might be more accurate for them to think of films as vehicles for the delivery of images of the body in extreme circumstances. The inherent voyeuristic nature of film makes it a commodity that works by visualizing for viewers the body in attitudes that are otherwise difficult to see. Few people in quotidian life see couples making love on a regular basis, while that experience is routine to filmgoers. Likewise, in peacetime, most middle class people rarely see dead, mutilated, bleeding bodies, while the average viewer has no shortage of such images.

So films, one could say, are a streamlined delivery system that produces dramatically these bodily images in exchange for a sum of money (as soft drinks can be said to be part of a system for delivering caffeine and sugar or as cigarettes are really time-release delivery systems for nicotine administration). As novels were seen to be mechanisms for the cultural production of normativity, so films have to be seen in the same regard, with the addition that the phantasm of the body is particularly subject to these normativizing activities.

Films enforce the normal body but through a rather strange process. The normal body, which had been invented in the nineteenth century as a departure from the ideal body, shifted over to a new concept—the normal ideal. This normal ideal body is now the one that we see on the screen. It is the commodified body of the eroticized male and female stars. This body is not actually the norm, but it is the fantasized, hypostatized body of commodified desire. In order to generate this body and proliferate its images, films have constantly to police and to regulate the variety of bodily differences. These bodies are the modern equivalents of the nude Venuses, and to keep them viable, to encourage viewers to think on and obsess about them, the Medusa body has constantly to be shown, reshown, placed, categorized, itemized, and anatomized. In short, we cannot have Sharon Stone without Linda Hunt; we cannot have Tom Cruise without Ron Kovic; we cannot have the fantasy of the erotic femme fatale's body without having the sickened, disabled, deformed person's story testifying to the universal power of the human spirit to overcome adversity. As Norden points out when films about disabled people are made, more often than not the disabled characters get cured by the end of the film. The tension between the whole and the fragmented body, between the erotic complete body and the uncanny incomplete body, must be constantly deployed and resolved through films.

The film *Boxing Helena* provides some interesting ways of seeing these tensions worked through. In the film, Nick (Julian Sands), a surgeon, amputates the legs of Helena (Sherilyn Fenn), the bitchy, sexualized woman with whom he is obsessed but who rejects his advances. He performs the amputation initially to save her life after a car accident but then goes on to amputate her arms as a way of keeping her and containing her—of rendering her helpless so he can take care of her.

A replica of the Venus de Milo decorates Nick's family mansion. The statue is used as a double symbol. In one aspect, it is an illustration of the former beauty of the dismembered Helena, its marmoreal glaze representing the still and ever beautiful Helena. But, it also represents idealized female beauty (in its wholeness) and is associated with Nick's mother, whose blatant sexuality was used to humiliate her son when he was young. The filmmaker wants us to see the dismemberment partly as an act of revenge against the castrating mother, whose legacy shows up in Nick's premature ejaculation syndrome (which in that sense renders him disabled). The mother, who has died, later returns to Nick's gaze, seen from the back as the naked and armless Venus, and the statue itself at one time falls on

Nick and in another moment explodes from within, thus illustrating the repressed reality of the fragmented body.

The salient point is that when Helena's limbs are amputated, that is, she becomes the Venus, she becomes desexualized—merely idealized. Whereas before her dismemberment she is a fantasy of ravenous female sexuality unencumbered by the traditional female values of caring, nurturing, or sweetness, after her dismemberment, she loses her sexuality. In a typical ableist moment, she says after her amputation: "How can I ever look at myself and think of myself as worthwhile?" Her worth in this case is her sexuality, which is lost. Her disability is actually created and owned by Nick.

In another instance of bourgeois, ableist celebration of the discursivity of sexuality, both she and Nick regain their sexual function (thus becoming undisabled) through eros. He buries his head in her lap, which of course despite all the mutilation leads us to realize that everything that is conventionally part of female sexuality is still intact—and in a moment of his fantasy she comes alive sexually, a trope that is equated with her suddenly having arms and legs. She caresses his head, walks, and whispers the answer to Freud's question, "What do women want?" telling him how women want to be made love to. Her whispered erotic litany begins to release the bad dream of disability. But it is only he, as the owner of her body, who can fully accomplish this release, and so she begs him: "I want to feel like a woman. Give me back what you've taken away." The supplement that has been missing is returned like the Lacanian phallus by Nick through a very Lacanian moment. As Helena watches through a semiopened door, Nick makes love to another woman (who in the credits is called "fantasy woman"), and we see that he is no longer sexually dysfunctional. Helena's self is reconstituted through a triangularization of desire in which her mirror imago of the whole body is recreated by viewing the desire of the Other. The other woman represents her wholeness, and the entire issue of functionality is blurred into sexual ability.

Although the director, Jennifer Lynch, is presenting an unusual story about a disabled person, she cannot separate herself from traditional views of people with disabilities. Never does the surgeon have to change a bedpan or a tampon; more tellingly, Helena is never allowed to be shown both naked and disabled—although her body was openly revealed before her amputations. Her double-amputated body is partly held up as an object of beauty, but it is not an object of sexuality—and therefore it can never be seen naked, as it was revealed to the camera's gaze before the operations. Unlike Mary Duffy or Jo Spence, Lynch cannot allow herself to show us the naked, disabled body. This would be too great a primal-scene moment in which the true nakedness of disability, its connection with the nakedness of the unwhole fragmented body, would be unavoidable and unable to be repressed.

The film ends with the revelation that the entire narrative has been, of course,

Nick's dream. Helena was hit by a car, but in actuality she was taken to the hospital, and she remains intact physically at the end of the film. Disability is just a bad dream, as Helena herself had called it in her outcry at first discovering that her legs had been amputated. She is cured.

The film returns to the whole, untarnished body because that is always seen as the norm. In general, when the body is mentioned in literature or depicted in drama and film, it is always already thought of as whole, entire, complete, and ideal. In literature, central characters of novels are imaged as normal unless specific instruction is given to alter that norm, and where a disability is present, the literary work will focus on the disability as a problem. Rare indeed is a novel, play, or film that introduces a disabled character whose disability is not the central focus of the work.[29] More often, the disability becomes part of a theme in which a "normal" person becomes romantically involved with a person with a disability and proves that the disability is no obstacle to attractiveness. At its most egregious, this theme is taken up in works like Somerset Maugham's *Of Human Bondage,* in which the character's sexual life is cleared of problems only when the disability is removed. With an only slightly more enlightened perspective, films like *My Left Foot* confirm the character's inner worth when he attracts a wife at the end of the film. And *Boxing Helena* is simply part of this genre.

In art, photography, film, and other media in which the body is represented, the "normal" body always exists in a dialectical play with the disabled body. Indeed, our representations of the body are really investigations of and defenses against the notion that the body is anything but a seamless, whole, complete, unfragmented entity. So, in addition to the terms of race, class, gender, sexual preference, and so on—all of which are factors in the social construction of the body—the concept of disability adds a background of somatic concerns. But disability is more than a background. It is in some sense the basis on which the "normal" body is constructed; disability defines the negative space the body must not occupy; it is the Manichaean binary in contention with normality. However, this dialectic is one that is enforced by a set of social conditions and is not natural in any sense. Only when disability is made visible as a compulsory term in a hegemonic process, only when the binary is exposed and the continuum acknowledged, only when the body is seen apart from its existence as an object of production or consumption—only then will normalcy cease being a term of enforcement in a somatic judicial system.

NOTES

1. S. E. Browne, D. Connors, and N. Stern, eds., *With the Power of Each Breath: A Disabled Women's Anthology* (Pittsburgh, PA: Cleis Press, 1985), 147.

2. Browne, Connors, and Stern, *With the Power of Each Breath,* 155.

3. Anne Finger, "Comrade Luxemburg and Comrade Gramsci Pass Each Other at a Congress of the Second International in Switzerland on the 10th of March, 1912." *Ploughshares* 22, no. 1 (Spring 1997): 74.

4. Michael Oliver, *The Politics of Disablement: A Sociological Approach* (New York: St. Martin's Press, 1990), 27.

5. *New York Times,* 27 October 1994, sec 22A.

6. The pairing of beauty with ugliness is further carried out in Venus's marriage to Vulcan, who is himself both ugly and lame. Lameness tends to be associated in an ableist way with impotence—as it is, for example, in W. Somerset Maugham's *Of Human Bondage.*

7. Kenneth Clark, *The Nude: A Study in Ideal Form* (1956; reprint, New York: Pantheon, 1964), 5. Most future references will be made parenthetically in the text.

8. Lynda Nead, *The Female Nude: Art, Obscenity and Sexuality* (London and New York: Routledge, 1992), 1.

9. Ibid., 17–18.

10. Kaja Silverman, "Historical Trauma and Male Subjectivity," in *Psychoanalysis and Cinema,* ed. E. Ann Kaplan (New York: Routledge, 1990), 114.

11. Nead, *The Female Nude,* 19.

12. Peter Stallybrass and Allon White, *The Politics of Transgression* (Ithaca, NY: Cornell University Press, 1987).

13. Clark, *The Nude,* 91.

14. John Barrell, "'The Dangerous Goddess': Masculinity, Prestige, and the Aesthetic in Early-Eighteenth-Century Britain." *Cultural Critique* 12 (1989): 127.

15. Ibid.

16. The Medici Venus has been reconstructed, so the eighteenth-century men did not have to face the incompleteness of their erotic subject.

17. Walter Benjamin, *Illuminations* (New York: Schocken, 1969), 223–24.

18. Jacques Lacan, *Ecrits: A Selection* (New York: Norton, 1977), 2. All future references will be made in the text.

19. Elie Ragland-Sullivan, *Jacques Lacan and the Philosophy of Psychoanalysis* (Urbana, IL: University of Illinois Press, 1987), 21.

20. Ibid., 27.

21. Robert Graves, *The Greek Myths* (1955; reprint, New York: Penguin, 1957), 49.

22. In "Communication Barriers between 'the Able-bodied' and 'the Handicapped'," in *Psychological and Social Impact of Physical Disability,* ed. Robert P. Marinelli and Arthur E. Dell Orto (New York: Springer, 1984), Irving Kenneth Zola pointed out that people with disabilities are mostly born into "normal" bodies. Thus they are socialized into an ableist culture and have to adopt their disabled identity. "We think of ourselves in the shadows of the external world. The very vocabulary we use to describe ourselves is borrowed from that society. We are *de*-formed, *dis*-eased, *dis*-abled, *dis*-ordered, *ab*-normal, and most telling of all an *in*-valid."

23. Sigmund Freud, "The Uncanny," in *Studies in Parapsychology* (New York: Collier, 1963).

24. Nead, *The Female Nude,* 78.

25. Jo Spence, *Putting Myself in the Picture: A Political, Personal, and Photographic Autobiography* (London: Camden Press, 1986).

26. David Hevey, *The Creatures Time Forgot: Photography and Disability Imagery* (London: Routledge, 1992), 54.

27. Ibid., 53.

28. Ibid., 57.

29. For extended discussion of the image of the disabled in literature, film, and journalism see Alan Gartner and Tom Joe, *Images of the Disabled/Disabling Images* and Michelle Fine and Adrienne Asch, *Women with Disabilities: Essays in Psychology, Culture, and Politics.*

Disfigurement and Reconstruction in Oliver Wendell Holmes's "The Human Wheel, Its Spokes and Felloes"

David D. Yuan

Susan Reynolds Whyte, summarizing Henri-Jacques Stiker's monumental history of the discourse on bodily abnormality in the West, *Corps infirmes et sociétés*, writes that after World War I "a broad paradigm shift" occurred in Europe and the United States: now "damaged people" were to be "rehabilitated," that is, they were to be "returned to a real or postulated preexisting norm of reference, and reassimilated into society"; "[w]hereas earlier epochs situated the infirm as exceptional in some way, the modern intention (or pretension) is that they are ordinary and should be integrated into ordinary life and work."[1] From this perspective, the quintessentially modern concept of rehabilitation began as a strategy for winning "professional control over the damaged bodies" of World War I veterans and preventing old war wounds from hindering the post–world war economy.[2] For Stiker, this move was critical, as it marked the "beginning of the denial of difference" that is "characteristic of our time."[3] But this "broad paradigm shift" in the treatment of the disabled, as singular as it may have seemed in the wake of the almost unimaginable carnage of World War I, was not entirely unprecedented: many of the tenets of the new ideology (rehabilitation, reassimilation, the social "invisibility" of the disabled) had in fact been anticipated during the aftermath of the American Civil War.

Regarding military technology and strategy, the importance of the American Civil War as a precedent for World War I has been widely acknowledged: the Civil War, after all, introduced ironclad warships, repeating rifles, telegraphy, and the importance of controlling the railways to Western war making. Because weapons technology outstripped medical technology between 1861 and 1865, the Civil War was one of the most injurious wars in history: over 600,000 Americans died as a direct consequence of the Civil War, more than died in both world wars, the Korean War, and the Vietnam War combined.[4] In addition, the Civil War produced more amputees than any other war Americans have fought in; three out of every four operations performed on Union soldiers were amputations, and altogether 130,000 men were "scarred or disfigured for life" during the war.[5]

Thus it is not surprising that the Civil War and Reconstruction not only redefined war but also helped to redefine disability for the modern state.[6] Looking past the war that was still convulsing the country, Oliver Wendell Holmes

Sr.—physician, poet, inventor, and futurist—was one of the first to propose that, in effect, rehabilitation and reassimilation should become critical components of a new paradigm for the treatment of the disabled (albeit Holmes, already in his fifties by the start of the war, sometimes shrank from his own vision of the future). But equally important to the modern history of physical difference, Holmes adumbrated what might be called a nationalist body aesthetics whose implications went well beyond the practical task of rehabilitating disabled workers. For Holmes, it was important not only that the disabled citizen be rehabilitated into the workforce but also that his or her body—like the bodies of all citizens—properly emblematized the body politic. For Holmes, the disabled body was not a correct emblem for the Reconstructed United States.

Holmes published his seminal article on disability and prosthetics, "The Human Wheel, Its Spokes and Felloes," in the *Atlantic Monthly* in May 1863. By then any illusion that the Civil War would be brief and casualties few had long been shattered. Holmes writes at the start that the raison d'être for his article is the sudden, alarming ubiquitousness of the amputee.

> The starting point of this paper was a desire to call attention to certain remarkable AMERICAN INVENTIONS, especially to one class of mechanical contrivances, which, at the present time, assumes a vast importance and interests great multitudes. The limbs of our friends and countrymen are a part of the melancholy harvest which war is sweeping down with Dahlgren's mowing-machine[7] and the patent reapers of Springfield and Hartford. The admirable contrivances of an American inventor, prized as they were in ordinary times, have risen into the character of great national blessings since the necessity for them has become so widely felt. While the weapons that have gone from Mr. Colt's armories have been carrying death to friend and foe, the beneficent and ingenious inventions of MR. PALMER have been repairing the losses inflicted by the implements of war.[8]

The American inventor B. Frank Palmer (whom Holmes surmises was aptly named for the inventive Benjamin Franklin), an amputee from childhood, designed his own prosthetic leg, allegedly because he was disgusted with the simple "peg leg" that he had worn since childhood. The "Palmer leg" was designed to replace an entire limb—including the complex knee joint. Unlike the peg leg, the Palmer leg was carefully shaped to resemble a natural limb from thigh to foot. Most important, the artificial knee was articulated, thanks to an intricate system of springs and pulleys hidden inside the prosthesis, allowing the amputee to walk much more naturally (see fig. 1).

While the Palmer leg is Holmes's ostensible subject, "The Human Wheel" also includes a brief lecture on human locomotion, another on the mass production of boots and shoes, and, to conclude, a chauvinist harangue on American ingenuity.

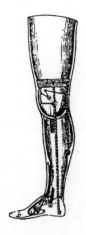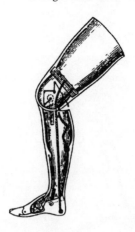

Fig. 1. The Palmer leg was modeled on an actual leg, including the complex knee joint, and allowed the amputee to walk more naturally than its predecessor, the peg leg. Engravings from "The Human Wheel, Its Spokes and Felloes," by Oliver Wendell Holmes, *Atlantic Monthly*, May 1863, 575.

The essay's title refers to the then recent discovery of the true nature of human locomotion, a discovery that could not be made, according to Holmes, until the advent of instantaneous photography made it possible to freeze each moment of the marvelously integrated process that is the act of walking. Instantaneous photography revealed that "Man is a *wheel*, with two spokes, his legs, and two fragments of a tire, his feet. He *rolls* successively on each of these fragments from the heel to the toe" (see fig. 2); "Walking, then, is a perpetual self-recovery. It is a complex, violent, and perilous operation, which we divest of its extreme danger only by continual practice from a very early period of life . . . We discover how dangerous it is, when we slip or trip . . . or overlook the last step of a flight of stairs, and discover with what headlong violence we have been hurling ourselves forward" (571). Like much of Holmes's writing, "The Human Wheel" has allegorical overtones. By 1863, the Civil War, already far from the brief affair that the young recruits had expected, could be allegorized as a national Fall, a Fall that revealed with what headlong violence the young nation had been hurling itself into the future.

The photograph (like the microscope) has the power to reveal the invisible; we would not know that "Man is a wheel" without photography. But the goal of the Palmer leg is a kind of invisibility: its goal is to fool the observer into thinking that the amputee is not an amputee. The highest compliment that Holmes can pay the Palmer leg is that "No victim of the thimblerigger's trickery was ever more completely taken in than we were by the contrivance of the ingenious Surgeon-Artist" (577). Holmes, who begins his essay by making visible the hitherto invis-

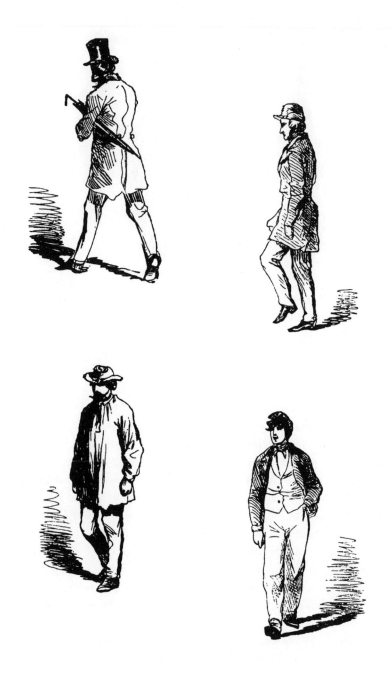

Fig. 2. Holmes uses these four views of men walking to
illustrate the process of human locomotion. "Man is a *wheel*,
with two spokes, his legs, and two fragments of a tire, his feet.
He *rolls* successively on each of these fragments from the heel to
the toe." (Engravings [based on stereoscopic views] in Holmes,
"The Human Wheel," 570.)

ible act of human locomotion, concludes by championing the Palmer leg, a device intended not so much to improve the amputee's mobility as to improve his appearance by rendering his injury invisible: "counterfeiting its aspect so far as possible" (575). Holmes insists that for "polite society" the sight of the "odious 'peg'" is simply intolerable: "misfortunes of a certain obtrusiveness may be pitied, but are never tolerated under the chandeliers" (574). In other words, polite society does not wish to see certain realities, and Holmes recognizes that American ingenuity exists not only to reveal truth but also to hide it.

Holmes, summing up, writes that the United States finds itself in an "age when appearances are realities"; thus the technology of disguise becomes crucial. The fact that the Palmer artificial leg does not quite achieve a perfect illusion of normalcy (see 576) is beside the point. "The Human Wheel" implies that eventually the amputee will be able to "pass" for a whole-limbed person with the aid of an ever-improving American technology: "As we wean ourselves from the Old World, and become more and more nationalized in our great struggle for existence as a free people, we shall carry this aptness for the production of beautiful forms more and more into common life" (578).

"The Human Wheel" recalls the dilemma of photographers who sought to capture the sights of the Civil War. Even as the advent of photography helps to reveal the true nature of war and deconstructs the glamorous image that had long protected society from war's horrors, it provokes the question, To what extent is it desirable to know the truth about war? For Holmes it seems enough for the revelatory photograph (the photograph that reveals the mundane violence of locomotion) to return the secrets of human anatomy and physiology to the realm of the invisible: if the Civil War is reaping a "melancholy harvest" of limbs, then American ingenuity is just as rapidly replacing them with its prostheses. And if the war's devastations can be reversed in this way, then the extent to which the war appears to inflict permanent damage is mitigated. As Timothy Sweet has argued, the very notion of "harvest" that is promulgated by Holmes and others suggests the hopefulness of renewal and rebirth, a rebirth to follow the holocaust of the war.[9]

Holmes's other analogy for the war is the bloody but lifesaving surgical operation: "We are in trouble just now, on account of a neglected hereditary *melanosis*"; we must "eliminate the *materies morbi*" if the body politic is to be cured (580). Like the pastoral analogy, the medical analogy was very popular with intellectuals who sought to explain the Civil War's necessity.

Anticipating a Union victory and the postbellum society that will follow, Holmes finds that not only is the Civil War a kind of surgery but that the prosthesis will assist in a kind of social reconstruction even as it completes the body's reconstruction. Undisguised limblessness is simply not to be tolerated in the postbellum society. But it requires a new technology to create an artificial limb that will convincingly disguise the intolerable fact of the incomplete body. Holmes understands well the broader implications of the problem: "Reconstruction," in all senses of the term, will require new technologies of disguise. Reconstruction will require a national ideology that privileges the new, while disguising or even displacing the past. Holmes even theorizes why Europeans tolerate the sight of the peg leg while Americans do not: it is the fineness of the "national eye for the harmonies of form and color," the superiority of the American's visual aesthetic (578). In short, appearances matter more in America than they do in the Old World.

In an earlier article, "The Doings of the Sunbeam," Holmes reveals the mysterious process of production at a commercial photograph factory.[10] In "The Human Wheel," Holmes seeks to convey Palmer's extraordinary achievement by dissecting what Holmes calls an *Autoperipatetikos*, a "walking" automaton, which Holmes gleefully exposes as an impostor. One *Autoperipatetikos* in particular has become famous because she "toddle[s]" behind a shop window, attracting great crowds of spectators.

> An autopsy of one of her family which fell into our hands reveals the secret springs of her action. Wishing to spare her as a member of the defenseless sex, it pains us to say, that, ingenious as her counterfeit walking is, she is an impostor. Worse than this . . . duty compels us to reveal a fact concerning her which will shock the feelings of those who have watched the stately rigidity of decorum with which she moves . . . *She is a quadruped!* Inside of her great golden boots, which represent one pair of feet, is another smaller pair, which move freely through these hollow casings . . . Her movement, then, is not walking . . . it is more like that of a person walking with two crutches besides his two legs. (572)

Holmes's ostensible point here is to highlight the ingenuity of the Palmer prosthesis by revealing the automaton's failings, but the very act of comparing the automaton and the amputee-with-prosthesis suggests the conflation of humans and machines, an idea that Holmes explicitly evokes later in the essay: "gradually the wooden limb seems to become, as it were, penetrated by the nerves, and the intelligence to run downwards until it reaches the last joint of the member" (576–77). Moreover, the conflation of machine and person is further suggested by the way in which Holmes goes on to "dissect" B. Frank Palmer in much the same way as he dissects and explains the prosthesis and the *Autoperipatetikos*: analyzing Palmer's exterior and interior, extracting his motivation and character. Holmes explains Palmer's motivation, imagining the emotional burden of Palmer's "unsightly appendage" (his peg leg) during "adolescence" and how this misery proved to be the source of his inventiveness (574). Then Holmes explicates and evaluates both the mechanics of Palmer's novel prosthesis as such (the "ingenious arrangement of springs and cords in the *inside* of the limb") and the mechanics of inventor and invention (amputee and prosthesis) in combination: "He puts his vegetable leg through many of the movements which would seem to demand the contractile animal fibre. He goes up and down stairs with very tolerable ease and dispatch. Only when he comes to *stand* upon the human limb, we begin to find that it is not in all respects equal to the divine one" (576). If this man-machine hybrid does not perfectly imitate the divine creation, it is a better illusion than the "walking" automaton, which transfixed the crowds gathering around the shop window.

What "The Human Wheel" offers, as Holmes is well aware, is a vision of American society in the near future for which the boundary between bodies and machines has become ambiguous. In other words, Holmes anticipates the "machine culture" (or "prosthetic culture") that was to become dominant in the latter nineteenth century, a culture whose paradigmatic issue is "the problem of the body."[11] Holmes's use of the feminized *Autoperipatetikos* anticipates what Mark Seltzer identifies as the naturalist novel's exploration of "the mechanism of the feminine."[12] Furthermore, Holmes's interior and exterior dissection of Palmer (the psychoanalytic pursuit of "what makes Palmer tick" alongside the analysis of how he physically moves) coupled with his dissection of the female automaton anticipates the postbellum assumption *"that bodies and persons are things that can be made."*[13]

As noted, production fascinates Holmes. Holmes, who was delighted with the primitive assembly line used by the E. T. Anthony firm to produce thousands of photographs in a day, visits the Palmer factory where "legs are organized," expecting to see another example of machine-driven efficiency (577). But at the Palmer factory, Holmes is surprised to discover that the shaping of the wooden limbs "is all done by hand".

> We had expected to see great lathes, worked by steam-power, taking in a rough stick and turning out a finished limb. But it is shaped very much as a sculptor finishes his marble, with an eye to artistic effect,—not so much in the view of the stranger, who does not look upon its naked loveliness, as in that of the wearer, who is seduced by its harmonious outlines into its purchase, and solaced with the consciousness that he carries so much beauty and symmetry about with him. (577)

Holmes's expectation of steam-powered lathes evokes not only the changing face of Northern industry (like the textile factory) but also the role of steam power in the Civil War, with armored steamships skirmishing in the bays and rivers and steam locomotives hauling supplies by rail to the front lines. Melville wrote derisively of the Monitor's battle with the Merrimac: "all went on by crank / Pivot, and screw." Melville recognized that the Civil War had ushered in a new kind of combat, as well as a new kind of soldier: "War yet shall be, but warriors / Are now but operatives."[14] Holmes himself has made the connection between a vital new mechanized industry and both the removal and the replacement of limbs, but here at the Palmer factory he is initially both surprised and gratified to discover that production is less an anticipation of the assembly line than a throwback to a vanishing era of handcrafted artisanship. Nevertheless, as we have already glimpsed, there is a disturbing subtext to "The Human Wheel": workers and soldiers seem to be not so much "operatives" as mechanical parts that are being operated. And because they are cogs in the war machine (human wheels), the implication is that they may be summarily repaired or replaced as needed. The Civil War, then, conflated the prosthesis and the soldier, as the industrial revolution conflated the prosthesis and the worker.

Henry Ford, writing sixty years after Holmes, dramatically expands the conflation of worker and prosthesis. Ford, writing about the Model T assembly line in his autobiographical *My Life and Work* (1923), notes that only 12 percent of the 7,882 work operations along the line required "strong, able-bodied, and practically physically perfect men." The vast majority of operations could be performed by workers who were less than "able bodied": "we found that 670 could be filled by legless men, 2,637 by one-legged men, two by armless men, 715 by one-armed men and ten by blind men."[15] Ford, like Holmes, is pondering the problem of reconstruction in the wake of a war of unprecedented mechanization and carnage.[16]

Ford's analysis suggests a future where the conflation of worker and prosthesis is virtually complete. The "worker" as such is no longer relevant; industry has become so specialized that it is now appropriate to speak of the laboring body part or function rather than the laborer.[17] What is striking about Ford's comment is the contrast it presents when compared to Holmes's argument in the "Human Wheel." For Ford, the literal prosthesis has become irrelevant. Instead of a worker needing a prosthesis to appear or perform as if whole bodied, he or she can dispense with this pretense altogether. Thus when industry begins to think of labor "prosthetically," the amputee laborer is liberated from the prosthesis; the 'incomplete" worker is redeemed. Appearances, so important to Holmes, seem to have lost their relevance for Ford, who is concerned with the part of each worker performing its discrete task rather than with the appearance of "wholeness."[18]

But while Ford, perhaps, felt that he was already living in a prosthetic culture, Holmes, in 1863, is somewhat nervously anticipating its arrival. Holmes unabashedly celebrates the triumphs of mechanized industry elsewhere (as in "The Doings of the Sunbeam"), but in "The Human Wheel" he seems to hesitate before its inexorable advance. At the Palmer factory, Holmes is deeply impressed by the fact that the Palmer leg is not purely an anonymous, machine-molded tool (like the weapons that had proved so proficient at removing limbs), calling it a "true artist's limb" (579). The Palmer leg is a commodity imbued with a soul. But Holmes's ambivalence toward the nascent machine-prosthetic culture is evident in the language he uses to describe the final phase of the Palmer leg's construction: "The hollowing-out of the interior is done by wicked-looking blades and scoops at the end of long stems, suggesting the thought of dentists' instruments as they might have been in the days of the giants" (577). Thus while the *exterior* shaping of the Palmer leg is done by hand, as "a sculptor finishes his marble," the *interior* of the prosthesis is prepared by the very sort of intimidating machines that Holmes had expected to see in the first place (there is a resemblance between Holmes's description of the factory machines and his earlier description of the peg leg [which is quoted later in this article]: the latter is "fearful-looking," the former "wicked-looking). Thus the Palmer leg is not simply useful sculpture, it is a peculiar combination of art and machine-produced artifact: the artist handing off the half-completed limb to the "wicked-looking" machinery to finish.

Holmes's mixed reaction to the Palmer factory is a sort of prototype for the ambivalence and confusion that would become a characteristic response as Americans confronted or evaded the implications of the body-machine complex. Like the responses of his later counterparts, Holmes's response to scenes of the "miscegenation of nature and culture," as Seltzer puts it, is itself mixed (21). Holmes is both eager and reluctant to gaze on the new society that machines are ushering into being, and he projects onto the hero of "The Human Wheel" this ambivalence in his very reading of the hero's name (B. Frank Palmer). Holmes initially draws out only the name's evocation of Benjamin Franklin, as noted. But later, Homes alludes to another Palmer "namesake": "We owe the well-shaped, intelligent, docile limb, the half-reasoning willow of Mr. Palmer, to the same sense of beauty and fitness which moulded the soft outlines of the Indian girl and the White Captive in the studio of his namesake in Albany" (578). The Albany namesake is Erastus Dow Palmer (1817–1904), the noted New York sculptor whose two most famous pieces are the *Indian Girl* (1856) and the *White Captive* (1858). Thus "B. Frank Palmer" signifies, for Holmes, the combined sensibilities of the artist and the scientist. The inventor is as much a hybrid as his invention.[19]

In another telling move, Holmes deliberately feminizes the prosthesis: the amputee is "seduced" into buying the beautiful limb, and he relishes its "naked loveliness" even though the public (which he intends to dupe with this counterfeit) will never see it, any more than they would see the naked loveliness of a genuine limb in a polite social context. A romantic description like this one softens the impression, given elsewhere in the essay, that the body itself has been reduced by medicine and technology to its mechanical essentials and that beauty and grace are no longer the body's most important attributes. Holmes's description represents an intriguing regendering of the Palmer leg from the obviously phallic (the Palmer leg "would almost persuade a man with two good legs to provide himself with a third") to the "feminine" as Holmes would define it (the leg is "well-shaped," "docile," and both "intelligent" and "half-reasoning" [577–78]). I will explore the political utility of this regendering of the prosthesis later on, but for now I only want to point out the range of examples of hybridity in Holmes's text: the "female" automaton, a counterfeit woman, is revealed to be a "quadruped"; "B. Frank Palmer" refers to two divergent antecedents; and the Palmer leg is a complex hybrid, emblematic of the complex nation that produced it. The Palmer leg is organic and inorganic, rational and romantic, masculine and feminine, intelligent and half-reasoning. Moreover, the Palmer leg becomes even more complex when it is conjoined with the amputee.

Holmes takes great pains to establish a stark contrast between the peg leg and the Palmer leg. The image of the former is grotesque, the amputee stumping about on the crude peg; the image of the latter is all symmetry and grace. Interestingly, the wound itself, the stump that marks the place where the natural limb should be, is not discussed (even though Holmes as a physician would be eminently equipped to discuss amputation and its aftereffects). It is not the absence of the limb that is grotesque or hideous; it is the peg leg's crudity, the rude transparency of its counterfeit, that offends. Or rather it is the *lack* of disguise that offends: the fact that the peg leg is actually no counterfeit limb at all but is simply a pragmatic response to the amputee's desire to move about. The Palmer leg's "naked loveliness" is enjoyed only by the amputee himself (in Holmes's imagining of it), but the nakedness of the peg leg is seen by all and disgusts all.

According to Holmes, B. Frank Palmer's leg was amputated when he was ten years old; Holmes does not give us the details of the accident, telling us only that the limb was "crushed." Holmes's truncated biography moves directly from the accident to Palmer's adolescence, because it is with the dawning of sexual possibility that the weight of Palmer's aesthetic disability begins to be felt.

> We can imagine what he suffered as he grew into adolescence under the cross of this unsightly appendage. He was of comely aspect, tall, well-shaped, with well-marked, regular features. But just at the period when personal graces are most valued, when a good presence is a blank check on the Bank of Fortune, with Nature's signature at the bottom, he found himself made hideous by this fearful-looking counterfeit of a limb. (574)

The peg leg is "hideous," "unsightly," and, perhaps most significantly of all, "fearful-looking." The horror of Palmer's condition is enhanced by the fact that he was otherwise a handsome, well-proportioned young man. Incongruity is a hallmark of the grotesque, and the incongruity of an otherwise thoroughly presentable young man stumping around on the rude peg makes this scenario not only pathetic but hideous. Indeed, the effect is so terrible that young Palmer could not tolerate it, and he abandons the peg leg for the "tender mercies of the crutch," as Holmes cryptically puts it. But the crutch is "at best an instrument of torture," pressing upon a "great bundle of nerves" in the armpit, distorting the figure, perhaps even "distempering the mind itself" (575). It seems remarkable that young Palmer would ever have thought the crutch a "tender merc[y]" for even a moment, but such is society's horror of "the odious 'peg'" that Palmer was driven to the attempt. Finally, the ingenious Palmer invents his superior prosthesis and resolves his aesthetic dilemma. Since it is allegedly the public appearance that counts in "The Human Wheel," it does not seem to matter that Palmer must still remove the artificial leg at night and expose his stump to plain view. Holmes is too discreet to imagine a Mrs. Palmer or how she might react to the real state of his bodily affairs.

Holmes's "The Human Wheel," like Thomas Jefferson's *Notes on the State of Virginia,* extrapolates from the individual to the national and addresses the place of the United States in the world scene. "The Human Wheel" is as much a reaction to the national crisis as it is to the specific plight of the amputee. Holmes, who is fond of offering readers the obvious analogy, fails to consider the Civil War as an amputation of the body politic: the nation losing its Southern half. But he does refer to the war as "a neglected hereditary *melanosis,*" which requires the elimination of "the *materies morbi*" (580). But what are the *materies morbi* for Holmes? The Confederate government? The institution of slavery? The blacks themselves? A "hereditary *melanosis*" suggests the origin of the national illness in the black slaves, but are they the cause or only the symptom of the disease?[20] Eliminating the *materies morbi,* in the medical sense, refers to the surgical removal of dead tissue; Holmes probably had the removal of a gangrenous limb in mind. Thus figurative amputation, like literal amputation, is for Holmes a beneficent, lifesaving procedure: the *materies morbi* are eliminated, and the patient survives. But an unsightly appearance in polite society is intolerable, and the scorn that a critical Europe might have for the struggling United States concerns Holmes. To European critics, Holmes offers a raw rebuttal: "We profess to make men and women out of human beings better than any of the joint-stock companies called dynasties have done or can do it" (580). Holmes will not allow Europe to believe that the United States itself is grotesque; the United States must not be viewed as a cripple among the nations nor a crude yokel whom genteel Europe finds intolerable.

Holmes blatantly uses the invention of the Palmer leg to refute the unexamined notion that Europe always surpasses the United States in the achievement of symmetry, harmony, and beauty. Holmes does not argue that American civilization is catching up with Europe, he argues that it is already surpassing Europe. Holmes proudly proclaims: "American taste was offended, outraged, by the odious 'peg' which the Old-World soldier or beggar was proud to show" (578).

Holmes's pride in the Palmer leg can be read as a remarkable evasion of the Civil War, which, after all, was the severest test that "American civilization" had ever faced. Holmes, in the middle of the most destructive war in history, finds in the very fact of unprecedented carnage the proof of American superiority. First, Holmes finds that the war is proving America's technical prowess: American ingenuity has produced both the best weapons for killing and wounding and the best prostheses. Second, it is not in spite of the war that "American civilization" aspires to a higher aesthetic plane, but, Holmes implies, partly *because* of the war: "As we wean ourselves from the Old World, and become more and more nationalized in our great struggle for existence as a free people, we shall carry this aptness for the production of beautiful forms more and more into common life" (578). The Civil War, then, is a continuation of the American Revolution; it is another milestone in the nation's growing up and away from the Old World. As most contemporary historians would be quick to agree, the Civil War was, as Holmes suggests, the introduction to a vast expansion of American nationalism. It is true that Holmes qualifies his cultural chauvinism a bit. He admits that "the national ear for music is not so acute [as Europe's]," but he insists that "the national eye for the harmonies of form and color is better than we often find in older communities" (578). The image of the peg-legged "beggar" (which is presumably more ubiquitous in the dynastic Old World than in democratic America) subtly invokes Poe's Europe of gothic horrors and grotesques: catacombs, plagues, madhouses, slums replete with the crippled and deformed.

But what is it that allows the European soldier to proudly display his peg, while the American soldier is ashamed to show his? Unlike the beggar's condition, whose meaning may be ambiguous, the veteran's wound is presumably a badge of courage and honor. Holmes implies that the American "eye" is not only more aesthetically refined and demanding but more democratic: America has less tolerance for the sight of the disfigured dregs of society. In the United States, the misshapen cannot be so cavalierly discarded and relegated to the interstices of polite society. American society has an obligation to recuperate the disfigured and offer them the opportunity to make themselves presentable. Importantly, Holmes refutes the idea that the democratic society drags the elite down to the level of the lowest denominator. Rather, it is the task of American technology and culture to raise the coarse and vulgar to the plane of symmetry and refinement—this is precisely what is involved in the process of weaning "ourselves from the Old World."

As an introduction to his analysis of the Palmer leg, Holmes presents Plumer's last: the shoe mold designed by the pioneering American podiatrist Dr. J. C. Plumer. Plumer last produced shoes and boots that conformed well to the actual shape of the human foot, in contrast to the typical nineteenth-century shoe, which forced the foot to do most of the conforming. The standard-issue boots supplied to the soldiers in the Union army were notoriously punishing, and it often took weeks of use before they could be worn without pain. (The Confederate soldiers were often not issued boots at all.) Along the way, the recruits were made uncomfortable, and some were even disabled by the boots—thwarting the men's morale and their readiness to fight. Dr. Plumer, the foot's great liberator, came to the rescue with his innovative last. Holmes applauds him as "the Garrison of these oppressed members of the body corporeal" and declares: "The foot's fingers are the slaves in the republic of the body. Their black leathern integument is only the mask of their servile condition. They bear the burdens, while the hands, their white masters, handle the money and wear the rings" (572). "[B]lack integument" here obviously invokes the slave's black skin, and black skin—to pursue Holmes's analogy—is a mask that helps to disguise the slave's essential humanity, thus justifying the misconception that the African

American is a separate species and is biologically suited for subjugation. (Holmes's discourse on toes as slaves and shoes as black skin is echoed later in the essay's closing description of the war as a "hereditary *melanosis*.")

Beneath the innocuous sheen of patent leather, the feet are performing the hardest labor in the republic of the body. Holmes's discourse on feet is comparable to his discourse on photography: in both discourses the overarching theme is the dis-covering of a hitherto invisible labor process. The wider implication of "The Human Wheel" is that medicine and physiology themselves may be understood in the same terms: they are the sciences dedicated to revealing how the body, which is a kind of organic labor process, or organic industry, is ordered and run. The feet suffer, in part, because we do not penetrate their "narrow prisons" to see how they labor. The feet, like the slaves, are de-formed by the severity of their labor and their harsh environment: "they grow into ignoble shapes, they become callous by long abuse, and all their natural gifts are crushed and trodden out of them" (572). The horror of slavery, then, is not simply that the slave suffers but that he literally becomes something grotesque and ignoble. It is not the "black integument"—the slave's physiognomy—that is grotesque, nor is the African American intrinsically benighted; it is the institution of slavery that deforms the slave.

Holmes's discussion of the body corporeal constantly evokes the body politic and vice versa; it seems he cannot investigate the one without investigating the other. As Holmes recounts it, Dr. Plumer began his research by "contemplating the natural foot as it appears in infancy, unspoiled as yet by social corruptions, in adults fortunate enough to have escaped these destructive influences, in the grim skeleton aspect divested of its outward designs" (572). Reading analogically again, it is not only the idea that the slave has been warped and corrupted that is conveyed here but also the idea that the master has been corrupted, which is a familiar, even predominant argument of the abolitionists. Holmes also returns to the contrast between appearance and the deep structures underlying appearance. The "grim skeleton" is "divested of its outward designs," and like the skull grinning in at the banquet that William James posits, the "skeleton" insists that we examine the true nature of our existence and our experience. Holmes directs the reader to dis-cover labor and production. Similarly, he asks the reader to look beneath the surface of the corporeal body and the body politic to view the complex stresses on bone and tendon, the delicate chemical negotiations occurring in the blood, and the despair attending a slave economy content to conduct business as usual.

Ultimately in "The Human Wheel," Holmes capitulates to the demands of appearance and the sanctity of socially approved disguise. But it is important to recognize the polarity in Holmes's thought: the tension between the tyranny of appearance and the need to deconstruct appearance (i.e., to estrange aspects of our experience in order to truly see and understand it). Thus toes are liberated by Plumer's last, but Palmer's wooden leg, schooled by the amputee himself, submits to the amputee's command, and the amputee himself—in wearing the Palmer leg—submits to the command of "American civilization" and conforms to the new code of public appearance.

> America has made implements . . . which out-mow and out-reap the world. She has contrived man-slaying engines which kill people faster than any others . . . She has bestowed upon you and the world an anodyne which enables you to cut arms and legs off without hurting the patient; and when his leg is cut off, she has given you a true artist's limb for your cripple to walk upon, instead of the peg on which he has stumped from the days of Guy de Chauliac. (579)

Holmes correctly anticipates a postbellum America that will lead rather than follow the other nations. Holmes's description recalls "Harvest of Death," Timothy O'Sullivan's famous photograph of corpses lying on the fields of Gettysburg. But this Civil War pastoralism (which Timothy Sweet correctly explains as an effort to make the carnage "natural" and thus more acceptable) is undercut by mechanoindustrial undertones ("implements" for mowing and reaping; "man-slaying engines"). Such language conveys the opposite idea of "unnatural" processes of production and destruction: farming as agribusiness; war and medicine as industry; the foreshadowing of the assembly line. Holmes seems reluctant to push the parallel he draws between harvesting/replanting and war/medicine (war removes limbs, medicine replaces them) to its conclusion. But what makes Holmes hesitate? Is it a reluctance to "naturalize" war, or is it a reluctance to recuperate a fallen America via the familiar naturalizing imagery?

The illustration of the human wheel that appears at the very beginning of the article, unlike the illustrations of walkers derived from photographs, is more than a diagram of human locomotion, it is an emblem of the essay's literal and metaphorical dimensions (see fig. 3). The human wheel emblem's evoking of the

Fig. 3. The human wheel, from which Holmes's article takes its name, can be seen as an emblem of the essay's metaphorical dimensions as well as a diagram of human locomotion. (Holmes, "The Human Wheel," 567.)

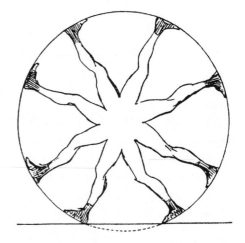

anthropometric studies of Leonardo da Vinci is probably intentional, and it serves to underscore one of Holmes's objectives: to provide a more accurate measure and definition of humanity—especially of humanity acting, of humanity moving, as opposed to humanity simply being.[21] As instantaneous photography allows us to understand human locomotion, so the arts of historical and cultural analysis allow us to trace the trajectory of the human species through time.

The human wheel as an emblem for the essay is appropriately paradoxical. The figure of the wheel suggests both returning and forward progress—and both ideas are powerfully attractive to Holmes, who is writing, despite his air of assurance, at a time of uncertainty and anxious confusion. Nevertheless, the surface of Holmes's text optimistically declares his dedication to forward progress. Holmes boasts that the "American Wheel is moving through the miseries of the Civil War to a better place in history, a place which will be envied by the great nations of the world." The amputee, the cripple, the grizzled veteran "stumping" around on his peg do not present the image appropriate to a young nation boldly on the rise. The "peg" is neatly opposed to the wheel in Holmes's essay: if America is the efficient, smoothly rolling wheel, then Europe is the splintery, inefficient, old peg.

The wheel does seem an apt metaphor for the United States—the Civil War was itself a demonstration on a vast scale of the wheel's power. First, the Civil War was "the first American conflict in which railroads played a major role."[22] The North's rail superiority was a key factor in securing its victory. Second, other innovative wheeled or wheel-like machines, from the field ambulance to the wheeled gun battery that was mounted on its own steel rails, were prominent during this war. And even as the war raged on, the transcontinental railway project was already underway; by 1869 the recently re-United States was spanned by rails from the Pacific to the Atlantic, greatly facilitating Easterners' migration to Western lands. (As the United States entered the twentieth century, the automobile allowed the wheel as national paradigm to continue to dominate the American landscape and imagination, replacing the railroad train as the quintessential wheeled machine.)

But while Holmes seems to believe that the future he envisions will come to pass, "The Human Wheel"'s subtext, as we have already seen, belies this rather bellicose optimism. Beneath Holmes's eager modernism is a deep desire to redeem the past and avoid the full consequences of the modernity Holmes sees hurtling toward him; Holmes hesitates before the prosthetic culture that he has insightfully anticipated. Even as Holmes professes the recuperation of amputees into society via the invisible prosthesis (the Palmer leg), he is compelled to confront the prostheticization of society, that is, the "dismemberment of the natural body" that Seltzer recognizes in Henry Ford's industrial "fantasy."[23]

We need to return to the most basic question about "The Human Wheel": why should Holmes demand that the prosthesis be invisible? The essay offers several explicit answers: America's highly developed aesthetic sense, the desire to demonstrate technical prowess, the stigma that the amputee must bear. But it is Holmes's stark maxim that "[a]ppearances are realities" that needs to be reexamined. The subtext of the maxim is that the visible prosthesis serves to remind us of the way in which prosthetic culture is enveloping all of society, not only the disabled and disfigured. Despite Holmes's huffing and puffing about the peg leg and the Old World, the visible prosthesis is as much an emblem of encroaching modernity as it is an emblem of the old order (like the human wheel, which stands for returning as well as for progress). If prostheses are invisible, then they do not exist; if we can convince ourselves that we are not living in a prosthetic culture, then we will not confront the political implications of the new order. Things will seem to be the way they have always been.[24] Holmes writes glowingly of liberation and freedom, but through his essay the reader may glimpse a rather different future American society: a society where no workers will be slaves but where workers will be not unlike the "well-shaped, intelligent, docile limb, the half-reasoning willow of Mr. Palmer" (578). The political expediency of Holmes's regendering of the phallic prosthesis is now clear: Holmes identifies as feminine the qualities of docility, gracefulness, and half-reasoning intelligence. And these are the qualities that should characterize the worker, who, like the willow limb, is "stupid until practice has taught . . . just what is expected" of him: this is what Holmes means by half-reasoning intelligence. If it is understood that the Civil War has conflated the soldier and the prosthesis, then it becomes apparent that the disciplinary strategies that served to order the soldier might also serve to order the postbellum worker. Like the well-disciplined soldier, the worker should be intelligent enough to perform assigned tasks but not intelligent enough to question them; the worker should be "free" yet subordinate.

NOTES

1. Benedicte Ingstad and Susan Reynolds Whyte, eds., *Disability and Culture* (Berkeley, CA: University of California Press, 1995), 270. Whyte, an anthropologist, suggests in her well-named essay "Disability between Discourse and Experience" that it is necessary to include both a historicizing discourse analysis and a thoughtful "appreciation of narratives and case studies" if one is to have a truly comprehensive disability studies (280). I concur with Whyte's integrationist view, and I would argue further that disability studies is not exclusively an inquiry into the construction of disability as it affects the disabled, but an inquiry into how the construction of disability affects and reflects an entire culture. To interrogate a culture's idea of disability is to interrogate that culture.

2. Ibid., 9.

3. Ibid., 270.

4. John Keegan, *A History of Warfare* (1993; reprint, New York: Vintage-Random House, 1994), 356. Over 400,000 Civil War deaths were the result of infection and disease

contracted after battle, often after surgery (antiseptic measures did not become standard medical procedure in the United States until after the Civil War).

5. Stewart Brooks, *Civil War Medicine* (Springfield, IL: Charles C. Thomas, 1966), 74, 97.

6. Hillel Schwartz has discussed the importance of the American Civil War in the history of prosthetics and has argued for a distinctive period of prosthetic innovation beginning in 1865 (Reconstruction) and culminating in 1920 (the post–World War I period). Schwartz writes that after the Civil War, "the United States became a leading innovator in the production and fitting of artificial limbs. These would subsequently be adapted and improved by the English, French and Germans during World War I" ("Torque: The New Kinaesthetic of the Twentieth Century," in *Incorporations*, ed. Jonathan Crary and Sanford Kwinter [New York: Zone Books, 1992], 102).

7. "Dahlgren's mowing-machine" refers to a devastating naval gun deployed by the Union Navy. Abraham Lincoln delighted "in the big splash eleven-inch shells made when fired into the Potomac by the great bottle-shaped Dahlgren guns" (Geoffrey Ward, *The Civil War: An Illustrated History* [New York: Alfred Knopf, 1990], 130).

8. Oliver Wendell Holmes Sr., "'The Human Wheel, Its Spokes and Felloes,'" *Atlantic Monthly*, May 1863, 567–80. Hereafter referred to as "The Human Wheel"; subsequent quotations from this work will be noted parenthetically in the text. All emphases in quotations from "The Human Wheel," unless otherwise indicated, are Holmes's.

9. Timothy Sweet, *Traces of War: Poetry, Photography, and the Crisis of the Union* (Baltimore, MD: Johns Hopkins University Press, 1990), 114.

10. Oliver Wendell Holmes Sr., "The Doings of the Sunbeam," *Atlantic Monthly*, July 1863, 1–15.

11. Mark Seltzer, *Bodies and Machines* (New York: Routledge, 1992), 3.

12. Ibid., 65.

13. Ibid., 152 (Seltzer's emphasis).

14. Herman Melville, "A Utilitarian View of the Monitor's Fight," in *Battle-Pieces and Aspects of the War* (1866; reprint, Amherst, MA: University of Massachusetts Press, 1972), 62.

15. Henry Ford, *My Life and Work* (Garden City, NJ: Doubleday, Page, 1923), 108–9.

16. The Ford Motor Company began building cars on the moving assembly line in 1913–14, at the same time as Europe was utilizing similar technological strategies to mobilize its armies (World War I is remembered as the first fully motorized war: the war that introduced the armed tank, submarine, and airplane). Holmes, writing in 1863, the year Henry Ford is born, anticipates the machine-driven (prosthetic) culture that would become so deeply associated with Ford in the twentieth century (the automobile, after all, is modern society's ultimate prosthesis).

17. Bill Brown has helpfully summarized the move by which labor is prostheticized: "Human labor is analytically and materially reduced to the operation of the body part, and the individual human functions only as a part, the 'conscious limb,' within the machine system" ("Science Fiction, the World's Fair, and the Prosthetics of Empire, 1910–1915," in *Cultures of United States Imperialism*, ed. Amy Kaplan and Donald E. Pease [Durham, NC: Duke University Press, 1993], 136).

18. Ford, as one might expect, is more concerned than is Holmes with the disabled

veteran's capacity to hold a factory job. Inside the factory's secure walls (and Ford always valued security), remote from the ballroom that is uppermost in Holmes's mind, the amputee's appearance would not matter as it would "under the chandeliers." The bold new ideology of the body that Holmes argues is peculiarly American is somewhat belied by Holmes's Old World attitude toward the disabled and work. When Holmes notes that Palmer's artificial arm (invented after Palmer's success with his artificial leg) "cannot serve a pianist or violinist" but "is yet equal to holding the reins in driving, receiving fees for professional services, and similar easy labors," he affirms the old notion that the disabled are incapable of performing complex or strenuous tasks (578).

19. I have found no evidence that B. Frank Palmer was actually named for Erastus Dow Palmer. I believe Holmes is simply using the coincidence of the two having the same name to amplify his point that the inventor has both technological ingenuity and a "sense of beauty and fitness." The patent that Palmer received in 1846 for his artificial leg (Patent No. 4,834) was granted to "Benjamin F. Palmer," suggesting that "B. Frank Palmer" was a variant he adopted later (Joseph Nathan Kane, *Famous First Facts* [New York: H. W. Wilson, 1981], 321).

20. While the *Oxford English Dictionary,* second edition, asserts that the primary meaning for *melanosis* in the mid-nineteenth century was "a morbid deposit or abnormal development of a black pigment in some tissue" (or hyperpigmentation), it seems more likely that Holmes had the more sinister secondary meaning of the word in mind here: a "black cancer" ([Oxford: Oxford-Clarendon University Press, 1989], volume IX, 576). "Black cancer" probably referred to what today is called melanoma: the highly malignant, dark-colored skin tumor that is often deadly if untreated.

21. And note that like Leonardo da Vinci, B. Frank Palmer and Holmes himself combine the roles of artist and scientist.

22. Eric Foner and John A. Garraty, eds., *The Reader's Companion to American History* (Boston, MA: Houghton and Mifflin Co., 1991), 907.

23. Seltzer, 157. The Palmer prosthesis, although admittedly imperfect, clearly represents Holmes's ideal (an ideal that I am calling the "invisible prosthesis").

24. This is the human wheel as conservative emblem (the human wheel returning). From this perspective, the object of Palmer's innovative invention is conservative: to return the body to its stainless antebellum state (Holmes, as indicated, already reads antebellum America as corresponding to a prelapsarian age in the national mythos). Thus missing limbs and other traces of conflict will be erased. Bill Brown, writing about nineteenth-century science fiction, describes the postbellum idealized male body as "a body on which history is not written but erased, a body without memory, a national body with no nation" (Brown, "Science Fiction," 155).

Defining the Defective ▶ Eugenics, Aesthetics, and Mass Culture in Early-Twentieth-Century America

Martin S. Pernick

From 1915 to 1918 Chicago surgeon Harry Haiselden electrified the nation by allowing the deaths of at least six infants he diagnosed as "defectives."[1] Seeking publicity for his efforts to eliminate those he considered "unfit," he displayed the dying infants to journalists and wrote a book-length series about them for the Hearst newspapers. His campaign was front-page news for weeks at a time.[2] He also wrote and starred in a feature motion picture, *The Black Stork*, a fictionalized account of his cases.[3]

In the unprecedented debate prompted by Haiselden's actions, hundreds of Americans took a public stand. A majority of those quoted in the press *opposed* preserving the lives of "defectives." They included public health nurse Lillian Wald, family law pioneer Judge Ben Lindsey, civil rights lawyer Clarence Darrow, historian Charles A. Beard,[4] even the blind and deaf reformer Helen Keller.[5]

Yet despite these dramatic events, media coverage of the issue faded rapidly during the 1920s. By the time similar proposals surfaced again in the mid-1930s, Haiselden and his actions appeared to have been almost totally forgotten.[6]

This story is important, not just for its novelty and drama but because it vividly demonstrates the crucial though little-recognized role played by mass culture in constructing both the meanings and the memory of the early-twentieth-century movement for hereditary improvement known as *eugenics*. (The term *mass culture* includes any productions made for a mass audience, whether or not they were demonstrably "popular" in origin.)

Eugenic leaders frequently attacked mass culture for what they considered its vulgar distortion of scientific ideas. Yale professor Irving Fisher complained, "Eugenics is one of the few cases in which a scientific term has come into popular use," but "it is subject to a great deal of misconception."[7]

Historians of eugenics focus on the movement's professional leadership, and many have implicitly adopted the leaders' views of mass culture. But I will argue that such an approach misses the vital role of mass culture as a battleground on which scientists, physicians, popularizers, journalists, censors, and audiences struggled to shape the meanings of "eugenics" and "heredity."[8]

The passage of time makes it easier to see the aesthetic, epistemological, and ethical values inherent in early-twentieth-century eugenics. But that should not be taken to mean that eugenics was either *uniquely* value laden or peculiarly influenced by mass culture. Nor am I arguing that mass culture corrupted "pure" genetic science by infecting it with "extraneous" aesthetic and moral concerns. Rather, I believe the history of eugenics is valuable because it makes so dramatically visible the cultural value judgments that are inevitably part of defining any human difference as a disease or a disability and identifying any specific factors as "the" cause.[9]

The role of aesthetic judgments in the definition of disease and disability is still a highly controversial issue today. Should laws protecting the disabled against discrimination apply to those who are simply judged unattractive? Should health insurance cover "cosmetic" surgery?[10] Do aesthetic values create disability in the same way that high stairs and other physical barriers do? Could changing such values create a more accessible culture? I believe that the history of eugenics shows the futility of trying to answer such questions by seeking a sharp line between "objective" physical diseases and "subjective" values. Any time a culture defines disease or causation, it is making a partly subjective, value-based judgment. Greater awareness of the inevitability of the value-based component of these debates might or might not help in reaching more satisfactory decisions. But pretending that such decisions can ever be made without values only delegitimates and prevents the necessary critical analysis of the implicit values at stake.

The American eugenics movement supported a very diverse range of activities, including advanced statistical analyses of human pedigrees, "better baby contests" modeled on rural livestock shows, compulsory sterilization of criminals and the retarded, and selective ethnic restrictions on immigration.[11] These efforts all were seen as "eugenic" because they all aimed at "improving human heredity." But the meanings of eugenics also depended on the answers to at least four related but separate and distinct questions.

1. What does "improvement" mean?
2. What does "heredity" mean?
3. By what methods should heredity be improved?
4. Who has the authority to answer questions 1–3?

This essay examines the role of mass culture in defining eugenics by providing one illustrative example of how that culture served as a battleground for competing answers to each of these key questions. In the first section, mass culture's representations of beauty and ugliness illustrate the construction of what counted as "improvement." The second example explores why in mass culture the meaning of "heredity" was not limited to traits caused by genes. The final section traces the debate over whether eugenic methods included death for those judged defective, and the ironic role of the mass media in creating a professional monopoly over such decisions.

In its heyday during the 1910s and 20s, eugenics was widely accepted as being an objective science, and when I use words like *defective* and *unfit,* I am quoting what eugenicists believed to be purely technical terms. But while eugenics claimed to be purely objective, this essay will show that subjective values, such as aesthetic standards of beauty and ugliness and moral attributions of responsibility, were central to eugenic constructions of hereditary disease and disability.

What Traits Are Good?
Eugenics and Aesthetics

Aesthetic values played a critical though little-known role in eugenic constructions of fitness and defectiveness. Eugenics promised to make humanity not just strong and smart but beautiful as well.

Efforts by leading scientists to explain the evolutionary role of beauty began in 1871 with Darwin's analysis of sex selection in *The Descent of Man.* Darwin's cousin Francis Galton, who coined the term *eugenics,* began his scientific career by compiling a "beauty map" of Britain, for which he calculated the ratio of attractive to plain and ugly women he encountered at various locations.[12]

But while these and other evolutionary scientists studied the aesthetic component of eugenic "fitness," aesthetic concerns appeared more frequently in the mass media.[13] One major eugenic popularizer, Albert Wiggam, saw an attractive appearance as the *best* external indicator of overall hereditary fitness. He regarded health, intellect, morality, and beauty as "different phases of the same inner . . . forces." "Good-looking people are better morally, on the average, than ugly people." Thus he concluded, "If men and women should select mates solely for beauty, it would increase all the other good qualities of the race." In the most extreme version of this view, aesthetic preferences were simply Nature's instinctive guide to finding the fittest mate, a view both Wiggam and Haiselden sometimes explicitly endorsed.[14]

But both eugenic leaders and popularizers were skeptical that truly healthy beauty could be recognized by the untrained eye. Scientists since Darwin found beauty problematic precisely because aesthetic preferences in choosing a mate often did *not* seem to favor other adaptive traits.[15] Thus eugenicists did not simply endorse existing cultural preferences but actively attempted to "improve" current standards. Fisher explained that careful propaganda was needed to "unconsciously favorably modif[y] the individual taste . . . in mate-choosing." Wiggam agreed, "If their ideals of human beauty are properly *trained,*" young people will "unconsciously reject the ugly" and will "fill their homes with beautiful wives and handsome husbands."[16]

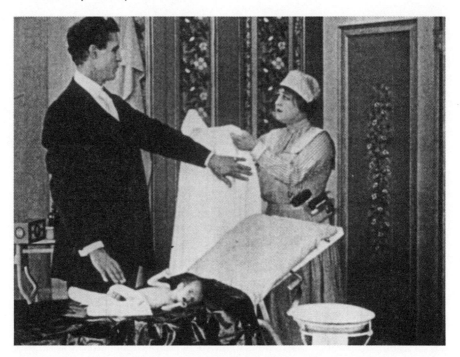

Fig. 1. Film still from *The Black Stork* showing the doctor refusing to operate on a disabled newborn. (University of Michigan Historical Health Film Collection, used with permission of John E. Allen.)

To illustrate the content of this aesthetic propaganda, I will focus on the only two surviving proeugenic full-length American motion pictures of the 1910s and 20s: *The Black Stork,* a feature film that dramatized Dr. Haiselden's crusade against saving impaired newborns, and the pioneering government-produced health education series *The Science of Life,* a twelve-reel survey of high school biology, distributed by the U.S. Public Health Service from 1922 to 1937.[17] In *The Black Stork,* Claude, who has an unnamed inherited disease, ignores graphic warnings from his doctor, played by Haiselden, and marries Anne. Their baby is born "defective" and needs immediate surgery to save its life, but the doctor refuses to operate (fig. 1). After God provides a horrific vision of the child's future of misery and crime, Anne agrees to withhold treatment, and the baby's soul leaps into the arms of a waiting Jesus.

Both films equated beauty with fitness. "An attractive appearance goes hand in hand with health," explained *The Science of Life.*[18] And both attempted to influence audience concepts of beauty. But each presented internally conflicting aesthetic standards, an ambivalent mix of modernism and romanticism.

The Science of Life emphasized stark mechanical images. It urged "THE

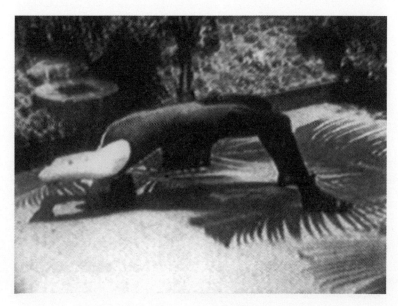

Fig. 2. Here, in *The Science of Life,* fitness is portrayed as modern hard-edged mass in efficient motion. (University of Michigan Historical Health Film Collection.)

WOMAN OF TOMORROW" to develop strength and beauty through vigorous exercises, demonstrated by a short-haired woman whose hard flat body was accentuated by stark black tights and knee-level photography (fig. 2). An attractive body also was explicitly equated with a sleek, streamlined locomotive, whose beauty became manifest in powerful motion and efficient function. Photographed in a low-angle tilt shot that swept upward from wheel level, the engine's sharp clean lines and powerful mass appeared starkly silhouetted against the sky. Motion pictures first made it possible to display the beauty of bodily action. The desire to depict the poetry and science of motion contributed to the development of cinema, while the use of film helped reshape modern beauty in terms of physiology, not anatomy, as active function, not just static form.[19]

But *The Science of Life* also promoted older romantic concepts of beauty. Intercut with the starkly modern images were scenes in which health and fitness were represented by a long-haired, round-cheeked, young woman in calm repose, photographed as glowing with cleanliness and natural sunlight in gauzy soft focus (fig. 3).[20]

The Black Stork emphasized the more naturalistic modernism of Thomas Eakins. Beauty was illustrated by athletic adolescents in outdoor settings: five naked boys diving into a swimming hole, a woman in a swimsuit doing handstands on the beach. The 1916 edition of *The Black Stork* explicitly *attacked* mechanical standards of beauty, using a speeding motorcar to represent not

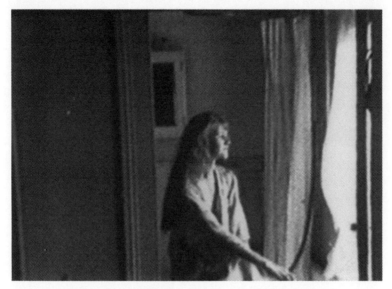

Fig. 3. This print from *The Science of Life* depicts fitness as soft-focus romantic beauty, cleanliness, and repose. (University of Michigan Historical Health Film Collection.)

modern aesthetics but the false allure of the "fast" life. Yet, when the film was rereleased in 1927, industrial modernism dominated. The sequence linking fast cars to loose living was deleted, while lengthy new scenes portrayed beauty as a massive new automobile, owned by a "professor of heredity."

This ambivalent aesthetic vision exemplified what Thomas Mann called "a highly technological romanticism." Eugenics promised to create a romantic utopia by means of modern science, and its aesthetic propaganda reflected this uneasy mix of goals.[21]

If eugenics equated fitness with beauty, it labeled ugliness a disability. "It was terribly ugly," Haiselden wrote of one baby. Such ugliness was not "light or superficial"; it was a true "handicap."[22] Both films selectively highlighted the repulsive ugliness of the "unfit," as in several scenes comparing them to cattle (fig. 4).[23] Again echoing Thomas Eakins, Haiselden described the case on which *The Black Stork* was based as "not a pretty one. It mars the pages of this book— as I intended it should mar them. It is better that the deformities of this tiny castaway should sear themselves into the minds of thinking men."[24]

Eugenic popularizers promoted definitions of ugliness that reinforced their judgments on other human differences, including gender, class, race, and nationality. Wiggam lamented:

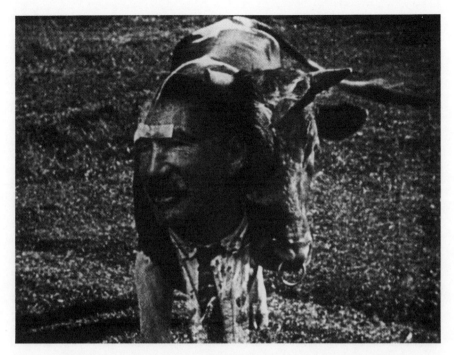

Fig. 4. In order to accentuate the ugliness of the "unfit," *The Black Stork* compares them with cattle. (University of Michigan Historical Health Film Collection, used with permission of John E. Allen.)

We want ugly women in America and we are getting them in millions. . . . [T]hree or four shiploads have been landing at Ellis Island every week . . . I have studied thousands of them . . . They are broad-hipped, short, stout-legged with big feet; . . . flat-chested . . . and with faces expressionless and devoid of beauty.

These "draft horses" were rapidly replacing "the beautiful women of the old American stocks, the Daughters of the Revolution."[25]

Both films linked aesthetics, disability, and race. The only identifiable blacks in each were photographed as repulsive defectives, as in this example from *The Black Stork* (fig. 5), and Haiselden repeatedly linked "blackness" with "ugliness."[26] Like race, economics also shaped the aesthetic distinctions between the fit and the defective. *The Science of Life* promised that both "health and success" awaited the visually attractive, and in both films, couples who illustrate "wise mating" wear tastefully conservative but up-to-date business suits and dresses on

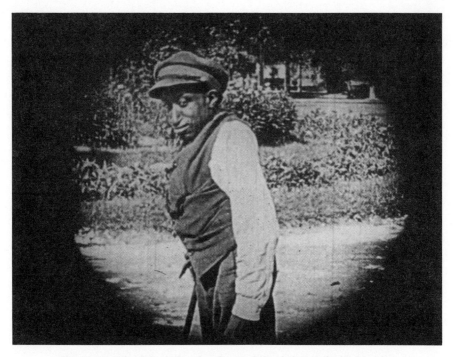

Fig. 5. In *The Black Stork*, physical disability is linked with race. (University of Michigan Historical Health Film Collection, used with permission of John E. Allen.)

their prosperously stout bodies. Portraying "others" as ugly was central to labeling them defective, while diagnosing "others" as diseased reinforced the perception of them as repulsive.

Eugenicists insisted that their diagnoses were based entirely on objective science. Even Helen Keller, the famed reformer who had become blind and deaf in childhood, believed that objective science could determine which mentally impaired infants should be eliminated. "A jury of physicians considering the case of an idiot would be exact and scientific. Their findings would be free from the prejudice and inaccuracy of untrained observation."[27]

Many eugenicists admitted that the distinction between "fit" and "defective" relied on aesthetic values, yet they denied that such classifications were therefore subjective or unscientific. They did not claim to be "value-free" but rather that their aesthetic values had been validated by objective scientific methods.[28]

Eugenic aesthetic judgments were based on broad cultural values that were not unique to eugenicists. But eugenics did not simply reflect cultural values indiscriminately. The movement's technocratic utopianism attracted mostly middle class, native born segments of the population who brought with them a specific set of values shared with others of their background, including their ambivalent romantic-modern aesthetic, and these selected preferences in turn shaped eugenic representations of beauty and ugliness.

Thus, eugenic popularizers promised to make people more attractive while they intervened in mass culture to selectively enhance the attractiveness of what they considered beautiful. They offered to eliminate ugliness while depicting as ugly everything they wished to eliminate. Their media efforts reveal the internal tensions and circular logic that characterized their constructions of the "fit" and the "defective."

These contradictions were heightened by the ease with which viewers found alternative meanings in such propaganda. For example, many reviewers of *The Black Stork* reported that the film's exhibition of deformed bodies evoked pity, or even fascination, rather than disgust. Disregarding the titles that labeled Claude and Anne's son an "abyss of abnormality" filled with "criminal desires," critics consistently praised the actor for making this character appealing, even noble.[29]

Others found that scenes intended to make disabled people look repulsive instead made the film itself "repellent" and "revolting." These critics often praised the film's educational and social value, but they found it aesthetically unacceptable: "grim," "depressing and unpleasant,"[30] "repulsive."[31] Louella Parsons complained that it was "neither a pretty nor a pleasant picture," because "it shows poor, misshapen bodies of miserable little children." Rival critic Kitty Kelly called it the "most repellent picture" she had ever seen.[32] Such reviewers concluded that anyone who wanted to see such films must be sick, suffering from a "morbid" perversion of the aesthetic senses.[33]

These unintended aesthetic responses were one important reason why films about eugenics were often banned.[34] Film censors went far beyond policing sexual morality, to include what I term "aesthetic censorship," much of which was aimed at eliminating unpleasant medical topics from entertainment films.[35] From the perspective of such aesthetic censors, both pro- and antieugenics films were unacceptably ugly. The powerful New York state film board banned both *The Black Stork* and *Tomorrow's Children,* a 1934 antieugenic melodrama, because eugenics was too "disgusting" a topic. They rejected *The Black Stork* in April 1923, not only for its "inhuman" position on euthanasia but for its "most unpleasant," "very distressing," "most revolting" depictions of disease. About *Tomorrow's Children* they concluded, "The sterilization of human beings is not a decent subject for public entertainment."[36]

Film censors shared the eugenicists' desire to pathologize and eradicate ugliness. They sought to ban the cinematic reproduction of ugly people, while eugenicists sought to ban their biological reproduction. But while eugenic publicists believed filming ugliness could help inoculate audiences against it, the censors feared that displaying ugly diseases would disseminate them, creating ugly-minded, diseased audiences. The attempt to make the disabled look ugly made eugenics seem repulsive as well.

What Is Heredity? Eugenics and
Moral Responsibility

Between the 1880s and 1910s, scientific concepts of heredity changed dramatically. The nineteenth-century "Lamarckian" view that environmentally caused changes in individuals could be passed on to their offspring was gradually supplanted by August Weismann's doctrine that individual heredity was permanent and unaffected by environmental forces.[37]

Yet in mass culture, the terms "heredity" and "eugenics" continued to be applied to traits that most scientists now attributed to environmental causes, from infections like tuberculosis and syphilis to bad prenatal care and malnutrition. For example, the only movie made by the "Eugenic Film Company," the 1917 film *Birth*, never mentioned genetics but simply provided detailed pregnancy and child care advice.[38] A 1917 feature, *Parentage*, was advertised as strongly "eugenic." It contrasted the families raised by good and by bad parents, explicitly conflating the effects of genetics and environment.[39]

Historians of eugenics usually attribute such examples to mass culture's scientific illiteracy.[40] But in doing so they miss a complex interplay among scientists, popularizers, and the public in defining "heredity." First, many scientists argued that Weismann's theory left room for environmental contributions to genetic disease; such views were neither unscientific nor limited to mass culture.[41]

Second, and most significantly, in mass culture and occasionally in the scientific literature, the term *hereditary* was not limited to genetics but meant that you "got it from your parents," regardless of whether "it" was transmitted by genes, germs, precepts, or probate. Thus *The Science of Life* defined a man's heredity as "what he receives from his ancestors."

Such definitions were not based on wrong science but on a different set of concerns. On this view, what defined "heredity" was the parents' moral responsibility for causing the trait, not the technical mechanism through which parental causation was transmitted. By this definition of "heredity," "eugenics" meant not just having good genes but being a good parent.[42]

Mass culture hardly ignored Weismann's science. At least a dozen films of the 1910s dichotomized heredity and environment, usually by portraying the life of a child whose foster parents differed radically from the biologic parents. Most such films concluded that key human differences were caused by environment, not heredity (at least for girls), but almost all presumed Weismann's radical disjuncture between nurture and nature.[43] Thus mass culture clearly reflected scientific concepts of heredity.

But in turn, leading scientists sometimes used "heredity" to mean "parental responsibility." The eminent British statistical geneticist R. A. Fisher argued that syphilis was a eugenic concern because it ran in families. "There may be something very much like inheritance [of syphilis], in the practical sense. Whether there is inheritance in the biological sense is not the only matter. We are anxious to make a more perfect mankind and we are interested in the practical side."

Even eugenic leaders who limited "heredity" to biological inheritance defined their movement as seeking good parenting, not simply good genes. New Jersey physician Theodore Robie declared at the Third International Eugenics Congress in 1932 that "it would . . . be conducive to racial improvement to sterilize even those feeble minded who do not necessarily fall in the hereditary group," since "*mental defectives tend to maintain inferior homes in inferior environments, and they quite generally rear their children in an inferior manner.*"[44] Whether or not all traits caused by parents were labeled "hereditary," any trait caused by parents was part of "eugenics." Identifying the parents as the cause made the parents morally as well as medically responsible.[45]

How to Eliminate the Unfit: Euthanasia and Eugenics

A few prominent scientists like German zoologist Ernst Haeckel favored death for the unfit as early as 1868, but prior to Dr. Haiselden's cases such ideas rarely won public endorsement from eugenic leaders.[46] Most advocated selective breeding, not the death of those already born with defects. Charles Davenport, perhaps the foremost American eugenic researcher of the period, insisted in 1911 that eugenics did "not imply the destruction of the unfit either before or after birth." Irving Fisher echoed Karl Pearson's "fundamental doctrine . . . that everyone, being born, has the right to live" but not the right "to reproduce his kind."[47]

Yet when Haiselden moved the issue from theory to practice, these same leaders proclaimed him a eugenic pioneer. Fisher now wrote to "emphatically approve" Haiselden's action. "I hope the time may come when it will be a commonplace that . . . defective babies be allowed to die." Davenport likewise now urged doctors not to "unduly restrict the operation of what is one of Nature's greatest racial blessings—death." If medicine prevented the death of defectives "it may conceivably destroy the race."[48]

Haiselden's attention-grabbing actions were a calculated effort to radicalize the eugenic leadership, a strategy anarchists of the time popularized as "propaganda of the deed." "Eugenics had a million theories . . . But it lacked drive," he explained. "[T]he times were crying for some one central deed—some decisive action that would draw together all these theories . . . into one definite crusade."[49] Haiselden was only one doctor, but by gaining extensive media coverage of his dramatic acts, he was able to reshape the leadership's definition of eugenic methods.

Ironically, while mass culture provided a key battleground on which competing groups struggled to define eugenics, many powerful figures in the film and journalism industries opposed public involvement in making these life-and-death decisions. The *New York Times* demanded that the power to selectively withhold treatment from impaired infants be "kept strictly within professional circles," free from "unenlightened sentimentality."[50] One common suggestion was to create special medical committees, what Helen Keller called "physicians' juries for defective babies." Mass culture thus played an important role in promoting the expansion of professional power.[51]

This media deference to professional expertise in turn contributed to the rapid decline in coverage of Haiselden's crusade and its erasure from public memory. Even people who demanded the death of the unfit opposed publicizing the issue. "I think all monstrosities should be permitted to die," wrote university president Frank H. H. Roberts, "but I do condemn the physician for making such a public ado about the matter." In an editorial entitled "He Forgets Silence Is Golden," the *New York Times* endorsed Haiselden's right to let infants die but denounced his use of media publicity. "If he is wise, as most doctors are, he settles the question for himself . . . and the incident does not become a subject of public discussion."[52]

This growing support for professional power and secrecy combined with the growth of aesthetic objections to eugenic subjects drastically curtailed media coverage of Haiselden's activities. By 1918, Haiselden's last reported euthanasia case received only a single column inch buried deep inside the *Chicago Tribune*, a paper that had supported him editorially and given front-page coverage to all his previous cases. Mass media preoccupation with novelty and impatience with complex issues clearly played a role in this change, as did the altered agenda of wartime and postwar politics. But in part, the disappearance of public debate appears to reflect a deliberate decision that the topic itself was unfit to discuss in public.[53]

And, as soon as the media attention flagged, eugenic leaders resumed their prior assertions that they opposed euthanasia, as if Haiselden had never existed. Irving Fisher started to distance himself as early as 1917, reiterating his earlier view that "eugenics does not require the old Spartan practise of infanticide" while simply ignoring his recent accolades for Haiselden.[54]

Thus, by 1930, Haiselden and his cases were not simply forgotten but intentionally erased from the history of eugenics. Both the immediate success and the eventual erasure of his efforts were the sometimes ironic product of the struggle to shape how mass culture portrayed the meanings of eugenics.

Conclusions

Mass culture was a battleground on which elite and other concepts of eugenics competed and interacted. Aesthetic and moral values played a key role in eugenic constructions of the hereditarily "fit" and the "defective," and these values were products of complex struggles to impose meaning on mass culture. Eugenic popularizers tried to use mass culture to promote their complex and circular aesthetic vision, but their efforts often had unintended consequences. The scientists' focus on the genetic mechanisms of heredity coexisted in uneasy tension with a broader, explicitly moral language in which hereditary causation meant parental responsibility. And while mass culture revealed wide support for empowering doctors to let the unfit die, it provoked even stronger opposition to talking about it in public.

NOTES

1. I am grateful to Peter Laipson for his many insightful contributions and to David Scobey for his helpful comments on the final draft. Marie Deveney's perceptive comments greatly helped sharpen my arguments. This essay is based on material from my book *The Black Stork: Eugenics and the Death of "Defective" Babies in American Medicine and Motion Pictures since 1915* (New York: Oxford University Press, 1996), used with the permission of Oxford University Press.

2. For easily accessible and/or unique accounts see the following. Bollinger: *New York Medical Journal* 102 (4 December 1915): 1132. Meter: *New York Times* (hereafter *NYT*), 25 July 1917, 11; *Chicago American* (hereafter *CA*), 24 July 1917, afternoon edition; *Medical Review of Reviews* (hereafter *MRR*), 23 (1917): 697–98; Werder: *CA*, 8 December 1915, afternoon edition; Grimshaw: *CA*, 28 December 1915, magazine page; *New York Call* (hereafter *Call*), 13 December 1915; Hodzima: *CA*, 13 November 1917; *New York Sun* (hereafter *NYS*), 13 November 1917; *NYT*, 16 November 1917, 4; *Chicago Herald* (hereafter *CH*), 20 November 1917; Stanke: *NYT*, 28 January 1918, 6. For cases prior to 1915, see *CA*, 23 November 1915, 3.

Extensive coverage may be found in newspapers nationwide, especially in the Midwest and East, for 12 November–30 December 1915; 5–7 February and 14–16 March 1916 (Bollinger, Roberts, Werder, and Grimshaw cases); 22–27 July and 12–20 November 1917 (Meter and Hodzima cases); 25–30 January 1918 (Stanke case); and 18–20 June 1919 (obituaries). *Note:* Unless otherwise stated all cited newspaper articles begin on page 1.

3. I found and restored the only viewable print, of the 1927 version. It is available for research use at the University of Michigan Historical Health Film Collection. An unprojectable fragmentary paper print of the 1916 version is at the Library of Congress Motion Picture, Broadcasting and Recorded Sound Division, Washington, DC (hereafter LC-MBRS), #LU-9978, Box 110.

4. Wald: *Independent*, 3 January 1916, 25; Lindsey: *CH*, 18 November 1915; Darrow: *Washington Post* (hereafter *WP*), 18 November 1915; Beard: *NYT*, 18 November 1915, 4. Darrow later repudiated eugenics in "The Eugenics Cult," *American Mercury* 8 (June 1926): 129–37.

I have identified 333 individuals who were quoted in the mass media on this issue. Of these, 167 (51 percent) opposed treating at least some types of impaired newborns, including 14 advocates of active killing. Another 32 favored leaving the choice up to the doctor, without saying what they thought the doctor should do. Only 116 (35 percent) said doctors should try to save all infants. Of course, this was not a scientific public opinion sample, but it does reflect the image of public opinion that was presented by the press. (Pernick, *Black Stork*, table 1)

5. Keller, in *The New Republic* (hereafter *TNR*), 18 December 1915, 173–74; and *Call*, 26 November 1915. Haiselden's critics initially cited her case to prove the social utility of preserving the lives of those with disabilities, for example, *WP*, 18 November 1915, 6; *NYS*, 18 November 1915; but Keller strongly supported Haiselden; so did at least one other spokesperson for the disabled, see *Detroit News* (hereafter *DN*), 18 November 1915, 25.

6. I could find only three references to Haiselden in the *NYT* and *Chicago Tribune* (hereafter *CT*) between 1920 and 1960.

7. Fisher, in National Conference on Race Betterment, *Proceedings* 2 (1915): 64. Irving Fisher and Eugene Lyman Fisk, *How to Live*, 12th ed. (New York: Funk & Wagnalls, 1917), 294.

For many similar comments see Mrs. Melvil Dewey, National Conference on Race Betterment, *Proceedings* 1 (1914): 349; Michael Guyer, *Being Well-Born: An Introduction to Heredity and Eugenics* (Indianapolis, IN: Bobbs-Merrill, 1927), 426; S. J. Holmes, "Misconceptions of Eugenics," *Atlantic*, February 1915, 222–27; Daniel Kevles, *In the Name of Eugenics: Genetics and the Uses of Human Heredity* (Berkeley, CA: University of California Press, 1985), esp. 58; William J. Robinson, *Eugenics, Marriage and Birth Control*, 2d ed. (New York: Critic & Guide, 1922), 91–93; *Fourth Annual Report of the State Charities Commission [Illinois], Institution Quarterly* 5 (June 1914): 65, as quoted in Patrick Almond Curtis, "Eugenic Reformers, Cultural Perceptions of Dependent Populations, and the Care of the Feebleminded in Illinois, 1909–1920" (Ph.D. diss., University of Illinois at Chicago, 1983), 91.

For the occasional less hostile view of mass cultural meanings see National Conference on Race Betterment, *Proceedings* 1 (1914): 272; *Good Health Magazine* 50 (1915): 485–88, and 51 (1916): 594–95.

8. For a few important exceptions see Mary Bogin, "The Meaning of Heredity in American Medicine and Popular Health Advice, 1771–1860" (Ph.D. diss., Cornell University, 1990); Robert W. Rydell, "Eugenics Hits the Road: The Popularization of Eugenics at American Fairs and Museums between the World Wars" (paper presented to the annual meeting of the History of Science Society, Chicago, December 1984); Dorothy Nelkin and M. Susan Lindee, *The DNA Mystique* (New York: W. H. Freeman, 1995); and the work in progress on eugenics in mass circulation magazines by Juan Leon.

9. Peter Steinfels, "Introduction" to issue on "The Concept of Health," *Hastings Center Studies* 1 (1973): 3–88; Charles Rosenberg, "Framing Disease," in *Framing Disease*, ed. Charles Rosenberg and Janet Golden (New Brunswick, NJ: Rutgers University Press, 1992), pp. xiii–xxvi; H. Tristram Engelhardt, "The Concepts of Health and Disease," *Evaluation and Explanation in the Biomedical Sciences* (Dordrecht: D. Reidel, 1975), 125–41; Sander Gilman, *Difference and Pathology* (Ithaca, NY: Cornell University Press, 1985). Pioneering work on these issues was done by Robert Veatch and Thomas Kuhn.

10. See, for example, T. R. B., "The Tyranny of Beauty," *TNR*, 12 October 1987, 4.

11. The literature on eugenics is vast. For an introduction to American eugenics, see Diane Paul, *Controlling Human Heredity 1865 to the Present* (Atlantic Highlands, NJ: Humanities Press, 1995); Kenneth L. Ludmerer, *Genetics and American Society* (Baltimore, MD: Johns Hopkins University Press, 1972); Mark Haller, *Eugenics* (New Brunswick, NJ: Rutgers University Press, 1963); Philip Reilly, *Genetics, Law, and Social Policy* (Cambridge, MA: Harvard University Press, 1977); Barry Alan Mehler, "A History of the American Eugenics Society, 1921–1940" (Ph.D. diss., University of Illinois, 1988).

To place the United States in comparative context, see Kevles, *In the Name of Eugenics;* Mark Adams, ed., *The Wellborn Science: Eugenics in Germany, France, Brazil, and Russia* (Oxford: Oxford University Press, 1989); Gar Allen, "Genetics, Eugenics, and Class Struggle," *Genetics* 79, suppl. (June 1975): 29–45; Jan Sapp, "The Struggle for Authority in the Field of Heredity 1900–1932: New Perspectives on the Rise of Genetics," *Journal of the History of Biology* 16 (1983): 311–42.

12. Cynthia Eagle Russett, *Sexual Science* (Cambridge, MA: Harvard University Press, 1989), 78–92; for Galton's "beauty map," see Kevles, *Name of Eugenics,* 12; Albert E. Wiggam, *The Fruit of the Family Tree* (Garden City, NY: Garden City Publishing, 1924); "Jackie Swims to Increase Beauty," *Call,* 24 November 1915, 5.

See also Lawrence Birken, *Consuming Desire: Sexual Science and the Emergence of a Culture of Abundance 1871–1914* (Ithaca, NY: Cornell University Press, 1989); Stephen Trombley, *The Right to Reproduce: A History of Coercive Sterilization* (London: Weidenfeld and Nicolson, 1988), 79; and H. G. Wells, *Modern Utopia* (London: Chapman & Hall, 1905).

13. Thus the aesthetic dimension of eugenics has often been overlooked. In addition, eugenicists' insistence on the objectivity of their science also made the movement seem hostile to emotions and art. Such was the view of James Joyce's Steven Daedalus, who contrasted "eugenics" and "esthetic" and accused eugenics of trying to reduce beauty to its biological functions. (James Joyce, *Portrait of the Artist as a Young Man* [1916; reprinted 1966, New York: Viking Press], quoted in Kevles, *Name of Eugenics,* 119)

Historians of Germany pioneered the recognition of the aesthetic dimension of eugenics, especially Sander L. Gilman, *Picturing Health and Illness* (Baltimore, MD: Johns Hopkins University Press, 1995); George Mosse, *Toward the Final Solution: A History of European Racism* (London: J. M. Dent, 1978), 2; George Mosse, *Nationalism and Sexuality* (New York: H. Fertig, 1985); Paul Weindling, *Health, Race and German Politics between National Unification and Nazism 1870–1945* (Cambridge: Cambridge University Press, 1989); Willibrald Saürländer, "The Nazis' Theater of Seduction," *New York Review of Books* 21 April 1994, 16–19; Hillel Tryster, "The Art and Science of Pure Racism," *Jerusalem Post International* 17 August 1991, 13.

14. Wiggam, *Fruit of the Family Tree,* 272, 279. For Haiselden see *CA,* 2 December 1915, 2.

This view still surfaces in media accounts of modern evolutionary studies. Natalie Angier, "Why Birds and Bees, Too, Like Good Looks," and "Not Just a Beauty Contest," *NYT,* 8 February 1994, B5, B8; Jane Brody, "Ideals of Beauty Seen as Innate," *NYT,* 21 March 1994, A6.

For more sophisticated current theories on the evolution of beauty, see David M. Buss,

The Evolution of Desire (New York: Basic Books, 1994); R. W. Smuts, "Fat, Sex, Class, Adaptive Flexibility, and Cultural Change," *Ethology and Sociobiology* 13 (1992), 523–42; and forthcoming work by Richard Alexander and Robert Trivers. I thank Bob Smuts for discussing these works with me and for saving me from my initial misrepresentation of Darwin's views.

15. Helena Cronin, *The Ant and the Peacock: Altruism and Sexual Selection from Darwin to Today* (New York: Cambridge University Press, 1992); Stephen Jay Gould, "The Great Seal Principle," in *Eight Little Piggies* (New York: W. W. Norton, 1993), 371–81.

In addition, many professionals among the eugenic leaders felt that "the mind is more important than the body" (*NYT,* 26 November 1915, 8). Sociology professor Franklin H. Giddings explained more bluntly: "The idiotic child should mercifully be allowed to die. The child with a good brain, however crippled otherwise, should be saved" (*Independent,* 3 January 1916, 23. For others with similar views, see *TNR,* 18 December 1915, 174; *NYT,* 18 November 1915, 4, and 25 November 1915; *CH,* 17 November 1915; *CT,* 18 November 1915; *New York American* (hereafter *NYAm*), 19 November 1915, 6; *New York Medical Journal* 100 (26 December 1914): 1247, 1249.

16. Fisher and Fisk, *How to Live,* 322; Wiggam, *Fruit of the Family Tree,* 275, emphasis added. See also Guyer, *Being Well-Born,* 438, passage retained from 1916 edition. For similar aesthetic efforts in German eugenics see Weindling, *Health, Race and German Politics,* 410–13.

The presumably unintended implication of communal living or polygamy in Wiggam's quote results from his diction, not my ellipsis.

17. Individual school districts continued to use *The Science of Life* for decades after 1937. For more on the film see Martin S. Pernick, "Sex Education Films, U.S. Government," *Isis* 84 (1993): 766–68. The last three reels focused on hygiene, human reproduction, VD, and eugenics.

I have identified over forty films shown in the United States between 1900 and 1930 that dealt with aspects of eugenics and/or human heredity. Most were short one- and two-reelers not yet subject indexed in any reference guide and so largely unknown to scholars. Almost all these films are now considered lost, though I have discussed and analyzed them from written records (see Pernick, *Black Stork,* chap. 7).

18. *Science of Life,* reel 12, *General Hygiene,* National Archives (hereafter NA), Motion Picture Division, College Park, MD, reel number 90.26. The following discussion is also based on two versions of reel 11, *Personal Hygiene for Young Men* and *Personal Hygiene for Young Women,* NA reels 90.24 and 90.25.

NYT, 15 November 1923, 10; *American Journal of Public Health* 12 (December 1922): 1033, and 13 (September 1923): 737; *Journal of Social Hygiene* 14 (January 1928): 14; New York State Archives, Motion Picture Division Scripts, Albany, NY (hereafter NYSA-MPD), Box 2565, Folders 12,471 and 12,493, including a clipping from the *New York Herald,* 15 April 1923; Records of the United States Public Health Service, NA, Record Group 90, File 1350. Thanks to Peter Laipson and Aloha South for locating the NA material.

19. Charles Musser, *The Emergence of Cinema* (New York: Scribner, 1990); Francois Dragognet, *Etienne-Jules Maret* (New York: Zone Books, 1992); Marta Braun, *Picturing*

Time: The Work of Etienne-Jules Maret (Chicago, IL: University of Chicago Press, 1992). Thanks to Rebecca Zurier for prompting these ideas.

20. This distinctive aesthetic mix reached its peak in *Way to Strength and Beauty,* a 1925 German film shown in the United States, which combined dramatically modern steep-angle cinematography with scenes of both classical and primitive Teutonic athletes. The film was produced by the UFA and is available from the Bundesarchiv in Cologne and the LC-MBRS. See also *Fit: Episodes in the History of the Body* (Straight Ahead Films, 1993); Lois Banner, *American Beauty* (New York: Alfred Knopf, 1983); and Martha Banta, *Imaging American Women* (New York: Columbia University Press, 1987).

21. Mann used the phrase to describe "the really characteristic and dangerous aspect of National Socialism," quoted in *New York Review of Books,* 30 January 1986, 21.

22. *CA,* 29 November 1915, and 30 November 1915, 2.

23. On photographic iconography see Martin Elks, "Visual Rhetoric: Photographs of the Feeble-Minded during the Eugenics Era, 1900–1930" (Ph.D. diss., Syracuse University, 1992). On the history of disability in entertainment film see Martin F. Norden, *The Cinema of Isolation: A History of Physical Disability in the Movies* (New Brunswick, NJ: Rutgers University Press, 1994); and Gaylyn Studlar, *This Mad Masquerade: Stardom and Masculinity in the Jazz Age* (New York: Columbia University Press, 1996), chap. 4. On disability in recent horror films see Paul K. Longmore, "Screening Stereotypes: Images of Disabled People," *Social Policy* 16 (summer 1985): 31–37.

24. *CA,* 2 December 1915, 2. In many ways Haiselden's approach to art mimicked that of Thomas Eakins. On art and disfiguration of the canvas, see Michael Fried, *Realism, Writing, Disfiguration* (Chicago, IL: University of Chicago Press, 1987). For other comparisons see Pernick, *Black Stork,* 60–71 passim.

25. Wiggam, *Fruit of the Family Tree,* 262, 273–74.

26. *CA,* 24 November 1915; 30 November 1915, 2.

27. *TNR,* 18 December 1915, 173–74.

28. Kevles, *Name of Eugenics,* 12. For Karl Pearson's insistence that his diagnosis of Jewish inferiority was based on "the cold light of statistical inquiry," not "prejudice," see his paper in the 1925 inaugural *Annals of Eugenics,* Karl Pearson and M. Moul, "The Problem of Alien Immigration into Great Britain, Illustrated by an Examination of Russian and Polish Jewish Children," *Annals of Eugenics* 1 [1925], 5–127, quoted by Stephen Jay Gould, *Hen's Teeth and Horse's Toes* (New York: W. W. Norton, 1983), 296–98. Wiggam, *Fruit of the Family Tree,* 272–79.

29. While the responses of ordinary viewers are hard to document, movie reviewers and film censors demonstrate that such "unauthorized" interpretations were common. *CT,* 2 April 1917, 18; *New York Dramatic Mirror* (hereafter *NYDM*), 17 February 1917, 32; *Wid's Film Daily,* 5 April 1917, 220; *Motion Picture News* (hereafter *MPN*), 24 February 1917, 1256.

30. *Exhibitors' Trade Review* (hereafter *ExTrR*), 24 February 1917, 836; *Motography,* 24 February 1917, 424. For similar mixed reviews see *NYDM,* 17 February 1917, 32; *MPN,* 24 February 1917, 1256.

31. *Wid's,* 5 April 1917, 220–21.

32. Parsons in *CH,* 2 April 1917, 11; Kelly in *Chicago Examiner* (hereafter *CE*), 4 April 1917, 8. *The Chicago Tribune* admitted the "ideas may be all right," but found the

film "as pleasant to look at as a running sore." Pursuing such clinical metaphors to the limit, *Photoplay* called Lait's screenplay "so slimy that it reminds us of nothing save the residue of a capital operation" (*CT*, 2 April 1917, 18; *Photoplay,* June 1917, 155).

33. The National Board of Review of Motion Pictures' advisors repeatedly used such language to describe the film's audiences as sick. See Andrew Edson of New York City's Education Department, 17 November; U. G. Manning, 18 November; Jonathan Dean, 18 November; Ernest Batchelder, 22 November; Maude Levy, 20 November; W. L. Percy, 21 November; and Robbins Gilman, 23 November; all 1916 and all in National Board of Review of Motion Picture Records, Controversial Film Correspondence, Rare Books and Manuscripts Division, the New York Public Library (hereafter NBRMP), Box 103.

34. *Chicago Daily News* (hereafter *CN*), 6 April 1917, 21.

35. The year it first rejected *The Black Stork,* the influential early Pennsylvania state film censor board adopted a list of aesthetic offenses that included any films about eugenics and a range of other medical topics (Pennsylvania State Board of Censors, *Rules and Standards* [Harrisburg, PA: J. L. L. Kuhn, 1918], 15–17). The first Production Code of the Motion Picture Producers and Distributors of America (1930), which synthesized this and similar state lists of forbidden topics, labeled "surgical operations" a "repellent subject" and included a catch-all restriction on all other "disgusting, unpleasant, though not necessarily evil, subjects" that was used to eliminate most other graphic or unpleasant depictions of medical issues.

Garth Jowett, *Film: The Democratic Art* (Boston, MA: Little, Brown, 1976), chaps. 5, 7, 10. Code of 1930 reprinted, 468–72. On precode films and the rise of censorship see also Francis Couvares, "Hollywood, Main Street, and the Church: Trying to Censor the Movies before the Production Code," *American Quarterly* 44 (December 1992): 584–615; Stephen Vaughn, "Morality and Entertainment: The Origins of the Motion Picture Production Code," *Journal of American History* 77 (June 1990): 39–65; Edward De Grazia and Roger K. Newman, *Banned Films: Movies, Censors and the First Amendment* (New York: R. R. Bowker, 1982).

For aesthetic censorship of Tod Browning's *Freaks,* see *NYT,* 9 July 1932, 7; Robert Bogdan, *Freak Show* (Chicago: University of Chicago Press, 1988); Leslie Fiedler, *Freaks* (New York: Simon & Schuster, 1978).

36. For censorship history of *The Black Stork,* see NBRMP, Box 103; NYSA-MPD, Box 2565, Folders 383 and 12,421. Quotations are from letter of disapproval, Commissioner to H. J. Brooks, 4 April 1923, NYSA-MPD, Box 2565, Folder 383.

In a private straw poll of community leaders from across the country conducted by a film industry voluntary rating agency, the National Board of Review of Motion Pictures, nine of the fifty-two respondents explicitly cited aesthetic objections as a major reason for not approving *The Black Stork,* NBRMP, Box 103.

On *Tomorrow's Children* see "Memo on Behalf of the Motion Picture Division to the Commissioner of Education," 4; and "Court of Appeals Brief for the Respondent," 6, both in NYSA-MPD, Box 333, Folder 28,361. The censors initially also declared the film "immoral" for showing audiences "methods that . . . prevent conception," but this argument was soon dropped; see letter of Irving Esmond, 24 August 1934, in Box 296, Folder 27,387.

For the role of VD and sex education films in the growth of film censorship, see

De Grazia and Newman, *Banned Films;* and Annette Kuhn, *Cinema, Censorship and Sexuality 1909–1925* (London: Routledge, 1988).

37. For the importance of this change see Carl Degler, *In Search of Human Nature* (New York: Oxford, 1991), part one.

The new definition meant individual heredity was unchangeable. For the first time, science viewed heredity and environment as distinct and exclusive categories, and selective reproduction now became the only mechanism for changing the future genetic composition of the population.

38. A scene script of *Birth* is in LC-MBRS copyright records #MU-835; quotes are from *Wid's,* 19 April 1917, 244–45. See also *Moving Picture World* (hereafter *MPW*), 28 April 1917, 609; *MPN,* 28 April 1917, 2687; *NYAm,* 8 April 1917, 7M, and 15 April 1917, 4M; *Motography,* 28 April 1917, 915; *DN,* 29 April 1917, 6, and 6 May 1917, 5. See also *New York Evening Journal,* 9 April 1917, 8, and ads 11–14 April 1917, movie page; American Film Institute (hereafter AFI), *Catalog of Feature Films, 1911–1920* (Berkeley, CA: University of California Press, 1989), 69–70.

See also the Children's Bureau film *Well Born: Child Health Magazine,* December 1923, 571–72, and September 1924, 407; *Educational Screen,* February 1924, 80; *American Journal of Public Health* 14 (1924): 276; *Bulletin of the National Tuberculosis Association,* January 1924, 4. Other Children's Bureau films of the 1920s are available at the National Archives, but no surviving copies of this one are known.

39. Quote from *Wid's,* 14 June 1917, 369–71. For promotion see *MPN,* June through August 1917.

40. Haller, *Eugenics,* 141–43; Kevles, *In the Name of Eugenics,* 100.

41. What were called environmental "germ poisons" were widely believed to cause inheritable mutations. Conversely, genetic factors might determine who was most susceptible to environmental damage. And some reputable scientists remained "Lamarckians" into the 1930s.

On germ poisons see *Popular Science Monthly* 88 (1916): 84–85; Allan Brandt, *No Magic Bullet* (New York: Oxford University Press, 1987), 14–15; *Eugenics in Race and State: Scientific Papers of the Second International Congress of Eugenics . . . New York 1921* (Baltimore, MD: Williams & Wilkins, 1923), 309, 346–47. Anti-Lamarckian prohibitionist John Harvey Kellogg gave extensive publicity to alcohol as a germ poison: *Good Health Magazine* 51 (1916): 75–76; 52 (1917): 502–3; 54 (1919): 164, 219–24, 273–78, 717. For a Lamarckian view of this research see Aldred Scott Warthin, *Creed of a Biologist* (New York: P. B. Hoeber, 1930), 57–58; Jean-Charles Sournia, *A History of Alcoholism* (Oxford: Basil Blackwell, 1990), chap. 7; L. Crowe, "Alcohol and Heredity: Theories about the Effects of Alcohol Use on Offspring," *Social Biology* 32 (1985): 146–61; R. H. Warner and H. L. Rosett, "Effects of Drinking on Offspring: An Historical Survey of the American and British Literature," *Journal of Studies of Alcohol* 36 (November 1975): 1395–1420.

On environmental susceptibility see René and Jean Dubos, *The White Plague: Tuberculosis, Man and Society* (London: Victor Gollancz, 1953), 28–43, 125–28; Robert N. Proctor, *Racial Hygiene: Medicine under the Nazis* (Cambridge, MA: Harvard University Press, 1988), 215–17; *Eugenics in Race and State,* 300–301.

For persistent Lamarckian beliefs in the 1930s see Warthin, *Creed of a Biologist.*

Thus eminent scientists like psychologist G. Stanley Hall considered germ fighting part of eugenics. His plan for a "Department of Eugenics" specifically included infectious diseases and milk inspection among its responsibilities (Dorothy Ross, *G. Stanley Hall* [Chicago, IL: University of Chicago Press, 1972], 362–63, 413. Thanks to Alice Smuts for this reference). Similar examples include Fisher and Fisk, *How to Live,* 293–94; *Good Health Magazine* 54 (1919): 658; *Social Hygiene Bulletin* 2 (January 1916): 3, and 3 (November 1916): 4.

42. Many motion pictures explicitly defined "eugenics" as meaning "fit to marry." *The Black Stork* itself was retitled *Are You Fit to Marry?* when it was rereleased in 1918–19 and in 1927. See also "heredity" in *Oxford English Dictionary* compact edition (New York: Oxford University Press, 1971).

On the link between causality and morality see Thomas Haskell, *The Emergence of Professional Social Science* (Urbana, IL: University of Illinois Press, 1977), esp. chap. 11; and Sylvia Tesh, *Hidden Arguments: Political Ideology and Disease Prevention Policy* (New Brunswick, NJ: Rutgers University Press, 1988).

43. Environment wins out in *Are They Born or Made?* (Warner, 1917), *A Daughter's Strange Inheritance* (Broadway Star-Vitagraph, 1917), *A Victim of Heredity* (Kalem, 1913), *The Power of Mind* (Mutual, 1916), *A Disciple of Nietzsche* (Thanhouser, 1915), and *The Red Circle* (Pathe, 1915).

Heredity wins in *Heredity* (Biograph, 1912), *Heredity* (Broadway Star, 1915), *Inherited Sin* (Universal, 1915), *The Power of Heredity* (Rex, 1913), and *The Second Generation* (Pathe, 1914).

One of the first commercial melodramas to be billed as an explicitly "eugenic" film was D. W. Griffith's *The Escape* (Reliance-Majestic, 1914). Following a prologue by Dr. Daniel Carson Goodman that called for breeding humans as carefully as livestock, it traces in gruesome detail the awful consequences of human "mismating." The fictional "Joyce" family compresses into two generations all the defects and deviance found among two centuries of Jukes and Kallikaks.

The film's conclusion may have been based on Lamarckian concepts of heredity (critics disagreed on this point—see *MPW,* 13 June 1914, 1515, versus *NYDM,* 10 June 1914, 42). The physician-hero cures a lunatic strangler surgically and redeems the lunatic's prostitute sister by marrying her. But whatever definition of heredity it was using, what made the film "eugenic" was its dramatization of the effects of bad parenting. AFI, *Catalog 1911–20,* 244; *Variety,* 5 June 1914, 19; *NYT,* 2 June 1914, 11; William K. Everson, *American Silent Film* (New York: Oxford University Press, 1978), 76; Robert Connelly, *The Motion Picture Guide: Silent Film* (Chicago, IL: Cinebooks, Inc., 1986), 74.

44. Fisher in *Eugenics in Race and State,* 318, 464–65. Robie in *A Decade of Progress in Eugenics: Scientific Papers of the Third International Congress of Eugenics* (Baltimore, MD: Williams & Wilkins, 1934), 202; for similar views of the American Eugenics Society in 1935 see Ellsworth Huntington, *Tomorrow's Children* (New York: John Wiley, 1935), 41–42, quoted in Barry Mehler, "Eliminating the Inferior," *Science for the People,* November/December 1987, 16.

45. These concerns retain their influence today, even among those leading the return to supposedly biological explanations. Thus Richard Herrnstein and Charles Murray assert

in *The Bell Curve,* (New York: Free Press, 1994), "If women with low scores are reproducing more rapidly than women with high scores, the distribution of scores will, other things equal, decline, *no matter whether the women with the low scores came by them through nature or nurture*" (emphasis added). Quoted by Malcolm Browne, *New York Times Book Review,* 16 October 1994, 1.

46. Ernst Haeckel, *The Wonders of Life* (New York: Harper & Brothers, 1905), 21, 114–20; Haeckel, *The History of Creation,* vol. 1 (1868; reprint, New York; D. Appleton, 1876), 170–71; I. van der Sluis, "The Movement for Euthanasia, 1875–1975," *Janus* 66 (1979): 134–37; Daniel Gasman, *The Scientific Origins of National Socialism* (London: MacDonald, 1971), 91. On Haeckel's follower Ploetz, Stephen Trombley, *The Right to Reproduce: A History of Coercive Sterilization* (London: Weidenfeld and Nicolson, 1988), 71.

Other eugenic professionals who advocated such views prior to 1910 included Hungarian welfare expert Sigmund Engel, British physicians Charles E. Goddard and Robert Rentoul, Chicago dentist Eugene Talbot, Yale law professor Simeon Baldwin, physicians William D. McKim and Edward Wallace Lee, Chicago surgeon G. Frank Lydston, psychologist G. Stanley Hall, and psychiatrist Walter Kempster. The first effort to legislate such proposals was introduced by Link Rodgers in Michigan in 1903, and similar bills were debated in Iowa and Ohio in 1906.

Sigmund Engel, *The Elements of Child-Protection,* trans. Eden Paul (New York: Macmillan, 1912). For Goddard, see O. Ruth Russell, *Freedom to Die: Moral and Legal Aspects of Euthanasia* (New York: Human Sciences Press, 1975), 59. For Rentoul, see Trombley, *Right to Reproduce,* 19. Simeon Baldwin, "The Natural Right to a Natural Death," *Journal of Social Science* 37 (1899): 1–17, quoted in Cynthia B. Cohen, "The Treatment of Impaired Newborns in American History: Implications for Public Policy" (Department of Philosophy, Villanova University, 1985), 87; Eugene S. Talbot, *Degeneracy* (London: Walter Scott, [1898]), 3–4. For other U.S. proposals to kill the mentally retarded, as early as 1883, see Russell Hollander, "Euthanasia and Mental Retardation," *Mental Retardation* 27 (April 1989): 53–61; William McKim, *Heredity and Human Progress* (New York: G. P. Putnam's Sons, 1900), 188–92; G. Stanley Hall, "What Is to Become of Your Baby?" *Cosmopolitan* 47 (April 1910): 661–68; Ross, *Hall,* 318–19; Philip Reilly, *The Surgical Solution* (Baltimore, MD: Johns Hopkins University Press, 1991), 37–38; for Lydston, see Stephen Louis Kuepper, "Euthanasia in America, 1890–1960" (Ph.D. diss., Rutgers University, 1981), 65; for Lee, see *New York Medical Journal* 100 (26 December 1914): 1251. On the Michigan plan, see Curtis, "Eugenic Reformers," 69–70; *CE,* 22 May 1903; *DN,* 22 May 1903; on Rodgers see *Michigan State Gazeteer* (Detroit: R. L. Polk, 1903); *DN,* 21 May 1903, 3. For Kempster, *NYT,* 26 January 1906; for Dr. R. H. Gregory, van der Sluis, "Euthanasia," 135.

Infanticide for reasons including elimination of sickly infants had been practiced in the ancient world and in many non-Western cultures.

47. Davenport, *Heredity in Relation to Eugenics* (New York: Henry Holt, 1911), 4, quoted in Kuepper, "Euthanasia in America," 62. For Fisher, see National Conference on Race Betterment, *Proceedings,* 1 (1914): 472, 475. For others with same point at the conference see *Proceedings* 1 (1914): 477, 500–501; (1915): 89–90 and addenda slip for 61.

48. *Independent,* 3 January 1916, 23. The same article also contained an endorsement from Raymond Pearl.

49. *Boston American* (hereafter *BA,*) 20 December 1915, 16; George Woodcock, *Anarchism* (Cleveland, OH: World Publishing, 1962), 328, 336, 462. For comparisons between Dr. Haiselden and Dr. Jack Kevorkian today see Pernick, *Black Stork,* 170–71.

50. *NYT,* 13 November 1917, 12.

51. Keller in *TNR,* 18 December 1915, 173–74. *CH,* 20 November 1915, 2, and 21 November 1915, 3. *Call,* 29 November 1915, 3. A Los Angeles proposal was reported as early as 20 November; see *CA,* 24 November 1915, 3. For Haiselden's use of consultants to confirm his nontreatment decisions, see *CA,* 22 December 1915, magazine page; *CE,* 24 July 1917; *NYT,* 16 November 1917, 4; *MRR* 23 (1917): 607; *CA,* 16 November 1917, 3. For modern parallels see Mary B. Mahowald, "Baby Doe Committees: A Critical Evaluation," *Clinics in Perinatology* 15 (December 1988): 789–800.

Occupational health pioneer Dr. Alice Hamilton noted the irony that mass culture demanded expanding the power of the profession. "Curiously enough it is not the medical profession which is seeking an extension of its rights; it is the laity which is trying to force upon physicians a power over life and death which they themselves shrink from." *Survey* 35 (4 December 1915): 266. But popular support for giving doctors this particular power itself depended on a broader progressive-era faith in the methods of science, a faith that was actively promoted by medical and eugenic leaders.

52. *Independent,* 3 January 1916, 26; *NYT,* 16 July 1917, 10. Although the *Times* changed its position on nontreatment, the editors consistently maintained that the "wise" physician should make such decisions silently. *NYT,* 18 November 1915, 8; 22 November 1915, 14; 29 November 1915, part 2, 10.

Columbia University sociology chairman Franklin H. Giddings applauded the death of "molasses-minded" mental defectives but felt it was a "question that should be considered soberly, thoughtfully and by rigorous intellectual processes. To put it up to the general public in all the emotional and imaginative setting of a photo-play is, in my judgment, an utterly wrong thing to do." A series of legal investigations upheld Haiselden's refusal to treat impaired newborns, but he was expelled from the Chicago Medical Society for publicizing his actions. *NYT,* 18 November 1915, 4, and Giddings to W. D. McGuire, 20 November 1916, NBRMP, Box 103.

53. *CT,* 28 January 1918, 12. See chaps. 6 and 9 of Pernick, *The Black Stork.*

54. Fisher and Fisk, *How to Live,* 12th ed., 294. Even Dr. William J. Robinson, one of Haiselden's most vigorous supporters in 1915–16, wrote in 1917 that "no eugenic considerations will induce us to adopt Spartan-like methods and to neglect or kill off the weak and puny . . . Every child that is born . . . is entitled to the very best of care." William J. Robinson, *Eugenics and Marriage* (New York: Critic & Guide, 1917), 138, see also 73–76. For similar disavowals see Wiggam, *Fruit,* 283; Eden Paul, "Eugenics, Birth Control, and Socialism," in *Population and Birth Control* (New York: Critic & Guide, 1917), 142.

In Search of Al Schmid ▶ War Hero, Blinded Veteran, Everyman

David A. Gerber

During an intense firefight at the Tenaru River on Guadalcanal in August of 1942, Marine Private Al Schmid, a Philadelphia metalworker, shared a machine gun emplacement with two other young marines: Johnny Rivers, a Native American from rural Pennsylvania, and Lee Diamond, a Jew from Brooklyn. During hours of night combat, as wave after wave of Japanese tried unsuccessfully to cross the Tenaru and overwhelm the thin line of American defenders, first Rivers was shot and instantly killed, and then Diamond was severely wounded. Furious over the death of his friend and fighting for his life, Schmid continued to ward off the enemy. Toward the end of the battle, he was wounded by a grenade fragment. One of his eyes was immediately destroyed and the other was greatly damaged. Now sightless, Schmid continued, with what little aid Diamond could provide, to fire the machine gun. Eventually he was credited with killing two hundred Japanese before his position was relieved in the morning. Schmid spent much of the next two years in military hospitals, where unsuccessful efforts were made to save what little sight remained to him and where he began the process of blind rehabilitation.[1]

Schmid's courageous conduct in battle, the blindness he sustained, and the ordinariness that he projected under the glare of wartime publicity combined to establish him as a type of authentic twentieth-century American war hero, like Audie Murphy and Alvin York. And Schmid's reputation, like those of Murphy and York, would accrete layers of cultural symbolism as the legend of his heroism was gradually constructed. His role at the Tenaru quickly became well known and was officially recognized in January 1943 when President Roosevelt awarded him the prestigious Navy Cross. Articles in the press chronicled the comings and goings of a man always described as a "hero" and "the slayer of 200." A *Life* magazine editor, Roger Butterfield, celebrated his courage, rehabilitation, and homecoming in a feature article that became the basis for a popular wartime biography, *Al Schmid—Marine* (1944).[2] The book became the basis for the 1945 Warner Brothers feature, *Pride of the Marines*, in which the formidable Hollywood star, John Garfield, played Schmid. Like the movies made about the lives of Murphy and York, this film gave millions access to a legend in the making.[3]

The transformation of Al Schmid, metalworker, marine volunteer, and blinded veteran, into Al Schmid, American war hero, was the product of a number of competing forces that contended to define the meanings of his life. The popular press, the Marine Corps, the Roosevelt administration, Warner Brothers Studio, the Hollywood Left, and activists in the American blinded veterans movement all sought to claim Schmid's life as the basis for various inspirational and ideological messages. In their efforts, we have access to the dynamics of the construction of a twentieth-century American hero. Most of these messages went well beyond the facts of Schmid's life and were inconsistent with Schmid's understanding of himself. Yet when Schmid failed to play out the parts assigned to him in scripts written by various hero-crafting interests, he himself was found wanting.

This essay analyzes the tension between the cultural process of creating legends and the ongoing life of a man who was the basis of a legend. Schmid's life illustrates the difference between a flesh-and-blood man capable of extraordinary courage and a culturally constructed hero whom we seek to make the embodiment of a variety of timeless, inspirational qualities. It is not my purpose to destroy the various legends inspired by Schmid by holding his life up before them. Rather I suggest that we seek to understand them as a series of scripts, parallel to the one he was crafting for himself, that might have guided his self-understanding. It was Schmid who rejected those scripts, opting finally for one of his own creation and in so doing seeking relief from the tension that the struggle over his identity caused him. The essay, thus, is also an analysis of the construction and representation of the self.[4]

The American Everyman as War Hero

Al was born in 1922. His German father was a brewery worker. His Irish mother died when he was ten. Al's father quickly remarried, but Al did not get along with his stepmother. He did poorly in school, which he quit at fifteen, and with his father's encouragement left home to work in New England. In this way, he bounded through the late depression years until 1940, when he returned to Philadelphia, and its war-driven economic boom, to work in a metal foundry. Al believed that the years he had spent on his own, supporting himself and doing demanding and at times dangerous work, toughened him. He took pride in his trade, because it required endurance as well as skill. Al was proud too of his considerable prowess as an athlete and a hunter. Butterfield portrays a man who wants to be regarded as tough and independent and who is somewhat wary in dealing with others, largely out of fear that they will seek to undermine his independence. Though he dated regularly, he showed no interest in sacrificing his independence, especially when he had the high wages to enjoy it. Sometime in 1941, he was introduced to a young office worker, Ruth Hartley. Ruth found Al an indifferent, egocentric suitor.[5] Yet, for all his blunt and standoffish qualities, she detected a gentle, vulnerable, and boyish side, which leads her now to sum up Al's character by saying that he was "a lover, not a fighter."[6] At several points in their months of increasingly steady dating before Al went into the marines, he seemed on the verge of proposing marriage. Just before he left the country for combat in the Pacific, he finally signaled his seriousness by sending Ruth an engagement ring.[7]

Al did not follow politics and was not old enough to vote in the elections of 1940 when U.S. intervention in the conflicts now spanning the globe was widely debated. Al admitted that he had not known where Pearl Harbor was when he heard the radio reports of the Japanese attack on Sunday, 7 December. He and Ruth spent the day pursuing their own amusement. His enlistment on 9 December came as a surprise to those who knew him. It was an impulsive act, prompted by the example of two workmates, whose liberation from the foundry Al envied. Al does not seem to have known much about the marines or anticipated the forward role they would be asked to play in the Pacific war. What initially impressed him about the corps was that the recruiters were "gentlemen" enough to let him keep his New Year's Eve date with Ruth when he told them she was "a blond."[8] It is doubtful, however, that most Americans were any more knowledgeable about politics and the war than Al. Without such knowledge, Al chose to fashion a sensibility for himself out of the masculine bravado that was part of the American popular culture of war making. As with many other twentieth-century American soldiers, much of what Al knew about how he should behave as a soldier and patriot, and then as a hero, came from oral traditions that soldiers, beginning in basic training, hand down to one another and from war movies he had seen. The war itself he conceived through movie images rather than political realities. From the beginning of his stay there, he related, Guadalcanal reminded him of a movie set.[9]

Though not politically engaged, Al hated the Japanese, and this, along with patriotic feeling, enabled him to align himself wholeheartedly with his country's cause. His attitudes toward them were shaped by racial prejudice, but this, too, hardly makes him unique. Of the men who ran outdoor concessions at Atlantic City, the only Japanese he came into contact with before the war, he told Butterfield, "They always looked slinky to me. Those slanty eyes they had would always get me. They just reminded me of some dirty little rat." Al said that he hated "everything about them." He seems to have seen the war, at some semiconscious level, as a sort of hunting expedition. He promised Ruth he would bring her home some Japanese "pigtails" (an aspect of *Chinese* culture) to put on the Christmas tree, just as he had once brought back hunting trophies from the Pennsylvania backcountry.[10]

If Al lacked seriousness and political understanding in the face of the epic spasm of violence of which he had become a part, it is not surprising that he also lacked discipline as a soldier. Here, too, it is difficult to see him as unique, and it is easy to see the cultural influences that shaped his response to military life. During basic training, he drank a lot and gained a reputation for being a prankster when he was tipsy. He was so drunk the night his unit left the United States that he had to be carried onto his ship and later awoke surprised to find himself on his way to war. But Al did take seriously those aspects of basic training that he knew would be vital for his survival, and he liked working with weaponry, which inspired his skilled worker's pride of craft and prompted his memories of hunting. He recalled feeling confident that he, Rivers, and Diamond were ready to do "the job," his metaphor for combat. Moreover, Al developed some of the esprit de corps by which the marines have established their reputation, though he manifested it less in formal obedience to his commanders than in loyalty to his buddies. That sense of solidarity came to override his own desire for comfort and safety, exactly as the Marine Corps desired. Early in his service on Guadalcanal, Al developed a serious foot infection, and he was told on 21 August that without immediate medical evacuation he might lose a leg. Al pleaded for one more day with his outfit, because they all believed a battle was coming and he wanted to be there alongside Diamond and Rivers. Al fought that night with blood poisoning in his swollen leg. For years, the lymph glands in the leg, which doctors barely managed to save, would bother him, and this contributed to his decision to retire from his factory job and move to Florida in 1957. It seems typical of Al, and also of the way Al liked to think of himself, that he stumbled into his moment of glory, yet somehow typical, too, that once there he not only did his "job" but performed it well.[11]

For Americans, there is much that is attractive in Schmid's self-representation, which became the basis of his post-Guadalcanal public persona. He has endurance, toughness, and courage. He is ruggedly independent, yet just below the surface gentle, "a lover." He is attractive to women and enjoys their company but is not desirous of being tied down. He is tongue tied when the subject has to do with "soft" things, such as emotional relationships or patriotic ideals, and appears lacking in seriousness. Yet, somehow, he is full of the right impulses. He is disengaged almost right up until the critical moment when he must act. But then he does not shrink from duty because of fear.

When Samuel Stouffer and the colleagues with whom he wrote *The American Soldier*, the comprehensive study of the behavior of American combat troops in World War II, came to list the traits that represented masculine courage for the men they studied, most of what we see in Al Schmid was present in their inventory. In general form, too, these are the traits of many American movie heroes. Specifically, Schmid's self-representation has much in common with a twentieth-century American type, the hero in spite of himself, that Humphrey Bogart personified so well as Rick Blaine in *Casablanca* (1943) and as Harry Morgan in *To Have and Have Not* (1944). This unheroic hero is modern in his psychological complexity and ambiguity of motivation. His character stands him in sharp contrast to the chivalric notions of honor, derived from noble aspirations, ideals, and deeds, that informed nineteenth-century American ideals of courage. Like these Bogart characters, Al cares nothing for political abstractions or ideologies. He responds instead to elemental feelings of personal loyalty. Then, he acts decisively, without concern for personal interests. John Garfield embodied some of these traits, both in himself and in the characters he liked to play. But while Bogart's characters were often cold and calculating, concealing their decency far below the surface, Garfield's creations were, as Robert Sklar says, "lively, like-able, vulnerable, [and] open," more the way Schmid chose to think of himself. To the extent that Al learned from movies how to conceive of himself as the heroic American everyman, it is not surprising that moviemakers, and Garfield, too, were attracted to him.[12]

Schmid's self-representation in the second half of Butterfield's book, which deals with his hospitalization, initial rehabilitation, and return to Philadelphia, also casts him in an attractive, conventionalized heroic mold. While in the hospital he initially demonstrated, according to the medical personnel, courage and cheerfulness. But his condition was hardly promising, and, though he tried to be optimistic, it was evident that it troubled him deeply. In 1943–44, navy doctors guardedly held out the possibility that very partial vision could be restored in his remaining eye. As it was, Al then had little more than some vague color and object perception. By war's end, even that had largely disappeared. He was de-pendent and indulged, which cast him in a role he hated. He was lonely, yet the prospect of being reunited with Ruth filled him with dread. His future as a wage earner hung uncertainly before him, as did the future for so many severely disabled veterans early in the war. The G.I. Bill had not yet been passed, and it was unclear what assistance would be available to them. Moreover, work was the key to Al's independence and self-respect, and the possibility of government benefits did nothing to make him feel any better about his future. He refused to allow Ruth to come to see him at San Diego Naval Hospital and, for a brief time, broke off their engagement. He did not want pity, he said. Neither did he want to saddle Ruth with the burden of a blind husband who could not support her on the strength of his own employment. He resisted coming to terms with his blindness, refusing introductory Braille instruction and recordings for the blind and learn-ing only those skills, such as eating and lighting his cigarettes, that made him independent of others' help with his primary needs.[13] Yet all through this intense personal crisis, as the story of his heroism spread, Schmid was being showered with gifts and letters of praise from strangers, lauded in the press, and com-mended in politicians' and military commanders' speeches. He was frequently taken to nearby Hollywood to meet leading entertainers, including (well before there were plans to make a movie of his life) John Garfield.[14]

Just after the war Schmid's life was a conflict between the public role to which he had been assigned and the private life to which he and Ruth aspired. The war bond rallies and awards ceremonies had accustomed the young man to speaking before large audiences and allowing himself to be used as a symbol in the service of the mobilization of people on behalf of the war effort and of the rehabilitation of the growing number of disabled veterans. During the first postwar years he continued to be a well-known public figure. He spoke publicly, with a vaguely liberal slant, on a few matters, such as union representation for blind workers in sheltered workshops, but in general sought to stand above partisanship and ideology.[15] So well-known had Schmid become that, without any political or administrative experience, he was nominated by the state Democratic convention of 1946 for Pennsylvania secretary of internal affairs. He lost in the Republican tide that swept the nation that year.[16]

Schmid's Rehabilitation

Schmid's initial reactions to his blindness also narrowed the range of roles he was willing to assume. His posthospital transition from sight to blindness was difficult, considerably more so than we would have predicted from Butterfield's upbeat book or from Al's cheerful public performances. Privately he did not act the role of stoical blinded hero well and could not accept his situation. In this he was not much different from most of the approximately 1,400 American service-men blinded in combat, or by accidents or disease, during the war.[17] The military services discovered what civilian medical practitioners and blind rehabilitation workers had long known: for many blinded adults, a period of acute depression, accompanied by feelings of helplessness, follows the loss of vision. At this stage, people may relearn various elementary personal care skills, but their rehabilita-tion focuses mostly on marshaling the psychic resources to face the future with an impairment that is regarded by the average sighted person as one of the most severe disabilities. The historically low status of blind people complicated the work of spiritual rehabilitation among the disabled veterans of World War II. The stereotypes of blind people as beggars and denizens of sheltered workshops and as helpless, pitiable, and dependent upon impatient families, as well as the verbal imagery of darkness used to depict the consciousness of the blind, exacerbated readjustment problems. Ordinarily this psychological malaise begins to lift within six months, opening blinded individuals to a more extensive rehabilitation that focuses on preparation to resume normal social roles through acquisition of compensatory learning skills, techniques of independent mobility, and job train-ing.[18] The related branches of the armed services (the army and air force; the navy, marines, and Coast Guard) each developed blind rehabilitation facilities.[19]

An adult's emotional resources and practical abilities for dealing with the onset of blindness depend ultimately on that individual's personality, education, skills, and family life prior to the loss of vision. In the case of a young man like Schmid, who had been self-sufficient and had valued independence from an early point in life, and who was trained for skilled industrial work, the challenge of blindness, and its association with the dependence and helplessness of compromised manliness, seemed overwhelming. For those, moreover, for whom there remained some hope that even very limited vision could be preserved or restored, the willingness to accept advanced rehabilitation was retarded by hope that they really did not have to prepare themselves for a life of sightlessness. All too often, as in Schmid's case, such optimism proved an illusion, just as his doctors at San Diego warned. Meanwhile, the longer rehabilitation is delayed, the more firmly implanted become habits that impede learning techniques of independent orientation and mobility by which the blind achieve practical independence.[20]

At San Diego Naval Hospital and later at Philadelphia Naval Hospital, Schmid at first rejected and then only grudgingly accepted rehabilitation. A fellow blinded Navy veteran at the Philadelphia facility remembers that Al, with his hopes of regaining his vision and his desperate effort to maintain his independence, was a particularly difficult case for rehabilitation workers. In one incident a civilian blind man came to the hospital as a representative of the American Foundation for the Blind to pass out Braille wrist watches, which give newly blinded people an opportunity to regain time orientation and which thus usually offer them an immediate psychological boost. Schmid rejected the watch, saying that it was for blind people, not for him. A symbol of courage among the general public, Schmid soon became a personification of resistance to rehabilitation for those blinded men at the hospital who themselves were inclined toward cooperation.[21]

Schmid developed his own priorities, however, and gradually fashioned a positive stance toward rehabilitation that focused on fulfilling his needs, as he himself defined them. Technique for using the long, white, metal cane as a guide in independent travel was developed systematically for the first time during the war as a means for assisting blinded soldiers. Blinded men were taught a series of cane maneuvers, which made use of touch and sound as aids in orientation. Cane technique requires coordination of mind and body that is demanding and years of extensive training and frequent retraining.[22] Schmid learned enough cane technique to get to and from his home to the streetcar that daily took him to his factory job. Lamenting the fact he had never finished high school, he decided to get a general education certificate. In San Diego, he had resisted attempts by hospital personnel to introduce him to Braille. But spurred on by his desire to make up for his educational deficiency, he eventually developed a competence in Braille, which he worked to extend during the balance of his life. He also learned to use a Braille typewriter.[23]

Beyond fulfilling these focused needs, however, he sought little rehabilitation and settled for a level of personal independence that, as we shall see, fell short of the high standards set by those men who emerged as leaders of the postwar blinded veterans movement. He let some of the skills he had developed at the

Philadelphia Naval Hospital lapse after he left the workforce. The coordinator of the Visual Impairment Services at the Veterans Administration hospital in Florida that Schmid used in retirement, until his death in 1982, does not remember ever having seen Al with a white cane, let alone traveling independently. It was consistent with the close, private relationship he and Ruth desired that he would come to depend on her for much of the guidance he needed in orientation and mobility, and this dependence no doubt grew after he retired. To be sure, he had hobbies that he pursued independently, such as playing the organ and accordion, operating a transmitting radio, and fishing, and he was active in his church. His principal relationship with the Veterans Administration system's services for the blind was through the prosthetics division, from which he could get the technology (Braille typewriters, tape recorders, etc.) that helped him to pursue his hobbies. But he was wary of those Veterans Administration blindness workers who were involved, for example, in counseling about advanced cane technique, fearing perhaps that they would question his dependence on Ruth and, in doing so, cast doubt on the integrity of the life they shared and on his capacity for manly independence. He did eventually develop a relationship with the Visual Impairment Services coordinator, who recalls that Ruth served as Al's guide when he went out into the world and the two were never separated.[24]

This was not an unusual type of marriage among Al's generation of blinded veterans, many of whom came to depend greatly on their sighted spouses.[25] But what might simply have been convenient in other relationships was, in Al's case, reinforced by a tendency toward denial of his blindness. Here, too, he would fall short of the standards developed by activists in the blinded veterans movement. He did not seek out the company of others who were blind, and he tried, often with Ruth's help, to pass for sighted in public. Perhaps Al was resisting being typed and labeled, which is probably what Ruth Schmid implies when she says that "Al didn't make a big deal of being blind." But the evidence also suggests that Al possessed negative feelings toward blindness. Ruth remembers that when they rode the streetcar in Philadelphia, and Al was without his cane, he was sometimes taken for drunk when he stumbled. Strangers would express their sadness to Ruth that she had so irresponsible a husband, especially when their child was with them. The two of them shared a private joke on such occasions.[26] That Schmid would have rather been taken for drunk than blind, however, suggests shame and disgust that are at odds with the brave acceptance of his situation that we might have expected on the basis of his public legend. Al continued to try to pass, or not be typed, in later years, too, though these attempts mixed with his efforts to meet other needs. In Florida, years later, some of their neighbors did not even know he was blind, both because of the manner in which he and Ruth functioned as a couple and because of Al's own capacity for independent action and masquerade. He went up to the roof alone to fix his radio antenna, which

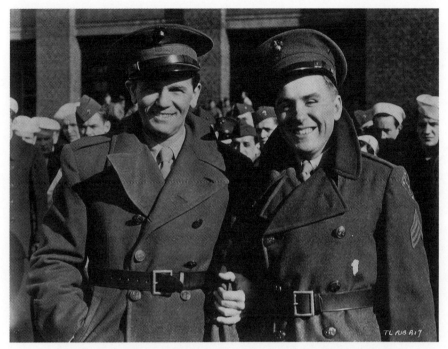

Fig. 1. This photograph of Al Schmid (right) and John Garfield was taken in the spring of 1945 by Warner Brothers studio for use in creating publicity for *Pride of the Marines*. The photograph documents Al Schmid's ability to avoid giving facial cues about his blindness. (Courtesy of the Museum of Modern Art/ Film Stills Archive, 53rd Street, New York City.)

allowed him, too, to assume a masculine "handyman" role. He made it a point in interactions with sighted people never to manifest any "blindisms"—body movements and facial expressions through which many blind people (especially the congenitally and long-term blind) unconsciously seek stimulation. Nor did Schmid (in sharp contrast to John Garfield playing him) show a blank stare. Indeed in some postinjury photographs Schmid looks directly into the camera or at some object in the foreground and smiles winningly. His prosthetic eye looks quite natural, while his remaining, natural eye, is not disfigured.[27] In casual interactions, with or without dark glasses and with Ruth at his side cuing him, Al might well have left the impression that he was not blind but rather a man who had left his glasses at home. The strategy that Schmid fashioned for dealing with his blindness involved limited and carefully chosen interactions with strangers and a strong dependence on Ruth, both of which reinforced their private, domestic lifestyle.

Blinded Veteran Activists Remember Schmid

In the efforts to cast Schmid as a hero and to evaluate the quality of his heroism most of these biographical matters either are never dealt with or are ultimately dealt with from a viewpoint other than Al's that finds Al himself wanting. A significant example may be found in the opinions of Schmid held by a number of the World War II veterans who have been activists in the Blinded Veterans Association (BVA). The BVA was founded in 1945 by a hundred blinded army men, the large majority of whom had together experienced hospitalization, followed by the army's intensive rehabilitation program. These men came from a wide variety of backgrounds, but social differences among them were overwhelmed by the common experience of injury and rehabilitation and by the resolve never to sink into the state of dependence and helplessness they associated with the civilian blind. They fashioned a program that combined self-help and public support: improvement of both military and Veterans Administration rehabilitation and benefit programs, open access to employment, and environmental accessibility for the blind. The BVA stood for the solidarity of all blinded veterans, welcoming blacks and Jews into its ranks from its inception. While at first the BVA depended on sighted advisors to administer its offices and programs, within a few years blinded men themselves ran the organization, not only nationally but in a growing number of regional offices, from which blind counselors traveled to the homes of frequently dispirited, isolated men who needed encouragement to resume rehabilitation and reenter the workforce.[28]

The BVA's early activists were mostly hardened combat veterans who wanted no pity for themselves, were impatient with self-pitying blinded veterans, and set high standards for what they considered to be successful rehabilitation. Russell Williams, an Indiana high school teacher blinded in combat, was one of the original BVA founders and has been a moving force in the blinded veterans movement since World War II. After the war, when the military rehabilitation programs gradually were phased out of operation to cut costs, the BVA made the creation of a permanent Veterans Administration visual impairment program a key demand. Williams, who became a blind rehabilitation worker after his injury, was chosen in 1948 to create the Veterans Administration program at the Hines, Illinois, VA Hospital. He soon established what was to that time probably the most systematic, rigorous blind rehabilitation program ever created in the United States. In the belief that independent orientation and mobility were the keys both to self-confidence and to practical, normalizing activities, especially employment, it placed heavy emphasis on cane technique. The program was uncompromising in the demands made for commitment to its methods and goals. Men had to leave their families for months at a time to live at Hines, where they spent their days in almost constant training that culminated in independent travel on public transportation around the Chicago area. Only when such tasks were mastered, Williams reasoned, was the veteran ready for vocational training and help in career planning.[29] At the heart of Williams's standard for evaluating success in rehabilitation was a vision of what he has called "respectability": personal independence, rejection of pity, and manly pride in the refusal to accept the dependent roles associated with the civilian blind and the gilded age of a federally subsidized retirement.[30]

When asked today about their recollections of Al Schmid, BVA World War II veterans, including Williams, speak with one, critical voice.[31] Schmid is not their idea of a strong, independent, blinded veteran, and, by way of proving it, he broke solidarity with them (and hence, to their minds, what they stood for) early in the BVA's history. Schmid was already known at Philadelphia Naval Hospital for his resistance to rehabilitation when he was placed on the first BVA Board of Directors in 1945. He was chosen because of his fame and because they wanted to provide a balanced representation from all the branches of the armed forces in the organization, which was at first dominated by army veterans. Schmid accepted the post but disappointed those who hoped he would be an activist. He failed to attend any board meetings and was not renominated when his term ended. He would never be active in the work of the BVA, though he remained a member.[32] Asked to explain Schmid's apparent indifference, early BVA leaders accuse him of being too ashamed of blindness to associate closely with those who were blind and of allowing himself to become the victim of his own fame. Schmid, one of them says, was "carried around on a chip"[33]—spoiled by well-meaning civilians who feted him, gave him gifts of cash, and nominated him for public office even though he lacked qualifications for an executive position in government. He thus soon lost his concern for the ordinary, less celebrated, blinded veterans. Moreover, they say, he absorbed messages that told him, in effect, that he did not have to be fully rehabilitated by the rigorous criteria of men like Williams, because some patron would always be there to take care of him.[34] These men speak of Schmid with enough bitterness that it is obvious he was a disappointment to them and a symbol of negativity marking the boundary between what was good and bad in the composition of the ideal blinded veteran's character.

Are such views of Schmid fair? Al did break solidarity with the BVA, and he was hardly the embodiment of their ideal. Yet few men actually lived up to that ideal, and under any circumstance, there does not seem to be only one way, sufficient in itself to last a lifetime, to deal with such a severely disabling impairment as blindness incurred in adulthood. Schmid had his own criteria for achieving rehabilitation, and while there was a degree of denial and masquerade in his response to blindness and a great dependence on Ruth, he, too, reentered the workforce, mastered Braille, pursued education, and developed hobbies and interests that kept him engaged productively after ill health forced him to retire. In his ongoing negotiations with blindness, he showed courage, creativity, and a capacity for growth.

In much of the rest of his postwar history, where some might detect self-imposed limitations, Al actually is not untypical of World War II blinded veterans. Because civilians widely believed that the loss of vision was among the most disabling and tragic wartime injuries, many of these men were "carried around on a chip." For many blinded veterans, such contacts with the sighted world beyond their families continued long after the war; like Al, blinded veterans had fewer interactions with blind people and more sighted friends than did the civilian blind of their generation.[35] Well over half of them had left the workforce within the two decades after the war to live on their generous benefits, some because they had reached the age of retirement but many others because of a lack of skills or, like Schmid, because of poor health, often related to combat injuries.[36] Neither Schmid's dependence on Ruth nor his selective use of rehabilitation services was unusual. The same blinded veterans who are critical of Schmid and his way of functioning as a blind man will also tell an interviewer today of the strong debt they owe their wives for years of practical and emotional support.[37] That Schmid let his cane technique lapse and used VA programs only on his own terms was not atypical either. As his VA blindness counselor told me, these patterns were common among most of the men she saw as they grew older. Blinded veterans became increasingly dependent on their wives as they let their cane technique decline: within two decades of the war, 83 percent of the blinded veterans surveyed said they used sighted guides (mostly wives), but only 31 percent reported ever using a cane. Finally, while not any more common among blinded veterans than among blind civilians, passing and denial are hardly unknown phenomena among blinded adults, among whom those representing themselves as having "some trouble seeing" or "eye problems" are a recognizable type.[38]

It would seem that the ethos that has guided Russell Williams and other BVA activists was a reflection less of widespread practice among blinded veterans than of the deeply felt need a proud, uncompromising segment of leadership in the blinded veterans movement felt to create standards that would mobilize the self-respect and the aspirations of blinded men. These activists were aware that by war's end many men had not taken full advantage of rehabilitation opportunities or had already begun to let their skills lapse and remained depressed and inert.[39] They would never achieve Williams's goal of "respectability." Yet many men who made quite acceptable lives for themselves fell short by Williams's criteria. The program he established at Hines has sometimes been criticized for insisting on the rightness of the one path to rehabilitation that "respectability" seemed to dictate. The familiar process by which standards become transformed from broad goals into the basis for belief that there is a single correct pattern of thought and practice helps greatly to account for the negative evaluation of Schmid by BVA activists. He did not live up to these standards and in their minds failed to act as a widely acclaimed blinded war hero should act. Decades later what they remember about him only is that he failed them.

Pride of the Marines

The consensus among diverse interests[40] on the need to draw ordinary citizens into identifying with official American wartime ideals and making personal sacrifices for the war effort led to the crafting of a particular type of wartime feature, of which *Pride of the Marines* is one of the purest examples. Wartime movies that emphasized recognition by ordinary Americans of the need for self-sacrifice and social unity on behalf of simplified, emotionally charged formulations of freedom and democracy appealed to each of these interests. This discursive message could be plausibly historicized in a narrative premised on the recognition that most Americans were like Schmid in thinking right up to 7 December 1941 that the United States need not become involved in the war and in being preoccupied with their private lives. Along with a number of other wartime Hollywood features *Pride of the Marines* was framed as a narrative of commitment, in which ordinary Americans came gradually to realize that they must surrender their parochial prejudices and private aspirations and become dedicated to a cause larger than themselves. If these movies focused on the home front, the cause was situated in the industrial workplace, in hospitals for wounded servicemen, or in the institutional contexts of volunteer war work. In a combat movie, the cause was placed in the dynamic context of the small fighting unit, with its mixture of ethnic, regional, racial, and social types. (*Pride of the Marines* would have the virtue of combining both combat and home front contexts, while Al's melting pot machine gun emplacement was the perfect symbol of pluralistic teamwork in the service of democracy.) These were also favorite themes in the popular periodical and newspaper press, which sought human interest stories revealing the roles, heroic and obscure alike, that ordinary individuals were playing at work and in the armed forces in determining the course of epic historical events. Butterfield's initial *Life* article about Schmid is an excellent example of this genre, which personalized the war for a mass readership.[41]

While Schmid's life seemed ideal for this sort of treatment, it did contain elements that the moviemakers came to see as inconvenient. This is clear in the formulaic happy ending Warner Brothers producer Jerry Wald and director Delmar Daves wrote into the screenplay, much to the strenuous but unsuccessful objections of Albert Maltz who wrote the script. A prominent Hollywood screenwriter, Maltz was a Communist Party member, and his politics colored his representation of Schmid's effort to come to terms with blindness. Maltz's script is vague about the exact nature of Al's injuries. Al has not lost an eye and had the other badly damaged, but he has nonetheless been blinded. The doctors are not encouraging, but they urge him to be patient and suggest he may need more surgery. The movie establishes that Al is impatient and bitter about his blindness and resistant to rehabilitation; and this was true. It also presents Al as reluctant to return to Philadelphia and to be reunited with Ruth (Eleanor Parker), which was also, briefly, true. Then, in the movie, Al is ordered, against his wishes, to return there to receive his medal, and he is tricked into meeting Ruth, neither of which was true. In the movie, following the ruse that brings the young couple together on Christmas Eve, Al comes to understand that he needs Ruth, and it is suggested that the commitment he knows he must make to her carries some of the same ethical imperatives about human solidarity that he has learned in fighting for his country and in discussing the future with Lee Diamond (Dane Clark) and other wounded combat veterans.[42] In the next sequence, the movie's last, Al and Ruth are about to hail a taxi following the impressive ceremony in which he has received the Navy Cross. Wald and Daves changed Maltz's script so that Al recognizes both the shape and color of a vehicle that, hence, he knows to be a typical red Philadelphia cab. The impression, which Maltz found objectionable because it was untrue and because it provided such a trite conclusion, was that everything has worked out perfectly for Al: he is universally revered, wiser, and secure in his love for Ruth, and now he is regaining his sight.

While Schmid actually did have some inconsistent color and object perception in his remaining eye at the time he received his medal, and the taxi incident was true, he told the press that he could not see the parade held in his honor or even the hand that pinned the medal on him. The doctors in San Diego had initially judged Al's chances of regaining even limited vision in that eye to be poor.[43] By the time the movie was released, Al had merely some light perception. But blindness is a terrifying disability in the imagination of the sighted, and Warner Brothers and the Marine Corps, which gave technical and marketing assistance to the project, seemed desirous of assuring people that, even in this war, not too much sacrifice need necessarily be required. Besides, by the end of the movie, with Al and Ruth reunited and Al acclaimed as a hero and established in our minds as a man of emotional strength as well as physical courage, the movie's hero-crafting function and its emotional catharsis had been achieved. To suggest that Al was going to face further difficulties and perhaps not handle himself well in confronting them was hardly desirable. The marines and the studio were no more honest about the issue in the publicity that accompanied the movie's release. A studio publicity poster showed Garfield, Parker, and Clark smiling and walking with arms linked, as if the movie were a musical or a romantic comedy. A publicity brochure for the press and community organizations, which was jointly published at the time of the premiere by the studio and the Marine Corps Division of Public Relations, states, only once, that Al had been "seriously wounded"

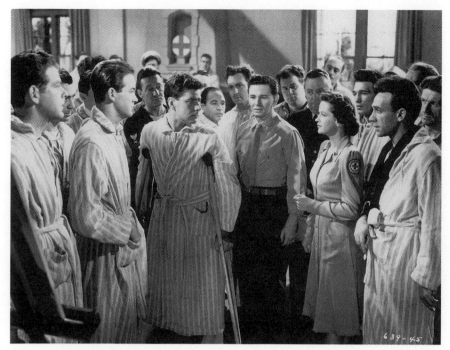

Fig. 2. In the center of the scene from *Pride of the Marines* is
Al Schmid (played by John Garfield) and at the right is
Lee Diamond (Dane Clark). The blank stare that John Garfield
often affected in the movie as a way of cuing Al's blindness
contrasts sharply with the engaging photo of Al made in the
spring of 1945. (Photo courtesy George Eastman House.)

but did not say in what way. It did not mention that Al was now blind and had no
hope of regaining his vision.[44]

Two scenes are essential to the political and disability discourses of the movie.
The most controversial of the two is set in the recreation room of the hospital
ward that Lee Diamond and Schmid share with other convalescing men. Here,
one afternoon, Al participates in a heated discussion about the future. The men
alternately reveal despair and hope about their prospects for postwar security and
dignity. Fears are expressed about the return of the depression and the likelihood
of future wars, and racially prejudiced statements are made by some and condemned by others. Also condemned is the prospect of, it is implied, corporations
and government "doing business with any new Hitler," which carried with it a
condemnation of capitalism. Maltz had his Lee Diamond character argue both
for humane and progressive American values in this scene and for hope for a
better postwar world. But the future, Lee argues, will only be won if veterans like

themselves struggle to preserve the spirit of unity and mutual concern occasioned by the war. Maltz whose Jewish identity as well as his politics came into play here, desired to take this opportunity not only for ideological expression but, in using the character of Diamond to speak for the American conscience, for combating the domestic influence of Nazi anti-Semitism.[45] Al is a bitter presence in this scene, gloomily predicting that he will have an impoverished, dead-end life selling pencils on a street corner. The debate about the uncertain shape of the postwar world is repeated later, though given a more personal and situational edge, in a scene on the train that is taking Al across the country to Philadelphia to receive his medal. Al is reluctant to return to his hometown but has been ordered to do so by officers who feel that he must remake his life there and that getting his medal in the city will be a good start for him. Lee has been ordered to accompany his friend. Schmid does not know that, against his wishes, Lee and Ruth are conspiring to have her meet them at the station and take Al to his coworker's house. Al is in the throes of self-pity, bitterness, and a fierce, masochistic determination to be independent of Ruth's love, which he suspects to be merely pity. Yet it is clear that he loves her deeply. The two men argue late into the night, with Diamond again expressing the values of solidarity and commitment. He criticizes Al for his self-pity, explaining that Al has indeed paid a heavy price but in a just and necessary cause and comparing Al's blindness to his own Jewish identity as a stigma. The only antidote for prejudice, Lee argues, is a humane Americanism that offers everyone compassion and fair play. Al is unconvinced. His mind remains fixed on his own grievance. There never is a point at which Al clearly articulates a commitment to Lee's way of thinking.[46] In surrendering finally to his need for Ruth, however, and adopting the hopeful and confident state of mind we find him in at the end of the movie, we are led to believe that he has opened himself to Lee's vision of the future.[47]

The ward scene, so offensive to anti-Communists during the early years of the cold war, is certainly plausible. We do not know if Al ever took part in such a discussion, but seriously wounded men would have been likely while hospitalized to discuss their hopes and fears for the future.[48] The scene is heavy handed in the deliberateness of its discursive messages, a few of which are delivered in brief dramatic monologues that seem to step out of the movie and are reminiscent of some highly affected moments in 1930s political theater. This is the way the scene struck wartime government censors at the Office of War Information, who liked the way Al "grew up" in the movie to become a more thoughtful and committed man but found the ward scene an example of "naive and immature" "home front propaganda."[49] The intense conversation on the train, however, is a conspicuous manipulation of Al's life. Lee did not accompany Al back to Philadelphia, let alone conspire to bring him and Ruth together. Diamond left San Diego Naval Hospital after three months, and he and Al never were to communicate again. Nor did Ruth ever communicate with or meet Lee.[50] Though Al had briefly broken off their engagement, he ultimately willingly returned to his hometown in anticipation of beginning with Ruth the private, family existence that he had been denied by the disruptions of his childhood and that he now knew was within his grasp. His Navy Cross and rehabilitation did await him in Philadelphia, but there proved no need for anyone to manipulate the situation to bring him together with Ruth. Al's hopes for the future did not depend on being won over to commitment to human solidarity. There is no evidence that he ever experienced a political revelation or conversion of any sort. His rejection of a future political role after the 1946 elections also seems a rejection of the script that Maltz projected for the balance of Al's life.

Guadalcanal Veterans Remember Schmid

For many years, the movie's celebration of Al's courage has served to alienate some of the Guadalcanal veterans, including Lee Diamond, from the legend of Al Schmid. Like the blinded veterans, these men, too, share a feeling of intense solidarity. It is rooted in the memory of lethal combat rather than the experience of lifetime impairment, but the bonds it has produced are just as tight as those found in the BVA. They remain haunted by the terrible costs of the Guadalcanal campaign, in which so many young marines, lacking combat experience, out-numbered and undersupplied, died to achieve victory. They do not trust any representation of Guadalcanal that suggests that one man, more than his com-rades, turned the tide of battle. How do we really know whose machine gun was responsible for any 200 of the 600 Japanese bodies found the morning after the Tenaru engagement? asks Harry Horsman, who also fought in that battle and is now the national historian of the Guadalcanal Campaign Veterans. Could Al have survived the night without Diamond's help? Horsman asks; and if not, why didn't Diamond get more recognition, beyond his own Navy Cross? Instead, after leaving the hospital, Diamond returned to active service, becoming again just another marine.[51]

Diamond himself seems completely indifferent to the matter of personal rec-ognition and instead overwhelmed still by the death and suffering he witnessed. Not long after the fiftieth anniversary of the Guadalcanal campaign he reflected on the unheralded deaths of so many young men, many of whom, he believes, could have delayed their exposure to combat by going to officer candidate school but chose out of a sense of duty to enter the marines and go to battle at the earliest possible point in the war. These thoughts have grown more, not less, burdensome for Diamond, who in 1993 told me that he had been watching videotaped docu-mentaries of the Guadalcanal campaign "over and over." On Memorial Day, 1993, as he pondered the experience of his generation, he became troubled by the thought that in a permissive cultural environment, in which, Diamond believed, the current commander in chief, President Bill Clinton himself, had deliberately avoided military service in a later war, an understanding of their devotion to duty could no longer be grasped.[52]

Thus, veterans like Diamond and Horsman have been crafting their own legend of Guadalcanal. It has led them to feel that Al broke solidarity with them. They are reluctant to criticize Schmid directly. They acknowledge his courage and speak with compassion of his injury. It is the movie they are quick to say that troubles them. They see the collusion of all the hero-crafting interests that cooperated in producing it. They may acknowledge the patriotic motives of these interests. But they are aware that the government and military placed them in harm's way, knowing that many of them were certain to be killed. They suspect, too, that even with the best of intentions, civilians can never conceive of the horror of their own experience of combat, least of all by watching Hollywood movies.[53] Diamond says dismissively of *Pride of the Marines* that it made him "uncomfortable," because "It was just p.r. for the war effort."[54]

Implicit in their criticisms of the movie is the view that Schmid allowed himself both to be used by those interests and to be placed above the men along with whom he was in combat. This is the source of the emotional distance one senses when they are questioned more closely about Schmid. It is perhaps for this reason, rather than simply a drifting apart in peacetime of men of different backgrounds artificially brought together by war, that after his own hospitalization in San Diego Diamond never sought to resume a relationship with Schmid, in spite of the intense experience they shared.[55]

Schmid also possessed this critical view of the heroic legend constructed out of his life. This was what caused him to protest publicly, even at the height of his fame, that he was just another one of the "gophers of Guadalcanal"; and it contributed to his decision to end the negotiations over his public role and image by returning to a more or less anonymous private life. While Al certainly profited from his heroic legend, it needs to be recalled that he was told that he was serving his country in becoming a public symbol. For a time, however, he broke faith with the combat veterans' ethos of remembrance, solidarity, and humility that has sustained these men for many years in confronting their memories. In consequence, it seems as if even in death the blinded hero can never be fully restored to their ranks.

NOTES

This is a revision of an essay, with the same title, that appeared in the *Journal of American Studies* 29, no. 1 (1995): 1–32.

1. Robert Butterfield, *Al Schmid—Marine* (New York: W. W. Norton, 1944), 94–106; Richard Tregaskis, *Guadalcanal Diary* (New York: Random House, 1943), 18, 127–

52, 215; Richard Frank, *Guadalcanal: The Definitive Account of the Landmark Battle* (New York: Penguin, 1990), 141–58; *Saint Petersburg Times*, 2 December 1982, obituary; Ken Pintwala, "Albert A. Schmid: Guadalcanal Hero," *Leatherneck* 69 (August 1986): 3207.

2. David D. Lee, *Sergeant York: An American Hero* (Lexington, KY: University Press of Kentucky, 1987); Don Graham, *No Names on the Bullet: A Biography of Audie Murphy* (New York: Viking, 1989); *New York Times*, 19, 20, 29 January 1943, 26 February 1943, 5, 11, 23 April 1943, 4 September 1943, 6 June 1944, 17, 18 October 1944, 28 March 1945, 23 May 1945; Roger Butterfield, "Al Schmid, Hero: Newly Blinded while Killing 200 Japs, He Has Returned to the Girl Who Waited for Him," *Life*, 22 March 1943, 35, 40–44; *Philadelphia Inquirer*, 11 November 1942, 6 May 1943, 11 October 1944, 7 December 1982, editorial; undated clippings, from *Philadelphia Inquirer*, *Philadelphia Record*, and *Philadelphia Bulletin* newspapers, in the Delmar Daves Collection, Stanford University Libraries (hereafter cited as DDC) and in the Al Schmid file, Marine Corps Historical Center, Washington, DC (hereafter cited as MCHC); *Pittsburgh Gazette*, 26 February 1943; *Albany Knickerbocker News*, 11 February 1943; *Washington, DC News*, 17 October 1944. Butterfield's *Al Schmid—Marine* closely follows the representation of Al's life that appeared as "Al Schmid, Hero," in *Life*.

3. The movies based on the lives of York and Murphy are *Sergeant York* (1941, dir. Howard Hawks); and *To Hell and Back* (1955, dir. Jesse Hibbs).

4. The influences on my conception of Schmid's story lie in recent, postbehaviorist, psychological literature, especially works on questions of individual agency and selfhood and on the narrative construction of the self. See Rom Harré and Grant Gillett, *The Discursive Mind* (London: Sage Publications, 1994); Jerome Bruner, *Acts of Meaning* (Cambridge, MA: Harvard University Press, 1990); Kenneth Gergen and Mary Gergen, "Narratives of the Self," in *Studies in Social Identity*, ed. Theodore R. Sarbin (New York: Prager, 1983), 254–73.

5. Butterfield, *Al Schmid—Marine*, 21–44; Virginia Pfeiffer to Ruth Hartley, 17 November 1942, DDC.

6. Telephone interview with Ruth Schmid, 3 August 1990 (hereafter cited as *RS, 3/8/1990*).

7. Butterfield, *Al Schmid—Marine*, 38–45; Al Schmid to Ruth Hartley, "Friday," [1942], DDC.

8. Butterfield, *Al Schmid—Marine*, 45–48; Butterfield, "Al Schmid, Hero," 41.

9. Butterfield, *Al Schmid—Marine*, 71, 73. On the influence of war movies on the imaginations of American young men, see Laurence H. Suid, *Guts and Glory: Great American War Movies* (Reading, MA: Addison-Wesley, 1978), 100–106.

10. Butterfield, *Al Schmid—Marine*, 48, 66, 83. On the pervasiveness of anti-Japanese racism among Americans, see John Dower, *War without Mercy: Race and Power in the Pacific War* (New York: Pantheon, 1986), 77–178.

11. *RS, 3/8/1990*; Butterfield, *Al Schmid—Marine*, 63, 89–93; *Saint Petersburg Independent*, 20 April 1957, 6 October 1957. On marine training philosophy and combat performance, see Gwynne Dwyer, *War* (New York: Crown Publishers, 1985), 104, 108, 114, 117–25.

12. Samuel Stouffer, *Combat and Its Aftermath*, The American Soldier, vol. 2 (Prince-

ton, NJ: Princeton University Press, 1949), 131–32, 150–51; Robert Sklar, *City Boys: Cagney, Bogart, Garfield* (Princeton, NJ: Princeton University Press, 1992), 163, 188.

13. Butterfield, *Al Schmid—Marine,* 113–29; *RS, 3/8/1990;* Virginia Pfeiffer to Ruth Hartley, 28 October 1942, 3, 4, 20 November 1942, 3, 8 December 1942; Al Schmid to Ruth Hartley, 31 October 1942; Virginia Pfeiffer to "Mrs. Schmid" [Al's sister-in-law], 4 November 1942, DDC.

14. *Philadelphia Inquirer,* 11 November 1942; undated clippings [1942], *Philadelphia Inquirer* and *Philadelphia Record,* DDC and MCHC; Virginia Pfeiffer to Ruth Hartley, 13, 17 November 1942; Al Schmid to "Everybody," 27 November 1942, DDC; Butterfield, *Al Schmid—Marine,* 126–28; *Pittsburgh Post-Gazette,* 4 August 1945.

15. *New York Times,* 23 May 1945, 29 January 1946, 7 June 1946, 22 October 1946; undated itinerary, "March" [1943?]; *Washington Star,* 13 March 1946.

16. *New York Times,* 22 May 1946, 7 November 1946; *Washington Star,* 13 March 1946.

17. Lloyd Greenwood, "The Blinded Veteran," in *Blindness,* ed. Paul A. Zahl (Princeton, NJ: Princeton University Press, 1950), 261.

18. Ibid., 264, 266–68; Hector Chevigny, *The Adjustment of the Blind* (New Haven, CT: Yale University Press, 1950), 228–30; Thomas J. Carroll, *Blindness: What It Is, What It Does, and How To Live with It* (Boston, MA: Little, Brown, 1960), 3–87; Robert Brown and Hope Schutte, *Our Fight: A Battle against Darkness* (Washington, DC: Blinded Veterans Association, 1991), 3–5, 11, 15, 35–41; Walt Stromer, "A Letter Too Late," *BVA Bulletin,* 45 (July/August 1990): 8.

19. Alan R. Blackburn, "The Army Blind in the United States," in *Blindness,* ed. Paul A. Zahl (Princeton, NJ: Princeton University Press, 1950), 272–87; and Merle Frampton, "Rehabilitation Procedures in the Navy, Marine Corps, and Coast Guard," in *Blindness,* 288–93.

20. Virginia Pfeiffer to Ruth Hartley, 8 December 1942, DDC; Ian Fraser, "The Service War-Blinded in Great Britain," in *Blindness,* ed. Paul A. Zahl (Princeton, NJ: Princeton University Press, 1950), 297–98; Chevigny, *The Adjustment of the Blind,* 228–30.

21. Butterfield, *Al Schmid—Marine,* 124, 128; Frances A. Koestler, *The Unseen Minority,* (New York: David McKay Co., 1976), 271–72; Frampton, "Rehabilitation Procedures," 288–93; telephone interview with Dr. Ed Glass, clinical psychologist and blinded veteran of World War II, 3 August 1990 (hereafter cited as *EG, 3/8/1990*).

22. Brown and Schutte, *Our Fight,* 15, 42–50; Richard Hoover, "The Cane as a Travel Aid," in *Blindness,* ed. Paul A. Zahl (Princeton, NJ: Princeton University Press, 1950), 353–65.

23. *RS, 3/8/1990; New York Times,* 23 May 1945.

24. Telephone interviews with Gloria Adalion, coordinator (retired), Visual Impairment Services, Bay Pines VA Hospital, St. Petersburg, Florida, 6, 15 August 1990, 13 June 1992. Ms. Adalion spoke to me about Al after obtaining Ruth Schmid's permission.

25. Telephone interview with Gloria Adalion, 13 June 1992; taped interview with Elaine Powers, coordinator of Visual Impairment Services, Buffalo VA Hospital, Buffalo, New York, 3 January 1990, in author's possession; taped interview with Edward Huyczyk, blinded veteran of World War II and early national board member of the Blinded Veterans Association, Amherst, New York, 14 August 1990, in author's possession (hereafter cited

as *EH, 14/8/1990*); Edward Lay, "Excuses and Blind Rehabilitation," *VIS View* (winter 1989): 9–10.

26. *RS, 3/8/1990.*

27. *RS, 3/8/1990.* Photos: Butterfield, "Al Schmid, Hero," 35; *Philadelphia Inquirer,* 6 March 1943; *Chicago Daily News,* 15 March 1944; *Washington Post,* 8 June 1944; *New York Times,* 22 May 1946; *Atlanta Journal,* 16 June 1946. *Saint Petersburg Independent,* 20 April 1957, 6 October 1957; *Saint Petersburg Times Independent,* 8 June 1972, 2 December 1982, obituary; studio publicity photographs, taken on location in Philadelphia during the filming of *Pride of the Marines* (Film Stills Archive, Museum of Modern Art, New York).

28. Brown and Schutte, *Our Fight,* 11–23; Koestler, *The Unseen Minority,* 380–88; *New York Times,* 26 June 1945, 20 January 1946, 9 June 1946, 9 August 1946, 27 November 1946, 7 September 1947, 13 March 1948, 13 April 1948, 8 August 1948, 3 September 1948, 20 October 1948; Greenwood, "The Blinded Veteran," 269–70.

29. Koestler, *The Unseen Minority,* 276–77, 279, 315–16; Brown and Schutte, *Our Fight,* 46–50; Chevigny, *The Adjustment of the Blind,* 245–46; *New York Times Magazine,* 19 May 1946, 56.

30. Russell Williams, "Some Historical Perspectives on VIST and Blindness," *VIS View* (winter 1984): 7; Russell Williams, "Believers," *VIS View* (winter 1989): 4–6; Ellen Papadimoulis, "Editorial," *VIS View* (winter 1989): 1–2.

31. *EG, 3/8/1990; EH, 14/8/1990;* and telephone interviews with Raymond Frey, first president of the BVA, 24 July 1990 (hereafter cited as *RW, 24/7/1990*).

32. *EH, 14/8/1990; RW, 24/7/1990; St. Petersburg Times,* 2 December 1982, obituary; Kathern Gruber, retired consultant to BVA, to David Gerber, [1991], in author's possession.

33. *RW, 24/7/1990.* Also, *RF, 24/7/1990,* who believes Schmid "might have rested on his laurels" for the balance of his life.

34. *RW, 24/7/1990; RF, 24/7/1990.*

35. *New York Times,* 10 September 1945, 3 October 1945, 15 November 1945, 21 November 1946, 15 January 1947; Greenwood, "The Blinded Veteran," 264; Brown and Schutte, *Our Fight,* 15. Robert A. Scott, *The Making of Blind Men: A Study in Adult Socialization* (New York: Russell Sage Foundation, 1969), 112–16.

36. Milton D. Graham, *851 Blinded Veterans: A Success Story* (New York: American Federation of the Blind, 1968), 74, 126–28.

37. *EH, 14/8/1990.*

38. Telephone interview with Gloria Adalion, 13 June 1992; Russell Williams, "Why Should I?" *VIS View* (February 1987): 12; Graham, *851 Blinded Veterans,* 66–68; Scott, *The Making of Blind Men,* 72.

39. Greenwood, "The Blinded Veteran," 266–68, 269–70; *The Long Cane* (training film, Veterans Administration, 1952).

40. *Pride of the Marines* was produced at Warner Brothers by Jerry Wald, one of the studio's leading executives, who was attracted to Butterfield's *Al Schmid—Marine.* Butterfield was consulted in the earliest stages of the adaptation of his book. The popular reception of Al, as reflected in the press, was studied by Wald, director Delmar Daves, and the writers during the adaptation process. A mainstream liberal in politics, Wald enthusias-

tically employed Left-oriented creative people on this and other projects, because he respected their talents in dealing with contemporary events. Alvah Bessie and Albert Maltz, two prominent Hollywood Communist Party members, were the key writers. Maltz was responsible for the final versions of the script, though Wald and Daves had the power to make changes in the script even when Maltz opposed them—a situation typical of the Hollywood studios system at the time. The Marine Corps gave the studio technical and marketing assistance. Most wartime movie scripts and movies that had any relevance to contemporary events were monitored by the Roosevelt administration's Office of War Information (OWI), which presented studios with evaluations and asked for revisions that might better serve the war effort. These elements are discussed subsequently; and also see Sklar, *City Boys,* 162–65; Charles Higham, *Warner Brothers* (New York: Charles Scribner, 1975), 144–71; Warner Brothers Pictures and U.S. Marine Corps, *Pride of the Marines* (n.p.: 1945; pressbook accompanying release of *Pride of the Marines*); Suid, *Guts and Glory,* 72–3, 92, Clayton R. Koppes and Gregory D. Black, *Hollywood Goes to War: How Politics, Profits and Propaganda Shaped World War II Movies* (Berkeley, CA: University of California Press, 1987); Ian Hamilton, *Writers in Hollywood, 1915–1951* (New York: Carroll and Graf Publishers, 1990), 191–283; Neal Gabler, *An Empire of Their Own: How the Jews Invented Hollywood* (New York: Crown Publishers, 1988), 311–60; Sklar, *City Boys,* 104–76.

41. Dana Polan, *Power and Paranoia: History, Narrative, and the American Cinema, 1940–1950* (New York: Columbia University Press, 1986), 86–96, 194–200, analyzes the movie (as "an exemplary case" of the juxtaposition of the themes of war and commitment) from the perspective of narrative theory. Reviews of Butterfield's *Al Schmid—Marine* laud the author for this personalization of the role of an ordinary man in the war; *Chicago Daily News,* 15 March 1944; *Philadelphia Record,* 10 April 1944.

42. *RS, 3/8/1990;* Butterfield, *Al Schmid—Marine,* 132–35; Albert Maltz, *"This Love of Ours": Suggestions and Criticisms,* 18 (typescript/memo, 2 December 1944), DDC. ("This Love of Ours" was an early, working title for *Pride of the Marines.*)

43. Butterfield, *Al Schmid—Marine,* 134–35; Virginia Pfeiffer to Ruth Hartley, 8 December 1942, DDC; *Pittsburgh Gazette,* 26 February 1943.

44. Warner Brothers Pictures and U.S. Marine Corps, *Pride of the Marines,* 9, 13, 14. Clive Hirshhorn, *The Warner Brothers Story* (New York: Crown Publishers, 1979), 179.

45. Maltz, *"This Love of Ours": Suggestions and Criticisms,* 9, DDC.

46. Maltz, *Suggestions for "Al Schmid—Marine"* 18–19, and idem, *"This Love of Ours": Suggestions and Criticisms,* 9–10, DDC; K. R. M. Short, "Hollywood Fights Anti-Semitism, 1940–1945," in *Film and Radio Propaganda in World War II,* ed. K. R. M. Short (Knoxville, TN: University of Tennessee Press, 1983), 166–68.

47. Cf. Sklar, *City Boys,* 164–65, which finds less political implication in the movie's depiction of Schmid's spiritual breakthrough but does not analyze it in the context of the crucial homecoming sequence that includes the argument between Al and Lee aboard the train. Peter Roffman and Jim Purdy, *The Hollywood Social Problem Film: Madness, Despair, and Politics from the Depression to the Fifties* (Bloomington, IN: Indiana University Press), 278–80, contend that the movie locates Al's problem squarely in his own "neurosis" and is without any apparent political implication, a reading that seems insensitive to the delicate ways in which Maltz chose to integrate politics into the script.

48. For evocations of the hospital ward culture of convalescing disabled combat veterans that confirm this plausibility, see, in autobiography, Harold Russell, *Victory in My Hands* (New York: Creative Age Press, Inc., 1949), 91–143, and idem, *The Best Years of My Life* (Middlebury, VT: Eriksson, 1981), 11–30; and, in autobiographically inspired fiction, James Jones, *Whistle* (New York: Delacorte Press, 1978).

49. Peggy Shepard, *Feature Reviewing—Pride of the Marines, July 11, 1945,* records of the Office of War Information, Record Group 208, Washington National Record Center, Suitland, MD.

50. *RS, 3/8/1990.*

51. Harry Horsman to David Gerber, 29 May 1993, 16, 19 June 1993. Other Tenaru River combat veterans also offered their opinions and evaluations of their own and Schmid's experiences: Lee Diamond to David Gerber, 2 June 1993; Fred Stewart to David Gerber, 26 July 1993, 10 August 1993. (All letters in the author's possession.) It is from these letters, and especially Harry Horsman's, that I have attempted to create a collective profile.

52. Diamond to Gerber, 2 June 1993.

53. Ibid. Horsman to Gerber, 19 June 1993. This state of mind is evoked very convincingly in Paul Fussell's controversial *Wartime: Understanding and Behavior in the Second World War* (New York: Oxford University Press, 1989), 52–65, 129–95, 251–97.

54. Diamond to Gerber, 2 June 1993. Horsman (19 June 1993 to Gerber) expresses himself in exactly, and even more precisely, the same terms. He focuses his search for the origins of the movie's conception on "the public relations office of the Marine Corps," which did indeed cooperate closely with Warner Brothers.

55. Ruth Schmid offered their difference in background as the explanation for this failure to revive their ties after the months in San Diego; *RS, 3/8/1990.*

Conspicuous Contribution and American Cultural Dilemmas ▶ Telethon Rituals of Cleansing and Renewal

Paul K. Longmore

On the 1989 Muscular Dystrophy Association (MDA) Telethon, the president of the firefighters association declared: "There are givers and there's takers in this world. Firefighters are givers. All those people who can hear me out there can be givers too." This differentiation, which recurs implicitly on all telethons, is more than a ploy to prod donations. It draws an important moral boundary. It contrasts humane concern for one's neighbors with selfish preoccupation with one's private interests. It distinguishes those who personally shoulder responsibility for the civic welfare from those who indulge in self-centered irresponsibility. This marking off of "givers" and "takers," a separation of sheep from goats, is a central symbolic task of telethons.

But as they draw the dichotomy between the compassionate and the selfish, telethons symbolically define not just two but three types of persons. There are not only givers and takers. It is necessary that there also be recipients of "giving." Invention of the third category is indispensable to creation and maintenance of the first two. These classifications have far-reaching consequences for the social identities and social careers of people with disabilities. They are the ones ceremonially defined as the natural objects of charity because, according to the telethons, they have been socially invalidated by disability. Telethons offer occasions for individuals to act upon genuinely compassionate regard for their fellow human beings, but this "caring" is inextricably intertwined with the social stigma inscribed on people with disabilities.

It is important to examine how and why these rites frame opportunities for interwoven compassion and contempt in the particular ways they do. The telethon, a late-twentieth-century American cultural invention, expresses distinctively American values and addresses peculiarly American concerns. It attempts to resolve a variety of historic and ongoing dilemmas within American culture. The telethon is, on one level, a response to a number of deep-rooted American cultural, ultimately moral, predicaments.

Beginning with the era of the Revolution, the founding moment when Americans set into orbit the constellation of values that compose their cultural universe, they have declared and celebrated the right of individuals to pursue their own personal happiness, their own private interests. The dynamic of individualism has functioned as one of the most powerful forces shaping American society, for good and for ill. It claims for each citizen the twin rights to equality of opportunity and equality of esteem.[1]

Yet individualism also has often seemed to Americans to eat away at the bonds of their community by setting individuals above that community and against it. From the beginning, Americans have feared this centrifugal effect of their commitment to an individualistic ethos. Their celebration of the value of the individual and their liberation of individual potentialities has simultaneously given free rein to privatistic and self-centered impulses. As American society emancipated individuals to advance their personal welfare, it also implicitly permitted them to ignore the public weal—and to feel justified in doing so.[2]

In response to this moral and political peril, Americans, throughout their history, have warned themselves that the success of their democratic experiment rests on the public virtue of the people at large. If citizens voluntarily put the common good above their private interests, free democratic society will flourish. But if they set selfish concerns ahead of the general welfare, democracy inevitably will fail. This belief in the necessity of public virtue has operated in tension, and even in competition, with the devotion to individualism.

In historical moments when self-centered, rather than public-minded, individualism seemingly has overtaken them and their society, Americans, with a tone of alarm, have preached to themselves the imperative to practice public virtue. That sense of alarm has grown acute in the late twentieth century as self-maximization seems to have become the credo of American culture. Pop psychologists and self-help gurus proclaim that individuals have first of all to take care of themselves. Social critics decry this as narcissism that spurns true human connection and communal responsibility. They charge that it teaches individuals to aggrandize themselves in disregard of authentic attachments and at the expense of other selves. In particular, some assert, the philosophy of capitalistic individualism teaches that one realizes one's self most fully through consumption. "Capitalism tells us that the meaningful life is the life that maximizes the self," writes Joel Kovel. "Whatever is 'me' has more, does more, achieves more; such is the good life, whether measured in terms of compact disks, muscles, orgasms, publicity, or cash."[3] Heeding such critics, many Americans fear that, getting and spending, buying and consuming, they have become takers, severed from any authentic community by an insatiable, self-centered pursuit of material possessions. At the least, they fear they may be accused of that sort of selfishness.

On one level of cultural meaning, telethon donation is a collective rite designed to enable Americans to demonstrate to themselves that they still belong to a moral community, that they have not succumbed to materialism, that they are givers who fulfill their obligations to their neighbors. The electronic display of charity is a communal response to the moral and social dangers of narcissism and materialism. The vast American audience uses telethon donation to reassure itself, individually and collectively, of *its moral health*.

As with Ebenezer Scrooge, Dickens's symbol of rapacious nineteenth-century capitalism, aiding Tiny Tim, the literal embodiment of neglected human need, telethon poster children are made the means by which nondisabled people can prove to themselves that they have not been corrupted by an egocentric and materialistic capitalist order. People with disabilities are ritually defined as dependent on the moral fitness of nondisabled people. While takers repudiate their duty to these helpless neighbors, the compassion of givers toward "the less fortunate" publicly verifies the givers' moral standing. Telethon giving demonstrates the persistence of public virtue. It confirms to individual donors their possession of that virtue by distinguishing them from both takers and the invalidated. It ritualistically enacts a reversal of everyday reality. The ceremonial counterimage to conspicuous consumption is conspicuous contribution.

The telethon ritual also proclaims as an important fact that givers practice their virtue voluntarily. This liturgy rests on the assumption that moral voluntarism, the decisions of individuals, freely and privately made, verifies the reality of public virtue, thus reassuring Americans of the viability of their democratic political order and capitalist economic system. Americans define these "free" choices of each particular donor to give for the common good as morally more laudable than a collective decision to provide for that common good by taxing themselves. The communal commitments of Western European societies to maintain comprehensive national health insurance systems implicitly seem to many Americans not only politically undesirable but morally suspect. Rather than regard such policies as implementing collective moral choices to ensure the common weal, Americans scorn them as state intrusion. Americans, among the most antistatist of peoples, gauge their devotion to the common good far less by the activities they require of their government "to promote the general welfare" than by the volume of their individual donations to private charities. The antistatism, individualism, and privatism so powerfully at work in American culture define the vigor of nongovernmental endeavors as the indicator of Americans' dedication to the general weal. Thus personal moral voluntarism and individual community volunteerism are made measures of the condition of American civic virtue.

From time to time, telethon participants, playing the role of moral leader, spell out this message of the telethon ritual. They proclaim that these efforts vindicate the moral superiority of American voluntarism and volunteerism. Year after year on the United Cerebral Palsy (UCP) Telethon, veteran national emcee Dennis James recites a poem about the special place in heaven reserved for volunteers. In 1993, Jerry Lewis proclaimed his "great pride" that MDA is not "government-oriented . . . We've never been subsidized by the government. We have done this ourselves, between you and me." On the 1994 Easter Seal Telethon, cohost Robb

Weller introduced someone who literally embodied American values, "the stunning young woman who will be representing the United States at the Miss Universe pageant, . . . Miss U.S.A." She would offer "some patriotic words about Easter Seals." Miss U.S.A. then delivered this "patriotic" homily: "Easter Seals typifies what America is all about: hard work, independence, and generosity. Generosity fills the heart of America, because when tragedy strikes, from Mississippi floods to California earthquakes, we Americans come together in the spirit of volunteerism, willing to give whatever we can to help our neighbors get back on their feet. But smaller tragedies happen every day. An auto accident costs a young mother her ability to walk. A stroke paralyzes a middle-aged father of three. A stray gunshot causes a high school senior to lose her sight . . . Easter Seals does all it can to help turn tragedy into triumph. So please, reach into your hearts and feel that truly American spirit of generosity."

The "generosity," the moral voluntarism, of charity volunteers aims to restore the "independence" of other individuals whose own competency for moral voluntarism has been compromised by "tragedies," physical and economic limitations resulting from natural catastrophes or physiological disabilities. The capacity to function as a true American, an independent moral agent, is predicated upon physical and economic self-sufficiency. Givers act to revalidate fellow Americans who have been rendered socially illegitimate by disability.

As ceremonies to certify the vitality of moral voluntarism, of public virtue, telethons are rites of American nationalism. In a centrifugal pluralistic society, the broadcasts are designed, in part, to fortify the national identity. Charity giving has long functioned to bolster patriotic Americanism.[4] In a sense, the only thing Americans have held in common, the only glue that has held them together, is a shared allegiance to what is regarded as a distinctive set of "American" values. The nationalistic telethon ritual marks off individuals who practice those values from those who fail to do so. It distinguishes "good," which is to say authentic, Americans from both bad ones and inauthentic ones, which is to say, from takers and those invalidated by disability.

Telethons sometimes convoke themselves as nationalistic ceremonies by stirring viewers with patriotic anthems. On the 1990 MDA extravaganza, live on stage, the venerable pop singer Ray Charles sang "America the Beautiful," and his young counterpart Michael Bolton, on tape at (perhaps predictably) a softball game, trumpeted "The Star-Spangled Banner." Sometimes the patriotic fervor turns militant. The 1992 Easter Seal rally heard country singer Eddie Rabbit proclaim in the song "I'm an American Boy": "I buy American. / I'll die an American." The 1991 UCP pageant occurred during the Persian Gulf War, so opera star Robert Merrill and the American Pilgrim Chorus offered a medley of patriotic songs that included "America the Beautiful" and "God Bless America," and a few minutes later that nationalistically named choir intoned "This Is My

Country." A few weeks later on the Easter Seal spectacle, Bobby Vinton sang "I'm Proud to Be an American."

Telethons are a combination of patriotic rally and religious revival. And so, a local Easter Seal host harangued viewers to phone in and make the light circle go all the way around. She proclaimed that Easter Seal was giving disabled people "a chance to step up and out and be a part of life like you and me! We take life for granted! Don't! These people don't!" Like a preacher in a tent meeting, she went on for several minutes, exhorting at the top of her voice. Some of the operators whose phones sat silent started to clap in unison. One of the male hosts also began preaching. The two hosts exhorted simultaneously. "We've got to do it!" they shouted. "I know you can do it! I know we can do it! I believe!"[5] Local hosts on some telethons entreat viewers to make the circle of lights go all the way around. They press watchers to call in so that the telephone operators can sit down. UCP emcee Dennis James will say: "I checked on the phones, and the phones are a hundred percent busy right now." It is a ritual exhortation to demonstrate commitment to moral community in a public way, to display civic virtue conspicuously.

Each year telethon hosts exhort viewers to help them top last year's total. "We have no goal," affirmed Dennis James on the 1993 UCP show and then proceeded to announce their goal. "We want to make as much or more than we made last year." "No telethon has ever gone lower than the year before," he explained significantly. "That's our measure of success. So I know that you're not going to let us down." Jerry Lewis agrees. He always declares his intention to get at least one dollar above the year before.

When the pace of pledge making lags, telethon hosts chide viewers, reminding them of their moral duty. "Sometimes we get to a point like this where I've got to be your conscience," James admonished the audience in a slack moment in 1994. "I've been saying that now for forty-three years on this telethon. I've got to be your conscience." "I hate to pound you," he said, "but I don't want to go off with any less than we had last year . . . It's your telethon. You're the ones who make the calls." During one pledge match on the 1989 Arthritis Telethon, cohost Larry Van Nuys exhorted: "You have to decide who you are and what you want to represent."

The annual increases in telethon donations are taken as another sign of the maintenance of public virtue. If the final totals dropped—or even stayed at the same level as the year before—it would evidence a decline in public virtue. Americans are legendary scorekeepers. They rate everything they do with numerical records. They measure their achievements by the stats. Telethon hosts note that many pledge makers like to phone in near the end of these protracted broadcasts. Telethon donation thus becomes a kind of competition, a sport, a game of reaching a new statistical high point. Are Americans more caring or less? More compassionate or more selfish? The figures flashing on the electronic tote boards will tell the tale of success or failure, of moral improvement or moral decline. To everyone's reassurance, the telethons' final totals are above last year's pledges. The numbers confirm that Americans still practice public virtue. "The generosity we're seeing tonight again proves that Americans are loving caring people," affirmed John Ritter on the 1995 UCP rally. "Let's see how loving, how caring," urged his cohost Henry Winkler. "Let's see the results." The two turned to the tote board. "We are a marvelous country of terrific people," declared Jerry Lewis on the 1989 MDA ritual, pointing to his telethon's tote board, "proof positive, people that care."

Telethon hosts repeatedly reassure viewers that Americans still "love one another," still sacrifice for "the less fortunate" and for the common good, still practice public virtue. At the wrap-up of the 1993 UCP rally, singer Florence Henderson concluded, "You know, I never cease to marvel at the warmth and generosity of the American people. And these are not easy times financially. We all know that. Yet year after year Star-athon reinforces my faith, and I know all of us, all our faiths, in the American spirit." Dennis James agreed. "I really believe that America's embarking, people, on a new era of giving something back to our country." This year, he added, the telethon would "go over the top."

Contrary to gloomy social critics, American public virtue, according to the telethons, is not in decline. In 1992 Easter Seal national cohost Mary Frann countered the Jeremiahs: "You know, we hear so much about the problems that we're facing as a society. Our economy is stalled. People are losing their jobs. And people say our values are declining. But I guess any one of those factors would seem like a reason to put off giving to Easter Seals. But thank goodness you decided that the reasons to give outweighed the ones not to. And that tremendous outpouring of goodwill says more about us as a society than any column or poll could ever say." UCP national cohost Nancy Dussault offered identical reassurance in 1994: "If we look at the headlines today, we are misled to believe that America is a nation of heartless, uncaring cynics. Nothing could be farther from the truth," she rebutted. "America is a land of thoughtful, caring, giving people, who do indeed love each other."

Easter Seal enlisted newly inaugurated President Bill Clinton in 1993 to proclaim the same comforting message from the "bully pulpit." The president told telethon viewers that there is "a new spirit" in the land. "There's a new sense of possibility," he claimed, "a new willingness to take on challenges, a new willingness to contribute, I think, a clear new understanding that we have to make strength and unity out of our many diversities as a society. We do have to go back to a community, to know that together we can do more than we ever can separately. So I want to congratulate the Easter Seals on its back-to-community movement. It's an important part of rebuilding the American community and securing the future for all of our people."

America, the historian Sidney Mead wrote, is "a nation with the soul of a church." Telethons are rituals of America's civic religion. They are moral allegories of cleansing and renewal. They symbolically represent individual and collective turning away from the self-centered conduct that is perceived as having undermined or ruptured the community. Although they ostensibly seek the physical repair of those socially invalidated by disability, they are more importantly rituals of moral restoration for nondisabled communicants. Telethons offer donors a momentary sense of the wholeness that comes with membership in a moral community. The broadcasts project a brief annual apparition of that community in a materialistic, competitive, atomized society.

All telethon hosts proclaim that their particular charity restores the sense of "caring" and "community." They call viewers to commit themselves to the telethon's mission. The hosts are not merely emcees but, more important, moral preceptors. And the ministry is the same for all the telethons: to help the needy, to aid "the less fortunate." "The Easter Seals way of caring," said one host in 1990, "is . . . one heart reaching out in love to another heart in need of compassion."

Giving to Get

In fact, of course, this "reaching out" of "one heart . . . to another" takes place only symbolically. The phone-in pledge makers do not directly come to know any particular person with a disability. The "caring" are connecting only with an image on their TV screens. It is a representation carefully fashioned within the telethon system and bearing little relation to the actual lives of people with disabilities. But this fictive reaching out to a contrived image is necessary to complete the verification of moral voluntarism and personal volunteerism on the part of givers. To function efficaciously, the ritual requires a class of persons defined as "needy," as socially invalidated.

In addition, the actual proportion of viewers phoning in pledges undercuts the claim that conspicuous telethon contribution demonstrates the vitality of American public virtue and community. Dennis James reported on the 1995 UCP Telethon that only two telethon watchers out of ten make pledges. It seems unlikely that other telethons induce much more than 20 percent of their audiences to respond. No more than a righteous remnant of the American people prove themselves to be givers.

Most important, a troubling feature of the telethon system subverts the self-proclaimed restoration of American community and sullies the vaunted virtue of givers. Telethons instantly taint the civic-mindedness they seek to renew by promoting the very materialism and self-centeredness they promise to exorcise. Even while telethon preceptors purport to call on viewers' sense of empathy, they often deliberately appeal to their avarice and self-aggrandizement.

During the 1980s and 1990s, telethons have drawn donations by offering bonuses and discounts, by putting up prizes and "free" gifts. The corporate sponsors of the telethon system promote a wide array of consumer products through special sales linked to the charities. Companies tell potential customers that they will be contributing to help the "less fortunate," even as those businesses urge individual donors to pursue personal economic advantage. A bold-lettered headline in Easter Seal's 1989 newspaper Sunday supplement urged consumers to join self-interest to condescension: "Save up to $8.00 and help us open doors for special people." In 1991, cohost Mary Frann counseled viewers: "You'll get a twofold benefit. You're gonna save lots of money, and you'll also help Easter Seals too by simply using these coupons." Telethons enable not just businesses to gain by giving but individual donors as well. The telethons and the manufacturers encourage consumers to profit under the guise of helping disabled people.

Hungry viewers can get discount coupons on food. In 1993, the marketing director of Little Caesar's Pizza, an Easter Seal corporate sponsor, described their two national promotional campaigns, a calendar and a coupon book available at Little Caesar's outlets. Customers would save money "on select Little Caesar's menu items." In 1994, a spokesman again touted the coupon books: "This is a great way for customers to save money on their favorite foods and help out this great cause." Friendly's Restaurants invites customers to give a dollar to Easter Seal and get something for themselves: a "free" ice cream cone or a discount coupon toward a meal. Consumers who aren't in the mood for pizza or ice cream can go to Wienerschnitzel. On the San Francisco Easter Seal broadcast (1991), a spokesperson announced the fast food chain's promotion: $5 coupon books for those who gave a dollar to Easter Seal. A local host immediately coined a sales slogan: "Eat a corn dog, help Easter Seals."

Local telethon segments offer most of the prizes. Viewers of one cutaway to the 1992 San Francisco Bay Area Easter Seal show could win a large floral bouquet if they were the eighth caller. Later in the broadcast, the first twenty callers would get a cookbook. And if they came down to the site of a remote telecast at a Safeway store in the East Bay, they might win prizes in several drawings: backyard barbecues, a set of roller blades, or hats. In 1994 and 1995 during various hours, anyone pledging fifty dollars or more would get, "free," a San Jose Sharks hat or a San Francisco 49ers cap or an Oakland A's or San Francisco Giants cap. And for a $75 donation, viewers got a Giants cap plus four tickets to a Giants game. During each hour, a different incentive lured pledges. On mid-1990s Easter Seal Chicago segments, a woman from the Honey Bear Ham Company was accompanied by "Mama and Papa Bear," two people wearing bear costumes. The first twenty callers pledging $100 would get Honey Bear's Easter basket with a glazed ham in it.

Likewise, the Bay Area segment of the 1992 Arthritis Telethon announced that donors could obtain celebrity-autographed items. And callers who pledged $200 or more would be eligible for a drawing for a diamond bracelet. At one point in the 1994 Arthritis show, the Bay Area host proclaimed that the next person to call with a $100 pledge would receive a green silk jacket from Bally's Casino and Resort in Las Vegas, the site of the national telecast.

Viewers of the Chicago portion of UCP's 1992 telecast could choose during various hours among an array of bonuses. In one hour, a pledge of $50 or more would garner from MCI a $25 certificate for long distance calls on any long distance carrier. In another hour, a contribution of at least $60 would yield a caller ID device supplied by Illinois Bell.

In 1992, JVC, a manufacturer of high-quality electronic equipment and a new MDA corporate sponsor, backed a promotional campaign at retail stores called "Help Jerry's Kids." Customers got an instant-win game piece on JVC video-cassettes. JVC offered as prizes $5 checks toward video rentals and "over $10,000" in JVC televisions. (The latter prizes amounted to a few dozen TV sets.) JVC also gave customers who donated to MDA free videocassettes and U.S. savings bonds.

Local hosts and participants dangle tickets of all sorts too. On the 1993 Easter Seal Chicago segment, a pro wrestler promised callers pledging $25 or more two "free" tickets to an upcoming wrestling match. Anyone pledging $200 during the 1992 San Francisco Bay Area Arthritis Telethon became eligible for two tickets to a Fred Travalena concert, while the Bay Area Easter Seal show that same year included a drawing for Oakland A's tickets.

The hosts of Easter Seal's 1989 Los Angeles segment announced a travel incentive to potential pledge makers. If callers pledged $52 or more, Uniglobe Travel, a corporate sponsor, would offer them a chance to win a free trip to Hawaii. Within minutes, dozens of $52 pledges flooded in. One emcee read a donor's name and exclaimed: "She may be going to Hawaii!" Another, sounding like a TV used car salesman, chimed in: "What a bargain! $52 works out to a dollar a week, first of all! That's not bad! A dollar a week for the next year is not bad! . . . Secondly, you're helping Easter Seals. You're helping people who need help here in Southern California. You're gonna feel good about it! And you might win the trip!"

Younger philanthropists can profit too. MDA's "hop-a-thons" offer non-disabled schoolchildren a selfish incentive. They can earn prizes while they hop "for those who can't."[6]

By using prizes and gifts and discount coupons to draw donations, telethons train nondisabled children and adults to regard people with disabilities not only as objects of their charity but as means for their personal aggrandizement. On the San Francisco portion of the 1994 Easter Seal Telethon, a local host asked one of the telephone operators about the caller she had just spoken with on the phone. "Somebody wants to know when the big screen TV is going to be raffled off," she explained. "Ah, well," said the emcee, a bit embarrassed, "they'll just have to wait on the big screen TV."

The offer of incentives—tickets and trips, big league caps and big screen TVs, and prizes for nondisabled kids who hop "for those who can't"—exposes a selfish motive behind the boasted public virtue. It reveals telethon donation as, for many givers, just one more means of personal gain, little different from buying a lottery ticket. Rather than being an American back-to-community effort, telethons often seem to be charity versions of another late-twentieth-century broadcast phenomenon, the home shopping networks.

The Sound of Trumpets

Even when the incentive is nonmaterial, the motive for giving promoted by telethons is still often self-centered.

Jesus Christ taught: "When you give alms, sound no trumpet before you, as the hypocrites do . . . that they may be praised by men . . . But when you give alms, do not let your left hand know what your right hand is doing, so that your alms may be in secret; and your Father who sees in secret will reward you."[7]

Andy Warhol foretold: "In the future everyone will be famous for fifteen minutes."[8]

Rather than follow the commandment of the Israelite teacher, telethons fulfill the prediction of the American prophet. Every donor gets a shot of celebrity. The national and local broadcasts feature an endless parade of check presenters. They represent labor unions and fraternal orders, schools and sororities, small businesses and, most visibly, large corporations. On national segments, corporate executives appear in the spotlight more frequently than any other type of check presenter. On some telethons, they display oversized mock "checks," and on all telethons corporate sponsors present their donations in several installments rather than one lump sum. All of this is designed to make the giving even more conspicuous. Sometimes corporate heads and union chiefs introduce employees, distributors, retailers, or members from around the country who have racked up the most pledges. The camera pans down the line, and the telethon hosts greet them. On the local segments, hosts call to center stage representatives of local companies, agencies, and service organizations who report how they raised the funds and present their checks.

Local telethon segments give particular recognition to donors pledging larger amounts. MDA has its "Star Patrons," Easter Seal its "Angel Boards," and the Arthritis Telethon its "VIP salutes." As the San Jose MDA segment host explained the Star Patron program in 1994, silver and gold stars were superimposed on the screen. Above the dollar value of each star was the phrase "Your Name Here."

But even the smallest contributors can get a few seconds of TV fame. Callers can hear their names and the amounts they have pledged read on the air or can see them roll across the bottom or top of the screen. On the national Arthritis, MDA, and UCP telecasts, hosts read the names of pledge makers from all over the country, giving their hometowns and the sums promised.[9] During the 1991 national MDA segments, the San Jose affiliate superimposed the following announcement: "If You Pledge $25 or More, Your Name Will Be Read in the Next Local Segment!" The 1993 Chicago-area Easter Seal broadcast made the same guarantee. The telethons' local hosts often promise to announce pledge makers' names no matter what the amount. As the phones ring, local emcees grab handfuls of pledge cards and reel off names and numbers: "Allen Baumann from West LA, $20. Mr. and Mrs. Gibbs from Reseda, $25. Joseph Withers in Long Beach, $15." And on and on. "Would you call now? We will read your name as fast as we possibly can."

On the 1993 MDA show, Jerry Lewis read the names and hometowns of people from all over the country who had been phoning in pledges. The amounts were of no consequence, he declared. "It demeans the program," evidently meaning that to announce how much individual callers had pledged would undercut the moral validity of the telethon. Immediately afterward, the broadcast cut away to the local stations where segment hosts read callers' names and the amounts of their pledges. If Lewis in fact disagreed with this practice of his own telethon, he certainly endorsed the principle of conspicuous contribution. "If you around this country want your name mentioned," he promised, "call up."

Local hosts introduce the telephone operators, sometimes individually, usually en bloc, and announce the group or company they represent. Sometimes the local TV crews are introduced, and Lewis always introduces the crew of the national MDA broadcasts. Every giver of money or time is made a celebrity. Conspicuous contribution by individuals parallels the conspicuous contribution of the telethons' corporate sponsors. Telethons invite all of them—each check presenter and phone-in pledge maker, each telephone operator and corporate executive—to perceive "the disabled" as the objects of their charity. With only rare exceptions, those doing the giving are nondisabled. Telethons furnish the setting in which nondisabled people can play the role of giver. And telethon hosts repeatedly urge viewers to call because "you're going to feel really good about yourself." Late in the twentieth century, many Americans confuse narcissism with empathy.

How many viewers, one wonders, would phone in a pledge if their names would not be announced? How many others would give if they could win no prizes or bonuses? How many fund-raisers would organize charity events if they could not present checks on camera? How many corporations would donate if their giving yielded no PR benefit or additional profits? The telethon makers make plain their answers to these questions.

Alluding to the prescient Andy Warhol, MDA's San Jose host pointed out in

1991: "We often talk about people having their own fifteen minutes of glory. You can have a moment of glory if you make that telephone call right now." Telethons encourage conspicuous charity partly because it stimulates donations. Americans will give if they know it will get their names or faces on the screen. A few dollars buys a few moments of celebrity.

Conspicuous contribution has a long history. Some early-twentieth-century immigrants found it a dismaying feature of American culture. For instance, a 1923 editorial in Chicago's *Sunday Jewish Courier* took the city's Jewish community to task for having adopted American ideas of "charity." Entitled "Too Much Charity—Too Little Tzdokoh," the column reminded readers that "tzdokoh means to give anonymously; charity is a matter of publicity . . . One can live in a large Jewish community in Europe for twenty years, and not hear a word about charity and institutions, but one can live no more than three days in a Jewish community in America without hearing a great to-do about charitable affairs, drives, institutions, etc."[10]

On the Los Angeles segment of the 1990 Easter Seal telethon, the hosts reported a surprising act. A man had called up and said he wanted to donate $10,000. He came over to the studio and wrote out a check but said he wanted to remain anonymous. He said to say it was "a gentleman from the Philippines." The hosts marveled at this secret act of generosity. The donation was unusual because one aspect of the Americanization of immigrants has been to teach them to authenticate their "American" identities by highly public charitable donation. To prove one's Americanness, to verify one's social legitimacy, one must publicize one's giving.

The traditional Jewish and Christian injunctions to give secretly have been supplanted by public and publicized donations. The transformation began in the 1920s and 1930s as a new brand of professional fund-raiser converted private and individual charity into public and mass philanthropy and made it a business. "What the scriptures had commanded to be done in secret," said one observer, "would before long be celebrated in public and shouted from the rooftops by a different name: philanthropy." "And the shouting would in time become shrill and incessant as it sought billions of dollars for welfare needs," wrote a historian of modern American fund-raising. "In this profound change from charity to public philanthropy the skilled fund raiser and high-pressure methods played a key role." Giving was made "a matter of published performance . . . a virtual tax with social penalties." Some donors, clinging to the traditional moral economy, objected, but publicity, as carrot and stick, as both personal incentive and social coercion, became established as a powerful central feature of fund-raising.[11]

But the professionalization of fund-raising is inadequate alone to explain the importance of publicity in twentieth-century American mass philanthropy and on telethons in particular. More is going on here than the showy display of generosity or the chance for charity volunteers to take a bow. There are deeper reasons that telethons parade donors across their stages and proclaim their names on the air. Telethons and other professional fund-raisers use the tactic so successfully because it touches upon dilemmas of fundamental concern to Americans. Conspicuous contribution ritually resolves distinctly American predicaments about virtue and community.

What strikes a late-twentieth-century observer is the earnest and unflagging energy with which Americans publicize their "giving." On the annual broadcasts and at fund-raising events throughout the year, they not only constantly put their charitable activities on display, they endlessly congratulate themselves for their generosity and seek public credit for it. They are, they proclaim, the most generous people on earth.

The purpose of conspicuous contribution is in part to reassure givers that they are not avaricious but altruistic, not materialistic but humane. They prove that they have escaped the taint of a culture of conspicuous consumption, that they have retained the public virtue necessary to maintain a democratic community. "It shows you care," declared an Easter Seal host in 1989. "It shows you want to help other people." "Let us read your name on the air," urged another local Easter Seal host in 1990, "so the rest of the world knows about it." The ritual display of charity verifies the social and moral validity of individual givers and the moral *health* of American society by dramatizing compassion toward those socially invalidated by disability or disease.

Predicaments of Identity and Status

Besides confirming the continuance of public virtue, conspicuous contribution helps symbolically to resolve other American dilemmas. It symbolically untangles predicaments of identity and status.

Conspicuous contribution bolsters the myth that America is a classless society that guarantees equal opportunities to all its members. The historian David Brion Davis noted that "beginning in the so-called Age of Jackson, white Americans of diverse backgrounds have anxiously tried to cast off any characteristics identifying them as members of a 'lower' class than the one with which they identify, precisely because they have believed in America as a land of opportunity—a land in which no fixed barriers prevent one from acquiring the skills, tastes, and demeanor, as shown in one's behavior as a consumer, that denote success."[12] Thus, even as they have denied the reality of class, Americans have unflaggingly practiced conspicuous consumption to demonstrate their upward mobility, socioeconomic success, and rising social status.

The fact of class has also been cloaked by the issue of race. Davis noted that one function of the American racial caste system has been to obscure the actual inequalities of class among whites, as well as the reality of disjunctures of class among America's racial groups. "The unacknowledged privileges and benefits most Americans derive from having white skin," wrote Davis, in part grew out of "the dialectical and historical connections between American slavery and American freedom, between the belief in an inferior, servile race and the vision of classless opportunity."[13]

Conspicuous contribution has functioned not only as the obverse of conspicuous consumption but also in a way similar to racial caste. The "dependent" are deemed another naturally servile caste. Even as charitable giving to aid the "less fortunate" marks class standing, it helps mask class distinctions. Philanthropy ascribes the distribution of good and ill fortune to personal effort, providence, or luck. The system of voluntary private charity helps camouflage the web of class by disguising it with myths of personal misfortune.

This fictionalization of life fortunes occurs where Americans least recognize it: in the tales they tell about individuals who become sick or disabled. Because disease and disability seem so self-evidently matters of biology, rather than sociology or public policy, the disadvantaging social and economic consequences endured by sick or disabled individuals are perceived as "natural," the inevitable social outcomes of biological "facts." But much of what Americans think of as the natural results of illness or disability are social and political artifacts.[14] This social construction is especially powerfully present in societal arrangements to provide financial aid to those who become sick or disabled. Establishment of universal, comprehensive health insurance and health care as social rights could prevent much of the financial and emotional devastation visited on American families, many times destroying them. Perpetuation of the system of private charity not only has proved inadequate to meet those needs, more pertinent to the point being made here, it helps sustain the American mythology of personal misfortune. That in turn upholds the corollary myth of classlessness.

Yet charity donation also silently fortifies class boundaries by serving as a visible symbol of status. Those who have succeeded register their upward mobility by giving to "help" the invalidated. The wealthiest and most successful give the most conspicuously at black-tie banquets honoring ones of their own. The second largest MDA fund-raising event (after the telethon itself) is the annual Mary and Harry Zimmerman dinner in Nashville sponsored by the Zimmerman-founded Service Merchandise Company. Each year a celebrity is given the Harry Zimmerman Award, and a million dollars is raised. A video report on this particular dinner is, of course, prominently featured on each year's telethon. Charity banquets such as this are staples of newspaper columns with names like "The Social Scene," through which America's upper crust displays itself.

In other ways, telethons diagram the American class hierarchy. Though telethon hosts emphasize that even the smallest pledges matter, the extra attention given to what a 1993 Chicago Easter Seal host referred to as "heavy hitters" makes plain that some donors matter more than others. Instead of *answering* calls from would-be pledge makers, corporate executive VIP volunteers exhibit their clout by *making* calls to friends and colleagues, soliciting larger donations and reading the names and amounts on the air. "Business and community leaders" in MDA lockups strut their status by phoning acquaintances to raise the $2,500 that will bail them out. UCP cofounder Jack Hausman reads the names of wealthy New Yorkers and of transplanted New Yorkers in Florida and Holly-wood, his personal friends, who donate $3,000, $5,000, $10,000, $25,000, $50,000. Every year on the night before the telethon, Hausman hosts a party for VIPs. At various times throughout each telethon, Dennis James refers to these parties and to some of the wealthy and important persons who attend. Hausman himself says his dinners included a "who's who of America" and mentions a couple of ambassadors. James chimes in with the names of bankers and philan-thropists. All of this conspicuous charity by high-status donors charts and bol-sters the American social hierarchy.

The telethon system urges average Americans to identify with these big givers by purchasing smaller scraps of the same status. The UCP Telethon's New York segment features a "Labor Cares" panel of union officers who read the names of individual donors and of locals and companies that have made contributions. The panel is the blue collar counterpart to Jack Hausman reading the names of his wealthy friends. And if middle class Americans cannot afford black-tie banquets, they can attend dinner dances and silent auctions and wine-tasting parties. Phi-lanthropy to aid people with disabilities thus helps obscure class lines. Small or big, all contributors are invited to place themselves symbolically on the validated side of a great social divide.

Telethons replicate the class structure in another way. The families affected by disability or disease who are exhibited on telethons are usually not poor and certainly not rich. They are middle class. They are overwhelmingly white, but whatever their ethnicity, they are middle class. That implicitly makes them, as one local Easter Seal host put it in 1992, "very deserving." MDA makes a point of announcing that it provides its services to families without requiring a means test. American public and private welfare has long operated on the premise that middle class families in crisis are morally worthy of aid. Means tests and moral evaluations are for the poor, who are inherently suspect and probably undeserv-ing of assistance.[15] Emcees locate telethon families in the social hierarchy by indicating to the vast, middle class audience, "They're just like your friends, your family, your neighbors."[16] One aim of the telethon ritual is to rescue middle class families from social invalidation.

Thus in several ways, conspicuous contribution buttresses, even as it helps to blur, the reality of social class. It disguises the socially and politically constructed causes of allegedly "natural" personal misfortunes. It facilitates display of the superior status of the most advantaged, thereby reinforcing their social power. It encourages ordinary middle class Americans to disregard the disadvantages and dangers to them under the private charity and for-profit health insurance system. Instead, middle class folks are prompted to identify with those who are wealthy enough that they will never need telethon charity.

But the American experience has involved more than a denial of the reality of class. It is much more complicated than that. The disavowed fact of social class is invisibly braided with the much noted fact of social fluidity. That intertwining has had profound and problematic consequences for American identities. Americans have celebrated the fluidity of their society without usually examining the specific nature of that fluidity. Fluidity is not the same thing as social and economic mobility, though for many white Americans it has included the possibility of such mobility. But that mobility might be downward as well as upward.

More troublesome, throughout much of American history the fluidity of American society has produced a disorienting shapelessness. Hurtling expansion, swift and ceaseless change, the relative newness of all institutions, and the ideology of egalitarian individualism together generated not only an exhilarating sense of boundless individual possibilities but sometimes a terrifying lack of personal and social boundaries. While the fluidity of the social structure opened enormous possibilities for individual development, it has also left a great many Americans adrift about who they are or what they should become. Americans have fashioned for themselves a society "in which," observed James Baldwin, "nothing is fixed and in which the individual must fight for his identity."[17] Liberated from rigid traditional social hierarchies, many white Americans have also felt dubiously emancipated from any clearly defined identity.

With every prospect seemingly available, no goal has seemed enough, and many Americans have found themselves drawn into an endless competition for status with no finish line, no resting place. As early as 1774, an observer noted that Americans were running "one continued race, in which everyone is endeavoring to distance all behind him, and to overtake or pass by, all before him; everyone flying from his inferiors in pursuit of his superiors, who fly from him with equal alacrity."[18] "People are not . . . terribly anxious to be equal," remarked Baldwin almost two centuries later, "but they love the idea of being superior. And this human truth has an especially grinding force here, where identity is almost impossible to achieve and people are perpetually attempting to find their feet on the shifting sands of status."[19] "There are no longer any universally accepted forms or standards," he pointed out, "and since all the roads to the achievement of an identity had vanished, the problem of status in American life became and it remains today acute. In a way, status became a kind of substitute for identity."[20]

In a society that vaunted itself as mobile, fluid, and egalitarian, how would individuals establish their personal identities and social status? And what criteria would the community—which is to say, those who labeled themselves "respectable"—use to measure the eligibility of individuals and groups for membership in that community, for equal citizenship? How would the majority simultaneously confirm their own validity, bar those they defined as socially invalid and therefore could justifiably exclude, and yet assure themselves of the openness and fairness of their society? How would dominant groups decide, as the historian Robert H. Wiebe noted, who was "qualified to participate in a democracy of free choices"?[21]

Between the Revolution and the Civil War, Americans devised answers to these questions. To solve the problems of selection and status, to gauge worthiness of social inclusion and attainment of social respect, they sketched a new picture of the social order. Doing away with the traditional conception of an organic hierarchy of stair-step ranks, they substituted "a simple separation," an uncomplicated "division between ins and outs."[22] They reduced the measurement of social validity—and thus of entitlement to equal citizenship—to a stark dichotomy.

That dichotomy grew out of the fluidity of American society, the individualistic ethos of Americans, and Americans' belief in the necessity of public virtue. Those features converged to define an authentic American as a person who was not subject to or dependent upon the will of another. A valid American was a property-holding and therefore economically, morally, and politically independent adult, white, able-bodied male. He was seen as economically and physically self-sufficient. Only a self-contained, self-sustaining person was capable of acting responsibly enough to uphold public virtue. Only such a person possessed the moral and political independence that would make the American democratic experiment viable.[23] Only such an individual was competent to claim and to realize the promise of democratic individualism. Only he qualified for inclusion and equality.

This myth of personal autonomy asserted the sovereignty of the individual over his destiny. Within acceptable society, it was claimed, each individual stood on an equal basis with every other individual, enjoying the same privileges and opportunities. The myth claimed that "everyone achieved a success equivalent to merit." And in a fluid, expanding economy, "enough abrupt falls and dramatic rises in fortune occurred to support the impression of a characterological justice in the world of affairs."[24]

Thus, individual character and status in large part came to be appraised according to personal economic success, a success mostly reckoned by conspicuous consumption. The capacity to consume served as a yardstick of who was "in." Monetary income and the material possessions and extraoccupational activities purchased by that income became primary measures of personal achievement, social standing, and qualification for inclusion. "Because money and the things money can buy is the universally accepted symbol here of status," said Baldwin, "we are often condemned as materialists. In fact, we are much closer to being metaphysical because nobody has ever expected from things the miracles that we expect."[25] With one another as audience, Americans have earned and spent and consumed, endlessly striving to verify their inner worth and social validity.

Conspicuous *contribution* also has served to verify one's place among the validated. Institutionalized charities manufacture "the less fortunate" as status-enhancing commodities. Telethon giving, like all charitable donation and volunteerism, is on one level a corrective of the morally and communally corrosive effects of individualistic consumerism. But the charities also have made donation a consumable product guaranteed to boost the buyer's social status and self-worth. "You're going to feel really good about yourself." If conspicuous contribution ritualistically reverses the consequences of consumerism, it simultaneously serves as another form of conspicuous consumption.

Putatively independent Americans thus have employed those they label "dependent" as a negative reference group against which to define themselves. Giving proves that the allegedly self-sufficient belong on the upper side of a great social divide that separates those designated autonomous from those branded dependent. Anyone resorting to public welfare or private charity is regarded as neither fully a person nor legitimately a citizen. The price of such societal aid in America is social invalidation.

The Sovereignty of the Self versus the Human Condition

But individual autonomy has meant more than exercising the capacity to get and spend and donate. Sovereignty over one's personal destiny came to include dominion over one's body, command of one's health. *Good* health and physical and mental fitness have been made measures of moral and social validity.

Traditional, Western Judeo-Christian cultures attributed health or disease to divine power. God punished or purified individuals with sickness or disability or allowed Satan for the moment to hold sway over them. Whatever the physiological and moral outcome, the entire course of events was determined by the inscrutable will of the sovereign deity. The human condition ultimately lay beyond the ken or control of finite creatures.

As Western societies modernized themselves, they inverted the order of the universe, commanding God to hew to rational laws that made sense to human beings and proclaiming the capacity of those humans not only to know the operating rules of the universe but increasingly to work the levers themselves. This transformation advanced most rapidly and most thoroughly in America, a society virtually born modern. Socially fluid, sloughing off "the dead hand of the past," future-oriented, American society proclaimed the competency of its people, collectively and individually, to shape human destiny.

Reflecting this long-term process, health reformers and fitness experts from the 1830s on have played a major role in American culture as prophets and pedagogues of individual control of the body and health. In the antebellum United States, disease and disability came to be regarded as resulting from violations of the laws of nature. But those laws were readily comprehensible. It did not require advanced medical or scientific training to know them. The rules of good health were accessible to all. Because those rules were accessible, good health and fitness became moral imperatives. Individuals usually achieved them, not accidentally or providentially or through esoteric knowledge, but simply through will power. Most persons could choose good health or reject it.[26]

Health and fitness thus often came to be taken as indicators of the appropriate exercise of the sovereignty of the self. They were made measures of a suitably American character. Antebellum "reformers assumed that a person could not behave in a morally responsible fashion unless his or her body was unfettered" from slavery "and uncorrupted" by bodily *infirmity*.[27] The assumption that disability corrupts one's capacity for responsible choices continued with the emergence of scientific medicine in the late nineteenth and twentieth centuries. Medical practice ostensibly forbears moral judgments against its patients, depicting disease and disability as biological processes, not divine chastisements. But in fact, moralizing about illness and disability persists, embedded in medical and societal discourse.[28] Sometimes this involves attribution of moral blame, for instance for contracting AIDs or acquiring a spinal cord injury while driving drunk. If traditional Western cultures took health or illness as signs of God's favor or displeasure, modern American culture has come to regard them as emblems of fulfillment or failure in meeting the requirements of democratic individualism. Since ill health supposedly results from individual negligence in following the principles of proper living, it is a distinctively modern form of moral failure: it is delinquency in the practice of individual self-control.

Twentieth-century medicine and allied social services also operate on a more far-reaching moral premise: the assumption that illness and, even more so, disability incapacitate individuals from participating in the democracy of free choices. Even if individuals are not culpable for their physical conditions, disabilities render them incompetent to practice the sovereignty of the self. So, whether they are morally blamable or the hapless victims of accidents or disease processes, they are unfitted for full and authentic citizenship. Disability evidences unwillingness or incompetency to practice self-determination.

As a result, in American culture personal health not only has affected the lives of individuals, it has far-reaching consequences for society. Insofar as impairment manifests the moral shortcomings of individuals, it exposes a negligence that threatens the viability of American freedom. Insofar as disability is a misfortune that befalls ill-fated souls, it subverts the very idea of a society of individuals in control of their personal destinies. Either way, the health of individuals will impede or perhaps even sabotage American social progress. Any dereliction of personal sovereignty, any incapacity for self-determination, calls democratic individualism into question. The presence of impairment raises a terrifying prospect: human beings may not be in control of their destinies after all. Disability imperils the American myth of the sovereignty of the self.

The fear evoked by the presence of people with disabilities has produced two simultaneous and predictable responses: they have been stigmatized, and they have been subjected to relentless exertions to fix them.

Stigmatizing disabled people has been a means of avoidance for the American majority whose identities and status and validity have been built on the myth of personal autonomy. Devaluation of people with disabilities has constituted an additional dichotomy that distinguishes the socially valid from the invalid. On one level, the dichotomy based on disability parallels the dichotomy based on race. Like racial prejudice, disability bias springs in part from what James Baldwin called the "social panic" of Euro-Americans, their "fear of losing status, [which] really amounts sometimes to a kind of social paranoia."

One cannot afford to lose status on this peculiar ladder, for the prevailing notion of American life seems to involve a kind of rung-by-rung ascension to some hideously desirable state. If this is one's concept of life, obviously one cannot afford to slip back one rung. When one slips, one slips back not a rung but back into chaos and no longer knows who he is. And this reason, this fear, suggests to me one of the real reasons for the status of the Negro in this country. In a way, the Negro tells where the bottom is: *because he is there*, and *where* he is, beneath us, we know where the limits are and how far we must not fall. We must not fall beneath him. We must never allow ourselves to fall that low . . . I think if one examines the myths which have proliferated in this country concerning the Negro, one discovers beneath these myths a kind of sleeping terror of some condition which we refuse to imagine. In a way, if the Negro were not here, we might be forced to deal within ourselves and our own personalities, with all those vices, all those conundrums, and all those mysteries with which we have invested the Negro race.[29]

Baldwin's insight about the origins of racial caste can help explain the fabrication of the disability caste. Disability too has functioned as a marker of where the bottom is in American society. Disabled people too have been invested with myths that have enabled the majority to avoid facing their own "condition." In the latter half of the twentieth century, the disability caste has become even more necessary. The civil rights movements of racial minorities and of women too have made it increasingly difficult to use belief in an inferior racial caste or a subordinated sex as a means of maintaining the myths of classlessness and boundless opportunity and of quieting the terror that one's status might plummet and one's identity might dissolve into chaos. At the same time, the myth of the self-contained, self-sufficient American individual more and more has clashed with contemporary experience. Americans cling to visions of absolute personal autonomy and unlimited individual possibility while, it seems to many of them, their power over their individual lives evaporates like a mirage.

As Baldwin pointed out, what human beings fear within themselves, they often attribute as the exclusive traits of some group they define as the opposite of them, their antithesis, the Other. White people have "need[ed] the nigger" to embody the traits that whites cannot tolerate within themselves. At the deepest level of American perception, " 'the Negro problem,' " contended David Brion Davis, "meant that blacks are associated metaphysically with everything that compromised or stood in the way of the American Dream—with finitude, failure, poverty, fate, the sins of our fathers, nemesis. In short, with dark reality."[30]

On late-twentieth-century American telethons, disability has implicitly been offered as a replacement for race. People with disabilities are ritually presented as the new mudsill, the bottom of the social ladder below whom "we" must never allow ourselves to fall. The myths about "the disabled" propagated by telethons reveal little about the daily lives of people with disabilities, but these phantasms do betray the night terrors of those who prefer to think of themselves as "able bodied," as whole. The myths assure that "they," not "we," are dependent, helpless, incomplete, inauthentic. This prospect of restricted powers terrifies Americans, because it means not just loss of control but loss of social validity within American society, loss of an American identity. Anyone who depends physically on others to carry out daily activities is seen as incapable of fulfilling the requirements for full membership in America. People with disabilities provoke anxiety and revulsion because they are defined as literally embodying that which Americans individually and collectively fear most: limitation and dependency, failure and incapacity, loss of control, loss of autonomy, at its deepest level, finitude, confinement within the human condition, subjection to fate.

To avoid confronting these fearsome inner and social demons and to protect their own social validity, nondisabled Americans must see themselves as autonomous, potent, in control. One means to do so is to display oneself as a giver. In America, it is not only better to give than to receive, it is a social necessity.

Thus, in America, giving must be public. It cannot be secret. Secretiveness would defeat one fundamental purpose of donating to help "the less fortunate." Contribution must be conspicuous for it to demarcate the radical difference between socially valid Americans and their counterimage, the invalidated, disabled Others.

But it is not enough to define people with disabilities as the inversion of authentic American identity. Merely invalidating them cannot adequately reassure those who are, for the moment, "healthy," because disability differs from race in one major respect: although white people cannot turn black, "healthy" people can and sometimes do get sick or become disabled. As the telethon hosts endlessly remind viewers, you or someone you love might in an instant be transformed—and invalidated. So, to sustain the myth that Americans control their destinies, the ritual invalidating people with disabilities must also attempt to revalidate them and thus reiterate the capacity of Americans to master fate.

At the beginning of the 1994 UCP Telethon, Dennis James explained that a few days earlier he had flown from Los Angeles to New York. He and his wife and son had just gone through the devastating Northridge earthquake. His house was a shambles. So was his son Brad's. On the flight east, he had reflected on "how unpredictable life can be, and how the forces of nature are at times so unexpected and so unaccountable. Now the flight to New York," he said, "gave me a chance to think, to think a lot about the reason why my family and I came to New York to do this annual telethon. It's a chance to once again meet, marvel, and appreciate the accomplishments of youngsters and adults who are disabled by cerebral palsy. When we see these accomplishments, I realize that it is literally within our power to do something about a force of nature which contributes to the birth of a brain-damaged child. Now we can't do anything about the force of an earthquake, but you can see what can be done about cerebral palsy's force. You'll actually see children, young people and adults who due to brain damage would have had a limited future, but because of the previous forty-two telethons . . . [you] have helped almost three generations to a maximum fulfillment of life."

The following year, James made the point again. He reminded the audience that last year just before the telethon the earthquake had hit Los Angeles. Now southern California was recovering from torrential rains, and there had been a devastating earthquake in Kobe, Japan. "It points out how unpredictable the forces of nature can be," he mused. "Now look, I'm not comparing an earthquake or a flood to the birth of a brain-damaged child," which was, of course, exactly what he was doing. "But the emotional trauma, the need for help and support, as in the case of California, our recovery shows me that we do have the power to do something about the force of nature, even with the birth of a brain-damaged child. When we meet the children, the young people and the adults, with cerebral palsy, you'll be thrilled to see their levels of accomplishment. Some who couldn't walk will walk this year. Some who couldn't talk will talk this year. Because of you." "Able-bodied" donors could reassure themselves; they could still master fate.

In a sense, a disability is more fearsome than an earthquake. An earthquake lasts a matter of seconds, and after that one can begin to rebuild. But disability is viewed as an ongoing catastrophe, a disaster that never stops. How can one build an American life on the shambles continuously being made by it? And given the American belief in the connection among health, personal sovereignty, and qualification "to participate in a democracy of free choices," disability endangers things more essential than property or even life. It imperils identity and status.

In the late twentieth century, seemingly intractable social problems have left many Americans feeling even more impotent than they feel when confronting natural disasters. At least after an earthquake or a hurricane, one can dig out and rebuild. Social ills often seem beyond anyone's ken or control. "When we read the newspapers or watch the news on TV," observed a Chicago-area UCP host in 1995, "we sometimes feel overwhelmed by problems that seem to have no solutions. It's a terrible helpless feeling." But people with disabilities can serve as vehicles to defeat that sense of helplessness. "United Cerebral Palsy offers everyone who wants to make a better world a way to solve problems that can be solved . . . Make it a better world. We can."

The medical model of disability presents disabled people as a means for Americans to escape the mood of futility and fatalism that has overtaken them. In a moment when the myth of the sovereignty of the self and of American dominion over destiny is under threat, the "power to do something about a force of nature," disability, reassures Americans that they can still transcend the human condition. Thus, fixing disabled people has become a cultural imperative. Americans can still bring fate to heel and master human destiny. Just as the telethon ritual reassures them about the viability of public virtue and moral community, it revalidates their American identities. All they have to do is take people with disabilities and make them over.

NOTES

1. Gordon Wood, *The Radicalism of the American Revolution* (New York: Vintage, 1992); J. R. Pole, *The Pursuit of Equality in American History* (Berkeley, CA: University of California Press, 1978).

2. Jack P. Greene, "The Limits of the American Revolution," in *The American Revolution, Its Character and Limits,* ed. Jack P. Greene (New York: New York University Press, 1987), 6–12.

3. Joel Kovel, *History and Spirit: An Inquiry into the Philosophy of Liberation* (Boston, MA: Beacon Press, 1992), 92.

4. Scott M. Cutlip, *Fund Raising in the United States, Its Role in America's Philanthropy* (New Brunswick, NJ: Rutgers University Press, 1965), 120–21.

5. Easter Seal Telethon 1989, Los Angeles segment.

6. Schools that sponsored hop-a-thons profited too. They got items like playground equipment.

7. Mt. 6:2, 4 Revised Standard Version.

8. James B. Simpson, *Simpson's Contemporary Quotations* (Boston, MA: Houghton Mifflin, 1988), 243, quoting from *Washington Post,* 15 November 1979.

9. On the 1994 Arthritis Telethon, cohosts Crystal Gayle and Sarah Purcell read from cards the names, geographical locations, and amounts promised by phone-in pledge makers, while Fred Travalena read the names, amounts donated by individuals, organizations, small businesses, and locations from a huge video screen. UCP had a series of revolving national announcers sitting in a "sky booth" who read the same information from pledge cards. On UCP's New York segments, labor leaders read the names of various donors and contributing union locals.

10. Editorial, *Chicago Sunday Jewish Courier,* 18 February 1923, quoted in Lizabeth Cohen, *Making a New Deal, Industrial Workers in Chicago, 1919–1939* (New York: Cambridge University Press, 1990), 59–60.

11. John Lear, "The Business of Giving," *Saturday Review,* 2 December 1961, 63, quoted in Cutlip, *Fund Raising,* 202; John R. Seeley et al., *Community Chest: A Case Study in Philanthropy* (Toronto: University of Toronto Press, 1957), 396, quoted in Cutlip, *Fund Raising,* 530; Cutlip, *Fund Raising,* 335–36.

12. David Brion Davis, "The American Dilemma," *New York Review of Books,* 16 June 1992, 13.

13. Ibid., 13.

14. William Roth, "Handicap as a Social Construct," *Society* 20 (March/April 1983): 56–61.

15. Edward D. Berkowitz, *America's Welfare State, from Roosevelt to Reagan* (Baltimore, MD: Johns Hopkins University Press, 1991), 91–93, 169; Theda Skocpol, *Protecting Soldiers and Mothers: The Political Origins of Social Policy in the United States* (Cambridge, MA: Harvard University Press, 1992), 118–20, 141–43, 148–51, 155–57, 467–68.

16. Easter Seal Telethon 1992.

17. James Baldwin, "The Discovery of What It Means to Be an American," in *The Price of the Ticket, Collected Nonfiction, 1948–1985* (New York: St. Martin's/Marek, 1985), 175.

18. Quoted in Wood, *The Radicalism of the American Revolution,* 135.

19. James Baldwin, "Down at the Cross, Letter from a Region in My Mind," in *The Price of the Ticket, Collected Nonfiction, 1948–1985* (New York: St. Martin's/Marek, 1985), 371.

20. James Baldwin, "In Search of a Majority," in *The Price of the Ticket, Collected Nonfiction, 1948–1985* (New York: St. Martin's/Marek, 1985), 231.

21. Robert H. Wiebe, *The Opening of American Society, from the Adoption of the Constitution to the Eve of Disunion* (New York: Alfred Knopf, 1984), 321.

22. Ibid., 327, 339.

23. Historians have omitted able bodiedness from the formulation of notions of American citizenship and identity, though it is often implicit. For general explanations of this formulation see Linda K. Kerber, "The Revolutionary Generation: Ideology, Politics, and Culture in the Early Republic," in *The New American History,* ed. Eric Foner (Philadelphia, PA: Temple University Press, 1990), 29; Wood, *Radicalism of the American Revolution,* 56, 178–79.

24. Wiebe, *The Opening of American Society,* 321–22.

25. Baldwin, "In Search of a Majority," 231.

26. Wiebe, *The Opening of American Society,* 160–63.

27. Ronald G. Walters, *American Reformers 1815–1860* (New York: Hill and Wang, 1978), 145.

28. Irving Kenneth Zola, "Medicine as an Institution of Social Control," *Sociological Review,* n.s. (November 1972): 491–92.

29. Baldwin, "In Search of a Majority," 232–33.

30. Davis, "The American Dilemma," 14.

PART 2 ► A History of Representations

Feminotopias ▸ The Pleasures of "Deformity" in Mid-Eighteenth-Century England

Felicity A. Nussbaum

Sarah Scott's *Millenium Hall* (1762) portrays a female Arcadia that is remarkably sensitive to the alignment of women's oppression with physical deformity. In this haven for the aged and the poor, the deformed and the disabled, dwarfs and giants live in a separate compound, a feature readers have found puzzling. An English counterpart to the seraglio that binds its mutes, eunuchs, and slaves to a female community, *Millenium Hall* plays on the structural kinship between domestic femininity and the perverse, the monstrous, and the deformed. For Scott, such so-called deformity may be both liberating and debilitating. In *Millenium Hall* the women, like the "monsters" they befriend, are "deformed" in the eyes of the men who observe them and who are persuaded to admire their eccentricity while affirming their womanhood.

I suggest that this connection between women's community and deformity in the novel reveals an aspect of its affinity to an orientalized feminotopia. *Feminotopia*, a term coined by Mary Louise Pratt, describes the "idealized worlds of female autonomy, empowerment, and pleasure" often found in women's travel narratives, some of which have a "decidedly orientalist flavor."[1] Feminotopias, "quests for self-realization and fantasies of social harmony," contest masculine versions of experience, even though they are often confined to the domestic sphere. In feminotopias, women thrive without men and find pleasure in living together without rancor or dissent. These exclusively female spaces share the mystique of being autonomous retreats impenetrable to masculine authority, happily sequestered from the larger patriarchal world of which they are an inevitable part. While the novel recognizes and explores the potential imprisonment of women in marriage, it offers an alternative to it. It is both a contest to male dominance over women and a testimony to its power.

An epistolary novel consisting of one lengthy letter written by a gentleman to his bookseller friend, *Millenium Hall* was actually written in the course of a month and published anonymously in October or early November 1762. In spite of virulently negative reviews, the book saw four editions between 1762 and 1778.[2] The book parallels Sarah Scott's life in that after a brief, unhappy marriage to George Scott, she lived in a close female friendship with Lady Barbara Montagu in Bath, where they conducted the sort of charitable activities that *Millenium Hall* fictionalizes.[3] While others have appropriately connected the novel to slavery and the West Indies via its sequel, *The History of Sir George Ellison* (1766), I would like to place *Millenium Hall* in the context of female community and its connection to monstrosity, the exotic, and the homosocial.[4] Sarah Scott describes the accomplished and dignified women through the appreciative but colonizing vision of the male observers of her feminotopia, Sir George Ellison and Lamont. The beginning of the novel is narrated by Ellison, who is accompanied by Mr. Lamont, the young son of an old friend, and who rediscovers his relationship to a long-lost cousin, Mrs. Maynard. Returning from Jamaica to England, Ellison is so much altered by his colonial stint that Mrs. Maynard, a founder of the Millenium Hall community, at first finds him unrecognizable.

The fiction suggests that the men's visit to Millenium Hall and its surroundings restores them from the fatigue of colonial travels. The impetus for their returning to England is to recover from the effects of twenty years in "the hot and unwholesome climate of Jamaica" and from the exhausting quest for mercantile gain. Possessed by a colonizing curiosity, "one of those insatiable passions that grow by gratification" (5), Ellison and Lamont happen upon the community of Millenium Hall. The "painful suspense" (72) that the occasion induces motivates the narrative.[5] In the idyllic woods that the ladies designed to surround Millenium Hall, the opposite of the colonial pertains and nature is protected: "Man never appears there as a merciless destroyer; but the preserver, instead of the tyrant, of the inferior part of creation" (17). Millenium Hall represents a respite from colonialism, from the travails of being a slave owner, and an alternative to the tyrannizing curiosity and rapacity of empire. Empire and colonization are ostensibly opposed to the domestic tranquility of the women's retreat.

The domestic enclosure of chaste, stubbornly nonsexual, English gentlewomen poses the apparent antithesis to the teeming sexuality of empire and its torrid zones. The core of the "amiable family" of women who have pooled their property and economic resources includes Mrs. Maynard, Miss Selvyn, Miss Mancel, Miss Trentham, Lady Mary Jones, and Mrs. Morgan, all dressed uniformly in clean white garments without ornamentation. Rather than a subculture, they represent a community that organizes its resources for mutual support while differing from the norm. Like Lady Mary Wortley Montagu's Turkish women in the baths, they resemble the Graces, and their community seems Edenic in its pastoral vision of an "asylum against every evil" (6) with its perfectly arranged flora and cattle lowing on the fields. Their rural simplicity recalls the mythic past rather than the present moment. In contrast the dissipated, fashionable observer Lamont rudely mocks the women's rusticity and well-regulated life.[6] The constant inquisitor, he queries the ladies' rigid routines, outmoded attitudes, and lack of concern for profit.

The women of Millenium Hall are thoroughly scrutinized by the two men, but the women attempt to control the terms of the viewing.[7] Lamont intermittently asserts himself against the female narrative, but the women triumph as he becomes educated to their value throughout the course of the novel. The men's voyeurism is motivated more from a curious, colonizing desire than from a sexual one, and the bucolic setting is a necessary preliminary to engaging the men's interest in the individual stories of the women.

In contrast to Hobbes's warlike society, Millenium Hall is a harmonious community of reason, reflection, and freedom to speak that is unattainable outside of its confines.[8] Miss Mancel launches into an argument against tyranny when Lamont wrongly assumes that the ladies keep wild beasts in an enclosed space. He asks: "What we behold is certainly an inclosure, how can that be without a confinement to those that are within it?" (19). Miss Mancel describes this community of refuge instead as one of mutual service and obligation for the poor, for dwarfs, and for gentlewomen who do not wish to marry. When Lamont protests, "You seem madam, to choose to make us all slaves to each other" (62), Miss Mancel counters that their female society is based on love and esteem rather than flattery or confinement. "What I understand by society," she says, "is a state of mutual confidence, reciprocal services, and correspondent affections; where numbers are thus united, there will be a free communication of sentiments, and we shall then find speech, that peculiar blessing given to man, a valuable gift indeed; but when we see it restrained by suspicion, or contaminated by detraction, we rather wonder that so dangerous a power was trusted with a race of beings who seldom make a proper use of it" (61). At Millenium Hall enclosure is distinguished from tyranny, and the disabled are enclosed without confinement to a benevolent servitude.

The household of six women at Millenium Hall, several times called a "family," is a feminotopia of domesticity that offers protection from unwanted marriage, pregnancy, and the disappointments and dangers of maternity. It provides daily sorority instead of isolation and a spiritual regimen to channel the women's sexual energies. The little histories of women are, in some sense, their sexual histories. Describing their rejection of marriage rather than their sexual performance constitutes an almost ritual induction into the community. Each woman first proves herself marriageable and is then freed from marital confinement. In turning to the community, the women steadfastly refuse to embrace heterosexuality while allowing that marriage is acceptable for others.

The novel redefines maternity so that it becomes something that the women can generously bestow upon each other. Scott's novel declares an opposition to the more traditional women of the previous generation who wanted their daughters to imitate their own coquettish, self-abnegating ways. In contrast to more traditional bourgeois domesticity, the women at Millenium Hall mother each other as well as becoming surrogate mothers to every fifth child among the poor families who surround their community.[9] The lack of a mother unites Miss Mancel and Mrs. Morgan (Lady Melvyn), both of whom are vulnerable to preying men and subject to the world's propensity to estrange women from women. The motherless Louisa Mancel was rescued from a dying aunt by Mr. Hintman, who agreed to adopt her. Sent to Mlle. D'Avaux's boarding school, Miss Mancel meets Miss Melvyn. Their great fondness for each other is couched in maternal terms: "Miss Melvyn . . . found great pleasure in endeavoring to instruct her; and grew to feel for her the tenderness of a mother, while Miss Mancel began to receive consolation from experiencing an affection quite maternal" (36). Though Louisa Mancel eventually discovers her lost mother in the American colonies, being motherless yokes these women together to nurture each other in a domestic economy. The various autobiographical accounts testify to the women's resistance to traditional socialization, "the little arts of behaviour which mothers too commonly inculcate with so much care."

> The first thing a girl is taught is to hide her sentiments, to contradict the thoughts of her heart, and tell all the civil lies which custom has sanctified, with as much affectation and conceit as her mother, and when she has acquired all the folly and impertinence of a riper age, and apes the woman more ungracefully than a monkey does a fine gentleman, the parents congratulate themselves with the extremest complacency in the charming education they have given their daughter. (181)

The novel supplants the scandalized renderings of lesbian relationships in female communities with an obdurate affirmation of nonsexual attachments, though an undercurrent of homoerotic bonding unsettles the narrative.[10] *Millenium Hall* actively resists the women's incorporation into conventional modes of marriage, maternity, and heterosexuality.

According to this cautionary tale, marital unions also endanger relationships among women and alienate them from each other. Miss Melvyn had been tricked into marrying the aged, unappealing Mr. Morgan to avoid being disgraced in the world. Her rank dictates her duty, and thus Miss Melvyn, like many of the other women in the autobiographical stories, is caught (in a predicament familiar to women) between two unappealing alternatives. Mr. Morgan's empire over her is complete, and she is forbidden the pleasure of female friendship with Miss Mancel, a friendship so troubling and intense that it challenges heterosexual arrangements.[11] Though the women of the community think of marriage "as absolutely necessary to the good of society," it is a "general duty" that they prefer to delegate to others. While Miss Melvyn selflessly marries an undesirable man, Miss Mancel fulfills her obligation in *refusing* to marry the man she loves, Sir Edward Lambton. Like Miss Melvyn, she uses rank as her alibi—she deems her fortune unworthy of him. In short, the crux for women is that few may expect to find happiness with a man.

The stories of Lady Mary Jones and Miss Selvyn resemble those of the first two women in that both appear to be left motherless at a very early age, though Miss Selvyn later discovers her mother, Lady Emilia. Pregnant by Lord Peyton, whom she loved, Lady Emilia had refused to marry him because of her oddly construed sense of propriety, and her illegitimate daughter had been adopted by Selvyn. As in the case of Miss Mancel, duty dictated an unhappy choice for Lady Emilia. Of course, the shame of premarital sex seems to a modern audience a misplaced guilt, but clearly this novel insists on the eradication of public apprehension about a woman's sexuality. Miss Selvyn's discovery of her mother allows her to redefine her mother's refusal to marry as a decision based on virtue, and it connects her with the repetitive theme that duty brings unhappiness to women.

The motherless but very handsome Miss Harriot Trentham ("beloved by her grandmother and Mr. Alworth, and hated and traduced by her female cousins" [183], Miss Alworth and the Miss Denhams) also recounts a plaintive story of feminine loss and antagonism. Harriot, who "never knew the blessing of a mother's care" (180), is the object of her female cousins' malice. In yet another testimony to the joys of asexual love, she desperately avoids marriage to Master Alworth. Contesting the notion of love as passion, the two celebrate "an affection calm and rational as theirs, totally free from that turbulency and wildness which had always appeared to them the true characteristics of love" (186) and are almost comical in their steady conviction to avoid the abhorred liaison of property and sexual intimacy that others urge them to accept. Belatedly, however, Alworth realizes that he does in fact possess violent passion for Harriot (not for his coquettish wife), and she flees from his newfound erotic desire. When Harriot conveniently contracts smallpox (like her creator Sarah Scott and "the youngest Miss Tunstall" in Scott's *History of Sir George Ellison*), she "acknowledged she was not insensible to this mortification; and to avoid the observation of the envious or even of the idly curious she retired, as soon as she was able to travel, to a country house which I hired for her" (199). Rather than becoming Alworth's wife, she instead derives pleasure from avoiding marriage and acting as a surrogate parent to his daughter rather than as a birth mother.

Although the novel outlines a radical political and social scheme, Scott is not proposing to overthrow the class system or to institute female governance beyond Millenium Hall. The women's domestic economy is not put forward as a serious model for the state economy, but Millenium Hall does make it possible for women to exercise both liberty and virtue within female sorority. Precise in its plans for economic well-being, it elaborates upon a feminine fantasy of self-governance and a woman's empire independent both of love's empire and of the masculine empire of imperial adventure. An empire without a monarch, female community and homosocial affiliation offer a feminotopia that rejects the despotic male empire of the seraglio. Millenium Hall provides an asylum for the various "deformed" who share the women's vision, and beyond that, it heretically makes possible taking genuine pleasure in that "deformity."

Defining beauty as a handicap and ugliness and deformity as agreeable, the women of Millenium Hall, like their deformed charges, are able to escape the sexual economy and its tropes. The visitors to Millenium Hall deflect their pity to admiration for the disabled because of the women's intervention: "Instead of feeling the pain one might naturally receive from seeing the human form so disgraced, we were filled with admiration of the human mind, when so nobly exalted by virtue, as it is in the patronesses of these poor creatures, who wore an air of cheerfulness" (21). The benevolent sentiment associated with philanthropic endeavors at midcentury extends here, as it had not yet in the society at large, to the handicapped.

Apparently the number of disabled people in eighteenth-century London was considerable. In Lady Mary Wortley Montagu's Turkish Embassy *Letters* she remarks that the streets of Rotterdam, in contrast to those of London, are free of the visual blight that she believes the handicapped create: "One is not shock'd with those loathsome Cripples so common in London, nor teiz'd with the Importunitys of idle Fellows and Wenches."[12] Dwarfs, giants, Siamese twins, hermaphrodites, and unusual beings with various physical deformities were regularly exhibited for profit in London in the early decades of the century. Those displayed included a Tartar with a horse's head, a man with a head growing out of his body, a man with breasts for thighs and legs, a girl without appendages, and a "midget negro" with his family at Charing Cross.[13]

Millenium Hall begins and ends with attention to deformity. Among the first group the narrator and Lamont happen upon at Millenium Hall is the colony of the disabled. The larger community includes five dwarfs "just three feet high," two giants, and a prematurely old man. In addition, the housekeeper has a maimed hand, the cook is on crutches, the dairymaid is deaf, and the housemaid has only one hand. However, these servants and others all are engaged in the arts or in other productive labor. A lame youth demonstrates his accomplishment at the French horn, and a nearly blind person plays the bassoon. In fact, disability is a *recommendation* for a position at Millenium Hall. The housekeeper's deformed hand means that "what had hitherto been an impediment was a stronger recommendation than the good character I had from my last place; and I am sure I have reason to value these distorted fingers, more than ever any one did the handsomest hands that ever nature made" (120). At Millenium Hall the culture's devaluation of deformity is reversed.

The "monsters," like the women saved from the marriage market, are taught to despise the profit they earned from being paraded as commodified spectacles. The community offers the deformed protection in exchange for their labor, and the women justify their segregation when attending church on the grounds of protecting them from gaping onlookers. The deformed (though they include both sexes) are gendered as women, and liberty is paradoxically achieved for deformed people, as for the women, in confining themselves within "so narrow a compass" (23), in avoiding the public sphere, and in refusing marriage. The deformed are not treated as slaves but rather as servants, since they are paid a small sum for their work. Nevertheless, when the visiting gentlemen ask Mrs. Morgan for an accounting, she has the case of the "monsters" on the tip of her tongue: "The maintenance of the monsters [costs] a hundred and twenty" (205) each year. Even as those at Millenium Hall contest tyranny in favor of harmonious community, the women themselves engage in establishing domain over the disabled.

The "monsters" of Millenium Hall are not unlike the exotic deformed, the emasculated eunuchs of the seraglio, who, in turn, resemble the assembly of women both in their failure to engage in reproductive sex and in being sublimely agreeable, even in their deformity. Deformity is often linked with race as well as with femininity, since the category of the monstrous in the eighteenth century loosely refers to the many varieties of unfamiliar beings. Black eunuchs supervised the women of the harem while white eunuchs guarded the sovereign, blackness in this case thus being associated with domestic femininity and whiteness with political authority. Deformity and racialist slavery united at the bottom of the masculine social scale in the black eunuchs who guarded the women's chastity and protected them from intruders. Deformity is commodified: "The black Eunuchs, who are brought out of *Africa,* much inferiour in point of number, are, as I said, much the dearer. The most deformed yield the greatest price, their extream ugliness being look'd on as beauty in their kind."[14] (Lady Mary Wortley Montagu remarks on the "natural deformity" of North Africans, a connection that derives in part from the belief that pygmies were believed to be apes.) Eunuchs themselves were classified as feminized monstrosities, though agreeably so, in a manner reminiscent of the dark, terrifying desirability of the sublime: "Of the many Thousands, of the Male Sex, who are there as 'twere in Prison, and have a dependance, one upon the other, none but the Prince himself has the sight of Women; for the Negro-Eunuchs, whom their deformity of body and countenance has, in a manner, transform'd into Monsters, are not to be admitted into the number of men."[15] Oriental tales such as Beckford's *Vathek* are populated with every imaginable deformity from the deaf to the humpbacked.[16] Alexander Pope too drew the connection between the East and his own agreeable deformity as Lady Mary embarked to Turkey in October 1716: "I am capable myself of following one I lov'd, not only to Constantinople, but to those parts of India, where they tell us the Women best like the Ugliest fellows, as the most admirable productions of nature, and look upon Deformities as the Signatures of divine Favour."[17] He thus aligns his deformity with the desirable exotic deformities of the East.[18]

Like Pope, William Hay, a member of the House of Commons, stood barely five feet high and was humpbacked, and he provides a kind of gloss on Sarah Scott's inclusion of the disabled within the female community. To counter the marketplace display of the deformed, Hay's seldom-discussed autobiographical pamphlet *Deformity: An Essay* (1754), on an "uncommon Subject," claims a subjectivity based on frank discussion of his very noticeable handicap, and he conceptualizes disability as an identity for the first time. Following Longinus's *Treatise on the Sublime,* Hay wishes "to write of Deformity with Beauty" (13) to reverse its association with the devil. Hay refuses the position of victim and eschews the self-pity that Burke in his *Philosophical Enquiry* assumed to be part of the definition of deformity. ("So if the back be humped, the man is deformed; because his back has an unusual figure, and what carries with it the idea of some disease or misfortune.")[19] Hay also believes that his oppression resembles racism, though by his account the plight of blacks is worse than of the disabled: his constituents, he writes, "are not like a venal Borough, of which there goes a Story; that, though they never took Exceptions to any Mn's Character, who came up to their Price, yet they once rejected the best Bidder, because he was a Negroe" (13).[20] A hierarchy of oppressions is emerging.

Clubs that segregate the handicapped—even well-meaning organizations such as the *Spectator's* "Ugly Club" or the "Short Club" (members of which included Isaac Newton and Christopher Wren) mentioned in Pope's letters to the *Guardian,* (25 June 1713 and 26 June 1713)—make a theatrical spectacle of deformity in Hays's opinion: "When deformed Persons appear together, it doubles the Ridicule, because of the Similitude" (14). But just as the *Spectator* recommends,[21] Hay possesses an inveterate cheerfulness about his deformity. In order to demonstrate that deformed people do not lack natural affection, Hay testifies to his own sentimentality: "If by natural Affection is here meant universal Benevolence, and Deformity necessarily implies a want of it, a deformed Person must then be a complete Monster. But however common the Case may be, my own Sensations inform me, that it is not universally true" (41–42). He traces his social uneasiness to taunts endured as a child that he has endeavored to overcome: "This Difference of Behaviour towards me hath given me the strongest Idea of the Force of Education; and taught me to set a right Value upon it" (10). Taunting persists when he enters a crowd: "When by some uncommon Accident I have been drawn into a Country Friar, Cock-pit, Bear-garden, or the like riotous Assemblies, after I have got from them, I have felt the Pleasure of one escaped from the Danger of a Wreck" (11). In spite of the taunting, Hay persistently redefines disability as advantageous. Drawing perhaps an ironic inference, Hay suggests that his treatise has in common with Hogarth's *Analysis of Beauty* that beauty "consists in Curve Lines." In his *Analysis of Beauty,* Hogarth argues that fitness, variety, uniformity, simplicity, intricacy, and quantity interact to produce beauty. Hay adds that after the initial prejudice against people of deformity, people sometimes "believe [the handicapped] better than they are" and may even take disability to be a sign of good luck. The modern term for this patronizing attitude is *handicappism*. Hay interprets the curved lines of his hunched back as the essence of beauty and disability to be "a Protection to a Man's Health and Person; which (strange as it may appear) are better defended by Feebleness than Strength" (27–28). He believes that a weak frame paradoxically encourages a man to be frugal with his energy, thus preserving it for a longer time. In giving deformity a subjectivity, Hay domesticates the exotic without sentimentalizing it, redefines deformity as beauty, and seeks transformation in societal attitudes toward the disabled.

Deformity is not the opposite of beauty but the "absence of 'the *compleat, common form*,'" according to Edmund Burke, an observation particularly relevant to our discussion of women, since the more perfect is also the more masculine.[22] Hay's essay sheds light on the confounding confluence of female subjectivity and disability because women, the disabled, and non-Europeans all are defined as lacking the complete, common form. The advantages of a fragile body, the transmutation of deformity into a thing of beauty, and the propensity to become the commodified object of public spectacle make the parallels acute. Scott's novel too, playing with the association between women and their deformed charges, emphasizes these advantages. Harriot Trentham's beauty was marred by smallpox, and Lady Mary Jones's face is disfigured, but all the women at Millenium Hall are "deformed" in the larger sense that none is involved with men in reproductive sex or consanguine motherhood, and they redefine beauty as a disadvantage. Miss Mancel's uncommon beauty made her the object of spectacle before she came to Millenium Hall, yet it threatened her economic survival because it prevented her from getting a position as a maid "since her beauty was the great obstacle to its being put in execution" (86). Beauty is an impediment, and deformity is meritorious in the terms of *Millenium Hall*.

A decade before *Millenium Hall* appeared, Sarah Scott had translated *La Laideur Aimable; ou Les Dangers de la Beauté* (1752), by Pierre Antoine de la Place, as *Agreeable Ugliness* (1754). Because Scott herself suffered the disfiguring effects of smallpox at seventeen, she played the ugly duckling to her beautiful sister, Elizabeth Montagu. In the translation of *Agreeable Ugliness*, the younger sister, "Shocking Monster," is morally superior to her beautiful and vain sister and ultimately finds a satisfying marriage by submitting completely to her father's will. She accepts the less interesting Dorigny, her father's favorite, to protect her from her passionate love for St. Furcy; but after Dorigny suffers a fatal wound, Shocking Monster is free to marry her original choice.[23] Like *Millenium Hall*, *Agreeable Ugliness* touts the perils of beauty that lead to dangerous liaisons and unsuitable marriages and connects femininity to disability.

Sarah Scott too converts deformity to advantage—literally in the case of smallpox but more forcefully with the "deformity" of not marrying, of refusing motherhood, and of living with and loving women. Unlike William Hay, women cannot overcome ugliness when competing in the marriage marketplace. Scott insists on the pleasures of deformity that women find outside reproductive sex in creating their own definitions and imagined alternatives. It is a crucial moment in history when women desiring women, women who do not wish to marry or reproduce, the deformed, and the exotic forge affinities in the novel in the name of resistance to their commodification in a mercantilist economy. Feminotopia newly envisages the connections between the homoerotic and the disabled in its orientalist idealization and defines female community as an autonomous women's empire.

In *Millenium Hall* an enclosure paradoxically brings freedom from tyranny through chastity, economic freedom, and mutual protection. Scott redefines the women's secluded community as a place of rational harmony and their reticence or refusal to marry as agreeable deformity. The novel also seeks to educate male observers to the opinion that feminotopias are not deformities but sites of beauty or self-defined sociability encompassing a range of female sexualities.

Yet Scott in her utopian vision replicates class differences and portrays women who engage in the charitable acts that are available to the privileged. *Millenium Hall* may be read as an addendum to the orientalism of women's narratives of the seraglio in that it shares the exoticism of the Eastern women's situation, imitating it even in the attachment of dwarfs and other deformed people to it. In fact, the women at Millenium Hall gain subjectivity and freedom in part by defining themselves as superior to the poor and to the disabled who depend upon them for benevolent, but colonizing, acts. *Millenium Hall* is uneven in its critique of eighteenth-century culture, as any representation of utopia must be. In creating a female empire, it empowers women of a certain class and nation, and it radically associates a fifth oppression—disability—with the more familiar quarter of race, class, gender, and sexuality. It thus participates in a qualitative break with the present, what might be called "the politics of transfiguration," emphasizing "the emergence of qualitatively new needs, social relations, and modes of association, which burst open the utopian potential within the old."[24] This articulation of an alternative to the existing, in spite of its limitations, makes historical and social change possible. Western feminist thought in particular needs to confront its relationship to deformity—racial, sexual, or bodily—as it constructs its histories. There is, of course, a need to be alert to the dangers of empowering the privileged to make something pleasurable, even a feminotopia, of another's vulnerability; but the resistance enacted through the sexual desire of women for each other, the agreeable ugliness that allows women to avoid marriage and its economy, and the hidden beauties of bodily deformity may be aligned across culture and chapter to build newly configured forms of collectivity.

NOTES

1. Pratt cites Latin American examples, such as Flora Tristan's utopian vision of the women in Peru and Maria Graham's description of women in Brazil and Chile, in *Imperial Eyes: Travel Writing and Transculturation* (London: Routledge, 1992), 155–71.

2. See the preface in Walter M. Crittenden, ed., *A Description of Millenium Hall,* by Sarah Scott (New York: Bookman, 1955), 5–22. All subsequent quotations of Scott's novel are from *A Description of Millenium Hall and the Country Adjacent Together with the Character of the Inhabitants* . . . (New York: Virago, 1987).

3. Sarah Scott lived with Barbara Montagu from 1748 until Montagu's death in 1765, and in spite of the usual historical caveat that brides often traveled with a female companion, their friendship may well have been sexual too.

4. See, for example, Moira Ferguson's *Subject to Others: British Women Writers and Colonial Slavery, 1670–1834* (New York: Routledge, 1992), 101–11. In *The History of Sir George Ellison* (London, 1766), written as Granville Sharp was pursuing his emancipation campaign, Ellison is a merchant and benevolent slave owner whose imperialist and racist activities are justified because of his kindness in conducting them. Ferguson harshly critiques the novel for promoting a sentimentalism that substitutes for political action and the eradication of slavery.

5. Mr. D'Avora, the Italian master to Misses Melvyn and Mancel, also possesses colonizing curiosity, "the curiosity of wisdom, not of impertinence" (*Millenium Hall,* 44), on his travels through Asia and Africa. George Haggerty, "'Romantic Friendship' and Patriarchal Narrative in Sarah Scott's *Millenium Hall,*" *Genders* 13 (spring 1992): 108–22, posits that D'Avora could be interpreted as a gay man who instructs the women in alternative sexualities or at least symbolizes them. D'Avora seems to me to occupy instead the place of the mediating eunuch of oriental tales.

6. In fact, however, instead of mocking the women, Ellison imitates the plan for a female academy in *The History of Sir George Ellison.*

7. In the introduction to the edition of *Millenium Hall* cited here, Jane Spencer notes that the novel is directed at men and is "primarily concerned with disabusing men of their errors about women" (xv).

8. Ruth Perry suggests that community is made possible in the novel by "the mix of self-sustaining labor and expressive pleasure, the balance between personal freedom and responsibility for others, the proper ratio between production for subsistence and production for art" and "a set of interventions in both the labor market and the marriage market." See Ruth Perry, "Bluestockings in Utopia," in *History, Gender, and Eighteenth-Century Literature,* ed. Beth Fowkes Tobin (Athens, GA: University of Georgia Press, 1994), 162–63.

9. This maternal relationship of the women to their charges is reinforced in George Ellison's later comment "that they could have better performed a mother's part they had evidently proved, without having stood in that relation to any one;" (*The History of Sir George Ellison,* 256).

10. Haggerty, "'Romantic Friendship' and Patriarchal Narrative," 113, finds that maternal relations in the novel are eroticized "as a way of challenging eighteenth-century assumptions concerning female subjectivity and the place of the mother in domestic rela-

tions." Treating primarily the Mancel-Morgan relationship, Haggerty associates lesbian narrative with breaking the bonds that heterosexuality and the cult of domesticity have held on women's alternative figurings of sexuality, but his argument for self-determination ignores important hierarchies that are necessary to the production of this feminotopia.

11. Their relationship is a counterexample to Lillian Faderman's claim in *Surpassing the Love of Men: Romantic Friendship and Love between Women from the Renaissance to the Present* (New York: Morrow, 1981) that even sensual romantic friendship was not regarded with concern because genital contact was unlikely.

12. To Lady Mar, 3 August [1716], in *The Complete Letters of Lady Mary Wortley Montagu*, ed. Robert Halsband, vol. 1 (Oxford: Clarendon, 1965), 249.

13. Aline Miller, "Sights and Monsters and Gulliver's *Voyage to Brobdingnag*," *Tulane Studies in English* 7 (1957): 20–82, cites the 1711–12 advertisement for the "midget Negro": "A little Black Man lately brought from the West Indies, being the Wonder of his Age, he being but 3 Foot high and 25 Years Old."

14. *A New Relation of the Inner-Part of the Grand Seignor's Seraglio. Containing Several Remarkable Particulars* . . . (London, 1677), 6.

15. Ibid., 79.

16. William Beckford, *Vathek,* ed. Roger Lonsdale (Oxford: Oxford University Press, 1983). The dwarfs in the harem sing and address Vathek in a "curious harangue," and objects of pity swarm about the Caliph: "At noon a superb corps of cripples made its appearance; . . . and the completest association of invalids that had ever been embodied till ten. The blind went groping with the blind, the lame limped on together, and the maimed made gestures to each other with the only arm that remained. The sides of a considerable water-fall were crowded by the deaf; . . . Nor were there wanting others in abundance with hump-backs; wenny necks; and even horns of an exquisite polish" (61).

17. *The Correspondence of Alexander Pope,* ed. George Sherburn, vol. 1 (Oxford: Clarendon, 1956), 364.

18. *A New Relation of the Inner-Part of the Grand Seignor's Seraglio* also describes the deformed in the seraglio: "The language of the Mutes, by signs, is as intelligible in the Seraglio, as if they had the liberty of speaking, and the Grand Seignor . . . understands it as well as any of them, as having been accustom'd thereto from his Infancy, and commonly discoursing with them" (87). Mutes were employed in the Turkish court to amuse the sultan but also to teach pages the sign language used to avoid distracting the monarch with the sound of voices. *The Present State of the Ottoman Empire* . . . , translated from the French manuscript of Elias Habesci (London, 1784), indicates that "such unfortunate beings, as thus 'curtailed of fair proportion,' have been, for ages, an appendage of Eastern grandeur . . . The dwarves are employed in the same manner as the mutes. If a dwarf happens to be a mute, he is much esteemed; and if likewise a eunuch, they esteem him as a great prodigy, and no pains or expense is spared to procure such a rarity" (164).

19. Edmund Burke, *A Philosophical Enquiry into the Origin of Our Ideas of the Sublime and Beautiful,* ed. J. T. Boulton (London: Routledge and Kegan Paul; New York: Columbia University Press, 1958), 103.

20. In another association between the monstrous and the African, "Alexander Carbuncle" writes in the *Spectator,* Tuesday, 20 March 1711, about the Ugly Club, a society of the deformed that mounts speeches in praise of the hunchbacked Aesop. He assumed that

Mr. Spectator would know nothing about the monstrous "unless it was your Fortune to touch upon some of the woody Parts of the *African* Continent, in your Voyage to or from *Grand Cairo*." Richard Steele, *The Spectator,* ed. Donald F. Bond, vol. 1 (Oxford: Clarendon, 1965), 76.

21. *Spectator,* Tuesday, 20 March 1711, 75: "It is happy for a Man, that has any of these Odnesses *[sic]* about him, if he can be as merry upon himself, as others are apt to be upon that Occasion . . . As it is barbarous in others to rally him for natural Defects, it is extreamly agreeable when he can Jest upon himself for them."

22. Burke, *A Philosophical Enquiry,* lxv.

23. Caroline Gonda, "Sarah Scott and 'The Sweet Excess of Paternal Love,'" *SEL* 32 (1992): 511–35, identifies the dangers of beauty and sexual attraction but focuses on the father-daughter relationship rather than the homosocial nature of ugliness and deformity.

24. Seyla Benhabib, *Critique, Norm, and Utopia: A Study of the Foundation of Critical Theory* (New York: Columbia University Press, 1986), 13.

"A Prisoner to the Couch" ▸ Harriet Martineau, Invalidism, and Self-Representation

Maria Frawley

"The ravings of the sick were the secrets of God," wrote Bram Stoker in the fin de siècle novel *Dracula*, summing up a century's attraction to all that was ill.[1] Just as Dracula's victims were drawn in their delirium to rant and rave, Victorians with more earthly kinds of sicknesses seemed led inexorably to write about their encounters with ill health and to view their sicknesses as, in some sense, heaven sent. Describing her first lengthy experience with illness, for example, Harriet Martineau—a Victorian journalist and intellectual who lived from 1802 until 1876—wrote in her autobiography: "I was patient in illness and pain because I was proud of the distinction, and of being taken into such special pupilage by God."[2] Pupil of God's or not, Martineau stayed in her sickroom, a self-declared "prisoner to the couch," for nearly six years.

Accounts of illness and recovery proliferated in Victorian England, an era fascinated like no other with the figure of the invalid and the spectacle of sickness. As Miriam Bailin has written, "the nineteenth-century sick were deeply concerned with their health and often obsessed with monitoring the body's vicissitudes."[3] While some scholars have emphasized the centrality of psychosomatic illness to the Victorian experience, others have focused on Victorian associations of physical health with spiritual excellence and, correlatively, of illness with moral failure. In *Somatic Fictions*, for example, Athena Vrettos concludes that "the process of *imagining* illness (or health) took on its own peculiar resonance for Victorian culture" (emphasis added).[4] Approaching the subject from a different angle, Bruce Haley writes in *The Healthy Body and Victorian Culture* that "Victorians used physical health as the model for a higher human excellence, a way of envisioning it."[5]

A recognizable feature of Victorian fiction, the sickroom scene entered the cultural landscape through a range of forms, not least of which were the many accounts authored by invalids. The Victorian period produced countless documents about illness by invalids, among them, for example, W. E. Henley's long poem *In Hospital*, S. Linden's "The Invalid Abroad: Sketches of Invalid Life in the High Alps," Alexander Shand's "The Pleasures of Illness," and anonymously written advice tracts such as *The Cup of Consolation, or Messages for the Sick Bed from an Invalid*. Such works are crucial to understanding the construction of the invalid in Victorian England. As Sheila Rothman has written, "The term [*invalid*] was as much a social as a medical category, defining the responsibilities of the sick even as it freed them from fault."[6] Victorian invalid narratives encompassed a wide spectrum of illnesses, ranging from the hypochondriac or neurotic to the consumptive or crippled. Constructed as a condition characterized not so much by specific disease or disorder but rather by one's loss of capacity for certain kinds of exertion, invalidism entailed a correlative focus on the psychological or emotional impact of extended illness and on what many Victorians represented as heightened imaginative *abilities*.[7] While recovery was a goal for some invalids, many lived under the assumption that good health would never again be experienced and that, in any case, one's essential "selfhood" was somehow forever altered. To apprehend the meaning of invalidism in the Victorian period, requires, among other things, attending to the ways in which those writing of their illnesses deal with issues of duration (e.g., through a rhetoric of "malingering" or "becoming inured") and, more generally, to the transformative potential of illness.

Narratives of invalidism thus become intriguing case studies of Victorian notions of the nature of subjectivity and of the public/private divide, for though autobiographical in orientation, many attempted as well a kind of objective accounting or "clinical frame" that physicians like Rita Charon associate with the medical establishment. Drawing on Bakhtin's notion of *heteroglossia*, Charon calls in her work on interpretive medical history for greater attention to the discursive strategies of the sick person, whose writings are shaped, she argues, by an elaborate grammar of selection, censoring, and editing. As Charon summarizes, fear, need, and the wish for a diagnosis, coupled with "the shame and humiliation that surround corporeal events . . . may transform a straightforward telling into a pressured, fragmented, resisted, and contradictory account."[8]

In this essay I will focus on Harriet Martineau's *Life in the Sickroom*, a work that, on its surface, shows little of the shame or humiliation that Charon would have us believe characterizes the sick person's story.[9] A close reading of *Life in the Sickroom* that attends to Martineau's implied audience and rhetoric of imprisonment and self-control reveals contradictions central to her vexed understanding of individual agency and, more generally, to the Victorian interest in illness. In doing so, Martineau's work highlights many issues of autonomy and self-reliance that are equally crucial to disability studies today. Indeed, when Foucault wrote in his preface to *The Birth of the Clinic* that "[t]his book is about space, about language, and about death; it is about the act of seeing, the gaze," he might well have been introducing Martineau's *Life in the Sickroom*.[10]

Published in 1844, Martineau's work belongs to the tail end of the period historians often associate with "premodern" medicine. As M. Jeanne Peterson has documented, the Medical Act of 1858 was a turning point in Victorian history, organizing the medical profession and enabling it to achieve some degree of "autonomy and self-regulation."[11] *Life in the Sickroom* was written in the oppositional period of medical history that predated the Medical Act and belongs to the culture of the invalid that prospered in the first half of nineteenth-century England concomitantly with a growth of movements organized around their confrontation with orthodox medicine.[12] In a sense, such movements empowered the individual to counter the presumed autonomy of medicine by usurping the right to limit medical intervention and to control treatment. *Life in the Sickroom* reveals a variety of strategies that Martineau deployed to distance herself from the "treatment" that would objectify her as patient and to establish instead her autonomy—and control—as invalid. As Alison Winter has summarized, "the work was unusual among sick-room literature and patients' testimonials for its intense focus on the invalid's experience of the room rather than a visitor's management of it."[13]

Martineau was well aware that her work was distinctively different from what she thought of as run-of-the-mill invalid literature. Excoriating what she called the "morbid appetite for pathological contemplation," she wrote in her autobiography:

> Tracts and religious books swarm among us, and are thrust into the hands of every body by every body else, which describe the sufferings of illness, and generate vanity and egotism about bodily pain and early death, rendering these disgraces of our ignorance and barbarism attractive to the foolish and the vain, and actually shaming the wholesome, natural desire for "a sound mind in a sound body." (vol. 1, 439–40).

Here as elsewhere in her autobiography Martineau stresses her intention to resist the representational norms of a culture that associates suffering with shame and proposes instead an alternative ideology of healthy illness.

Martineau's autobiography as well as her "autobiographic memoir," a self-prepared obituary, helps to situate her understanding of the relationship between health, authorship, and the relationship of private experience to public discourses. *Life in the Sickroom,* focusing as it does on the invalid's dual consciousness of her self and the self that others see, reveals the potential of disability to unravel traditional binary pairings such as those of sickness and health, mind and body, and reason and emotion. Illness provides Martineau with the raw material to explore the intersubjective nature of selfhood and of human experience more generally. In *Life in the Sickroom* she traces what she calls "an intense and growing self-consciousness" (182) and explores the ramifications of that "heightened sensitivity" (173) on her understanding of human history.

Martineau's study of the perspective of the sick subject, relying as it does on a rhetoric of interior control, exposes the inadequacy of traditional interpretations of doctor/patient relations that, following Foucault in *The Birth of the Clinic,* stress the "sovereign power of the empirical gaze" (xii). Martineau describes instead the ability of the invalid to achieve a distinctive kind of "autonomy and self-regulation," to use M. Jeanne Peterson's terms, not in the face of, but rather because of, illness. "You and I, and our fellow-sufferers, see differently," she wrote in her "Dedication" to *Life in the Sickroom* (xviii). Almost instantly dispensing with any pretense toward humility on the subject, Martineau goes on to proclaim the boundlessness of the "new insight" to which invalids have access: "We see the whole system of human life rising and rising into a higher region and a purer light" (xviii) and concludes, "This [is] our peculiar privilege, of seeing and feeling something of the simultaneous vastness, and minuteness of providential administration" (xix–xx).

Martineau's emphasis on the perspective of the invalid enables her to construct an ontology of invalidism, one that foregrounds the value of being, as opposed to doing, and that grants control to the invalid. In this way *Life in the Sickroom* sets itself against the ethos of an age that valued useful activity above all else and, in doing so, complicates the received image of Martineau as tireless public worker.[14] Finally, *Life in the Sickroom* counters a traditional history of medicine that, as Roy Porter and Dorothy Porter have argued, has been "strangely silent about the patient's role in the clinical encounter" and that has "reduced the patient to something akin to a corpse in a detective story."[15]

If *Life in the Sickroom* empowers the invalid with voice, it is a work nonetheless "strangely silent" about certain issues—particularly those having to do with diagnosis. One might read *Life in the Sickroom* in its entirety and not be sure of what disease or disability has confined Martineau to her sick space. Instead, she accounts for her retreat to what she calls her "couch of pain" (vol. 1, 438) in the "Fifth Period" of her autobiography, extending from roughly the age of 36 to 43. Excluding such an account from *Life in the Sickroom*, Martineau demarcates the boundaries of her study, implying that invalidism is constituted by what happens *within* the sickroom, not by the illness that has taken a person there.

The significance of what Martineau leaves out of *Life in the Sickroom* can be appreciated by gauging its function within her autobiography. Although she treats the onset of her first extended illness within a discrete section of the autobiography, her entire life story is framed by the encounter with prolonged sickness on which *Life in the Sickroom* was based, for in the opening paragraph of the autobiography she refers ominously to her "long illness at Tynemouth" (vol. 1, 1). Importantly, she implies at the commencement of the autobiography that her narrative, though undertaken as a duty, could not have been written if she were well.

Of late years, I have often said to my most intimate friends that I felt as if I could not die in peace till this work was done; and there has been no lack of

encouragement and instigation on their part: but, while I was in health, there
was always so much to do that was immediately wanted, that, as usually
happens in such cases, that which was not immediately necessary was
deferred.(vol. 1, 1)

Martineau situates the narrative as an example of "work" that had to be done
and, simultaneously, as something that could not have been done while there was
work to do.

Life in the Sickroom is similarly a product of contradictory attitudinal gestures. Martineau suggests in her autobiography that she had "accumulated a
weight of ideas and experiences which [she] longed to utter" and undertook the
study as a "mode of relief" that occurred to her as she reclined on the ubiquitous
couch (vol. 1, 456–57). Her rhetoric underscores the anxiety she experienced—
repeated invocations of her love of quiet and monotony notwithstanding—in her
retreat from activity. She continues by explaining that, having been informed by
"two able physicians" (vol. 1, 2) in London that she had a fatal disease and might
die at any time, she decided immediately to embark on her autobiography.

Martineau encourages her readers to interpret her autobiography as pathography. Her association of impending morbidity with the will to write her life story
exposes interesting assumptions about the value of her experience and the nature
of subjectivity. As Foucault explained in *The Birth of the Clinic:*

The perception of death in life does not have the same function in the nineteenth century as at the Renaissance . . . Now . . . it is constitutive of singularity; it is in that perception of death that the individual finds himself,
escaping from a monotonous, average life; in the slow, half-subterranean, but
already visible approach of death, the dull, common life becomes an individuality at last; a black border isolates it and gives it the style of its own truth.
(171)

When Martineau wrote *Life in the Sickroom* she had already begun to conceive of
her life as markedly different from the average—at least the average life of a
middle class woman—and to pronounce her individuality on this score. She
nevertheless seemed eager to retreat to Tynemouth from her hard-won fame and
public reputation as author and, in a gesture that seems to contradict Foucault's
paradigm, embraced the "monotonous," writing in her autobiography that "I
loved, as I still love, the most monotonous life possible" (vol. 1, 442). Yet,
Martineau argued that the tedium and uniformity of the sickroom and of illness
itself were the conditions that enabled her to achieve a distinct perspective, in
essence to realize the differences between her self and the self that others saw.

While Martineau makes references to her health throughout the autobiography, she is nearly 400 pages into her work before she gets to the Tynemouth

episode to which she alludes in the beginning. Evidently Martineau became ill while traveling on a continental journey that she undertook, ironically, "chiefly for the sake of escorting an invalid cousin to Switzerland" (vol. 1, 436) but also, as she explained in her "autobiographic memoir," to provide "rest and refreshment for herself" as well (vol. 2, 568). Once home, she retreated to a sickroom under the care of Dr. Thomas Greenhow, her brother-in-law, eventually moving to a conveniently located home of her own where she could be distanced from direct medical care but still reasonably accessible should she need it.

Throughout this episode of the autobiography Martineau intersperses anecdotes that help to constitute a brief health history and to endow her readers with the diagnostic capacity usually accorded to physicians: she describes, for example, her sleeping difficulties and fainting spells, in addition to mentioning briefly "an internal disease": "A tumour was forming of a kind which usually originates in mental suffering" (vol. 1, 442).[16] Here, as Diana Postlethwaite has argued, Martineau "echoes the medical opinion of her day, believing in a direct connection between the uterus and the emotions, and defining 'hysteria' as a distinctively feminine disease."[17] But she simultaneously counters medical opinion as well, citing additional sources of her suffering. She notes, among other things, her exhausting schedule of travels in America, the anxiety that accompanied her authorship of the novel *Deerbrook,* the shock of the death of two friends, and the general "domestic uneasiness" that resulted from caring for a blind mother whose "natural irritability" (vol. 1, 441) was often focused on her.

Throughout her account of her descent into invalidism, Martineau stresses the emotional and psychological dimensions of her condition, effectively teaching her readers about the inseparability of mental from bodily conditions and, correlatively, of private life from public life. She recognizes the compulsion to activity that drives her, seemingly against her will, to public performance and the psychic cost of that public role. Explaining the extent to which her nerves were "overstrained," she writes: "I had by that time resolved on the wisdom which I try to this day to practice:—longing for quiet, and yet finding it impossible in the nature of things that my life should be any thing but a busy, public, and diversified one,—*to keep a quiet mind*" (vol. 1, 428). Later she notes that she "was overworked . . . in addition to the pain of mind [she] had to bear" (vol. 1, 441–42). And describing her decision to stay confined for nearly six years, she writes:

Here closed the anxious period during which my reputation, and my industry, and my social intercourses were at their height of prosperity; but which was so charged with troubles that when I lay down on my couch of pain in my Tynemouth lodging, for a confinement of nearly six years, I felt myself comparatively happy in my release from responsibility, anxiety and suspense. The worst sufferings of my life were over now; and its best enjoyments and privileges were to come,—though I little knew it, and they were as yet a good way off. (vol. 1, 437–38)

With all the skill of a Victorian novelist enticing her readers to await the fulfillment of plot, Martineau restates here a thesis of *Life in the Sickroom*—that through a process of bodily and psychic transformation, the invalid comes to understand that his or her perspective in illness entails privilege. Just as Foucault called attention in *The Birth of the Clinic* to "the privilege of the consumptive," arguing that "in the nineteenth century, a man, in becoming tubercular, in the fever that hastens things and betrays them, fulfills his incommunicable secret" (172), so too does Martineau intimate that her illness has initiated her into a secret sanctum of opportunity. Invalidism, she argues, privileges sufferers with a unique subjectivity: "We see everything with different eyes," she declares (73).

It follows from Martineau's argument that the invalid's distinctive subjectivity results in different narrative abilities and demands different narratorial responsibilities. As narrator, the invalid's role is not to help other invalids achieve relief from their pain but rather to recognize the insights that come with their "condition of protracted suffering" (26). Martineau writes, "It may look like a paradox to say that a condition of permanent pain is that which, above all, proves to one the transient nature of pain; but this is what I do affirm, and can testify" (26). Constructing her self as experienced witness to pain, Martineau's closing "affirmation" underscores the connection between illness and selfhood. Her work suggests as well that the task of the invalid narrator is not to delineate stages along the process of recovery but, rather, to represent and analyze the experience of being incapacitated.

And, indeed, Martineau announces in the preface to *Life in the Sickroom* that her concern there is with the experience of "protracted unhealthiness" (xiv). Martineau's attention to the duration of illness helps her to establish the spatial and temporal dimensions of her subject and of pathography itself, what Alexander Shand referred to in his essay on "The Pleasures of Illness" as "the blessed borderland of convalescence."[18] "A day's illness may teach something of [the nature of 'permanent pain'] to a thoughtful mind," Martineau writes, "but the most inconsiderate can scarcely fail to learn the lesson, when the proof is drawn out over a succession of months and seasons" (26).[19] Through her emphasis on the prolonged nature of illness Martineau intimates a distrust of the medical establishment. Marginalizing such concepts as diagnosis, treatment, and recovery, she instead used *Life in the Sickroom* to treat topics that would help the healthy to understand the desire of the invalid to become acclimated to the sickroom and resigned to prolonged illness. Chapter headings emphasize the invalid's inner world: "The Transient and the Permanent in the Sickroom," "Sympathy to the Invalid," "Nature to the Invalid," "Becoming Inured," and "Power of Ideas in the Sick-Room."

In her distrust of medical treatment Martineau was also expressing the understandable desire to retain some degree of control over her illness. Arguably the most influential fictional study of early Victorian attitudes toward medicine, George Eliot's novel *Middlemarch* reveals a similar phenomenon through the encounter between the doctor Lydgate and his pneumonia-ridden patient Trumbull, a man tempted into believing that he might "make the disorder of his pulmonary functions a general benefit to society."[20] Trumbull "went without shrinking through his abstinence from drugs, much sustained by application of the thermometer which implied the importance of his temperature, by the sense that he furnished objects for the microscope, and by learning many new words which seemed suited to the dignity of his secretions" (491). Predictably, Trumbull recovers "with a disposition to speak of an illness in which he had manifested the strength of his mind as well as constitution" (491). Disease, Eliot implies, furnishes Trumbull with the stuff that selves are made of, and, if Trumbull is ultimately to benefit society, it will more likely be through his own words than through the success of Lydgate's public programs.

Like many of the fictional inhabitants of Middlemarch, Martineau resented the assurances of medicine. In *Life in the Sickroom* she acknowledged "quackeries of the time" (90) but argued for their "collateral good, whatever may be the express failure" (91). On the issue of mesmerism, a topic near and dear to her heart, she challenged her readers as follows: "Who looks back upon the mass of strange but authenticated historical narratives, which might be explained by this agent, and . . . will dare to say that there is nothing in it?" (91). Later referring in her "Autobiographic Memoir" to her "trial of mesmerism" she wrote sarcastically, "That she recovered when she ought to have died was an unpardonable offence" (44).[21] Gillian Thomas reports that when Martineau's brother-in-law published a pamphlet detailing his position on her recovery (titled "A Medical Report of the Case of Miss H------ M--------" and apparently giving a "detailed gynecological explanation of her symptoms"), Martineau "was appalled to find such a medical account of her problems 'in a shilling pamphlet—not even written in Latin—but open to all the world!' "[22]

Yet like the verbose Middlemarchian Trumbull, Martineau felt "disposed to speak" of her experience with illness and disability *and* she believed that in doing so she could benefit society—not as popularizer of medical beliefs, an ancillary role familiar to her, but rather by writing for a community of the ill. Although she dedicates *Life in the Sickroom* to a single, unnamed sufferer (Elizabeth Barrett Browning), she rhetorically expands her implied audience to other "fellow-sufferers." In her "Dedication" Martineau intimates her desire that her writing might perform restorative work: "I may have the honor of being your nurse, though I am myself laid low,—though hundreds of miles are between us, and though we can never know one another's face or voice" (xx).

Although utilitarian in its effort to serve a community of sufferers, Martineau's writing about personal health—*Life in the Sickroom,* "Letter to the Deaf," published in *Tait's Edinburgh Magazine* in 1834, and her "Letters on Mesmerism," published in 1845—is markedly different from much of her other writing, in which she, as Deirdre David has argued, aligns herself with a dominant ideology (usually patriarchy) and performs through her writing an ancillary role, what she thinks of as auxiliary service.[23] While Martineau understood the extent to which health was a matter of public concern (one of her last major writing projects was a campaign against the Contagious Diseases Acts), she identified her role as invalid narrator as helping the healthy public to understand the private experience of the invalid. Rather than embrace the subordination and debility entailed in invalidism, she argues for the superiority of the invalid's position in relation to the healthy, active, working world.

Thus, although Martineau claims in her "Dedication" to write to fellow-sufferers, her discursive strategies reveal otherwise, for much of the work is oriented toward a healthy readership whose limited experiences with illness have little prepared them to appreciate the perspective of the invalid. Throughout *Life in the Sickroom* Martineau distinguishes between her healthy and suffering readers. She occasionally directs her comments specifically to the unnamed subject of her dedication: "You, my fellow-sufferer, now lying on your couch, . . . are you not smiling at the thought that you have preserved, up to this time, more or less of that faith of your childhood—that everything that is in print is true?" (78). More typically Martineau assumes a healthy readership, as in the following passage: "Many will wonder at all this—will despise such sensitiveness to trifles, considering what deeds are done every day in the world. They do not know the pains and penalties of sickness—that is all: and it may do them no harm to learn what they are, while my fellow-sufferers may find some comfort in an honest recognition of them" (173). In its uneven construction of a narratee, *Life in the Sickroom* exhibits the kind of "pressured, fragmented, resisted, and contradictory" discourse that Rita Charon argues characterizes patient accounts.

If Martineau is consistent in *Life in the Sickroom* it is in her focus on the private, which she invokes both through her treatment of the physical condition of the sickroom and in her analysis of the invalid's interiority. Isolated from more public gathering spaces within the home, the sickroom functions, according to Martineau, as a "natural confessional" and a "sanctuary of confidence" that invites "spontaneous revelations" (196). Through her rhetoric, Martineau attempted to change the public perception of the invalid, not so much by countering perceived notions of the ill person's physical incapacities or dependencies but rather by emphasizing the unique psychological and emotional independence achieved within the sickroom. The invalid's physical surroundings nurture, she claims, special introspective abilities: "We may be excluded from much observation of the outer life of men, but of the inner life, which originates and interprets the outer, it is scarcely possible that in any other circumstances we could have known so much" (196). She invites her healthy readers to consider the invalid's privileged access to inner worlds but reminds them indirectly—and repeatedly— that their perspective has not been chosen, referring to other sufferers as "the sequestered" (178) or as "sick prisoner[s]" (60) and invoking the analogy of the sickroom itself as a prison.

Despite her rhetoric of confinement, Martineau constructs the sickroom as a kind of inverse panoptican, where the invalid, granted visionary power conferred by her unique access to death, defies what Foucault called "the empirical gaze."

> To us, whose whole life is sequestered,—who see nothing of the events of which we hear so much, or see them only as gleam or shadow passing along our prison-walls, there is something indescribably affecting in the act of re- garding History, Life, and Speculation as one . . . History becomes like actual life; life becomes comprehensive as history, and abstract as speculation. Not only does human life, from the cradle to the grave, lie open to us, the whole succession of generations, without the boundary line of the past being inter- posed: and with the very clouds of the future so thinned,—rendered so pene- trable, as that we believe we discern the salient and bright points of the human destiny yet to be revealed. (96–97)

Here Martineau returns to earlier themes, constructing herself as one granted "pupilage" by God and as God-like in her powers of penetration—what she at another point in the text designates as the invalid's "seraphic powers" (77).

Martineau's rhetoric of penetration and revelation is evidenced in her atten- tion throughout *Life in the Sickroom* to the function of the window. Her sick- room window marks the invalid's access to the wider world, but it functions symbolically as well to signify the meditative and visionary powers of invalidism. Martineau's window prompts her to discourse on the relationship between the liberty that the invalid has to observe and on the consequent responsibility to preserve others' rights to privacy; perhaps most importantly, it enables her to demarcate the boundaries between inner and outer worlds so central to her understanding of invalidism. All three functions are captured in an important passage in Martineau's fifth chapter, "Life to the Invalid."

> When I think of what I have seen with my own eyes from one back window, in the few years of my illness; of how indescribably clear to me are many truths of life from my observation of the doings of the tenants of a single row of houses; it seems to me scarcely necessary to see more than the smallest sample, in order to analyze life in its entirety. I could fill a volume—and an interesting one too—with a simple detail of what I have witnessed, as I said, from one back- window. But I must tell nothing. These two or three little courts and gardens

ought to be as sacred as any interior. Nothing of the spy shall mix itself with my relation to neighbors who have ever been kind to me. (93)

Martineau's visionary claims here—her ability to see the "truths of life" and "life in its entirety" from her observational post at one back window—echo other grandiose remarks made in *Life in the Sickroom* regarding the omniscience of sick vision. Yet she also collapses the distinction between the extraordinary and the everyday by constructing herself in the more mundane role of invalid ethnographer, filling volumes with what she observes, creating samples, and analyzing her findings. Her focus on interiors adds another level of complexity to the passage, for though she refers most obviously to the enclosed spaces on which she looks, they stand metonymically for the private lives of her neighbors and even for the "sacred" inner life of the invalid itself. Martineau's closing disavowal of her self as spy—after she has detailed the abundance of what she is able to see from her window—is also worth noting, calling attention as it does to the shifting boundaries of the public/private divide within the sickroom.

No single feature of the sickroom is comparable to the window, Martineau argues, in its capacity to provide the confined person with a necessary sense of liberty and access to the restorative elements of Nature. In "Nature to the Invalid," she explains the ways that access to the outside can facilitate recovery. Bemoaning the rooms "whose windows command dead walls, or paved courts," Martineau writes:

> I remember the heart-ache it gave me to see a youth, confined to a recumbent posture for two or three years, lying in a room whence he could see nothing, and dependent therefore on the cage of birds by his bedside, and the flowers his friends sent him, for the only notices of Nature that reached him. (59)

She then dons the mantle of professional invalid, writing:

> What is the best kind of view for a sick prisoner's windows to command? I have chosen the sea, and am satisfied with my choice. We should have the widest expanse of sky, for night scenery. We should have a wide expanse of land or water, for the sake of a sense of liberty, yet more than for variety; and also because then the inestimable help of a telescope may be called in. Think of the difference to us between seeing from our sofas the width of a street, even if it be Sackville-street, Dublin, or Portland Place, in London, and thirty miles of sea view, with its long boundary of rocks and the power of sweeping our glance over half a county, by means of a telescope. (60–61)

With her rhetorical question and prompt affirmation, Martineau again underscores the relationship between the perspective her illness has afforded her and her sense of autonomy. Her focus on the window position within the sickroom enables her to illustrate, if indirectly, the invalid's control of the perspective within the room. Although the eyes of the invalid's visitors—like the eyes of Martineau's readers—are turned toward her, the invalid, defying the "clinical gaze" of others, "commands" the view within her room, asking those around her to follow her eyes as she looks to the beyond. In essence, the sickroom becomes "A Room with a View," and others are implicitly invited to look *with,* not *at,* the invalid.[24]

Martineau's use of the window in her sickroom study to address larger issues of perspective might help to remind us in the end of the extent to which self-control permeates her understanding of illness, health, and authorship. In fact, self-control figured largely in Martineau's conception of public and private life. She began her autobiography with the unlikely claim that her public identity did not concern her: "I have no solicitude about fame, and no fear of my reputation . . . being injured by the publication of any thing I have ever put upon paper" (vol. 1, 2). Yet Martineau was nothing if not concerned with the way others would see her, a concern made particularly evident in her determination to control her public image by preparing her own obituary, the "autobiographic memoir" that originally appeared in the *Daily News* and was subsequently appended to her autobiography.

While *Life in the Sickroom* foregrounds Martineau's concern with self-control in a variety of ways, it also resists its own impulses as well, most especially in its effort to represent the passivity of the invalid and the cautionary tone it takes against active participation in human affairs. Although Martineau used the window to emphasize the observational propensities of the invalid and to draw her readers' attention to the subsequent complexities of perspective within the spatial configuration of the sickroom, her primary concern throughout *Life in the Sickroom* is with the metaphysical perspective of the sufferer. She implies, moreover, that passivity enables this perspective: "Nothing is more impossible to represent in words, even to one's self in meditative moments, than what it is to lie on the verge of life and watch, with nothing to do but to think, and learn from what we behold" (77). Martineau's emphasis on what she discovers through introspection is crucial to her construction of invalidism as a condition of mental activity, as opposed to physical disability. Indeed, Martineau's analysis of her own introspective processes in sickness led her, ultimately, to argue for an ontology of being.

> If I were asked whether there is any one idea more potential than any other over every sort of suffering, in a mode of life like ours, most hearers of the question would make haste to answer for me that there is such a variety of potential ideas, suited to such wide differences of mood, of mind and body, that it must be impossible to measure the strength of any one. Nevertheless, I should reply that there is one, to me more powerful at present than I can now

conceive any single idea to have been in any former state of my mind. It is this;
that it matters infinitely less what we *do* than what we *are*. (155)

The "most hearers" that Martineau refers to here are evidently the healthy
readers to whom she so often addresses her narrative. The passage is striking in its
evocation of the invalid's subjectivity. Martineau constructs a hypothetical audience of healthy skeptics in order to affirm her self and the "state of [her] mind."
Distinguishing again, if implicitly, between her self and the self that others see,
she argues for an identity constituted not by actions but by ideas. She performs
through this self-representational strategy, in other words, the "intellectual
work" that so much of her other writing valorized.[25]

No matter what Martineau's intellectual achievements may have been with
Life in the Sickroom, there is no escaping the fact that it is one of her works least
familiar to scholars today, despite the fact that in her own time "it was widely
hailed as her most important and influential work" (Winter, 598). It is difficult to
assess the substantive impact that Martineau's work may have had on its readers.
In his 1883 biographical essay on Martineau, the indomitably cheerful Samuel
Smiles marveled that "even when laid on her bed by sickness, she went on
writing, as if it had become habitual to her, and then produced one of her most
delightful books, her 'Life in the Sick-Room.'"[26] *Life in the Sickroom* will hardly
strike modern readers as "delightful," and yet it should be understood not as an
isolated instance of an illness narrative but rather as one manifestation of a broad
cultural tapestry that evidences and helps to elucidate the Victorian fascination
both with the invalid, a figure who in Martineau's estimation demonstrates the
triumph of self-reliance, and with invalidism, a condition that Martineau argued
nurtures self-transformation. Problematizing the notion of self-reliance by arguing for its compatibility with passivity and simultaneously making more complex
a cultural understanding of submission, Martineau undermined social, medical,
and religious constructions of invalidism. While the history of medicine has
become a cornerstone of Victorian cultural studies, these studies have focused
almost exclusively on perspectives offered by the medical establishment. Illness
narratives told by invalids—precisely because they are, as Rita Charon rightly
anticipates, "Pressured, fragmented, resisted, and contradictory"—provide an
alternative entrée into the rich complexity of the individual experience and help
to explain why Harriet Martineau was "proud of the distinction" (vol. 1, 440).

NOTES

1. Bram Stoker, *Dracula* (1897; reprint, New York: Signet, 1992), 113.
2. Harriet Martineau, *Autobiography. With Memorials by Maria Weston Chapman,*

vol. 1 (Boston, MA: Houghton, Osgood, and Co., 1877), 440. References are to this edition and will be cited parenthetically in the text by volume and page number.

3. Miriam Bailin, *The Sickroom in Victorian Fiction: The Art of Being Ill* (London: Cambridge University Press, 1994), 3.

4. Athena Vrettos, *Somatic Fictions: Imagining Illness in Victorian Culture* (Stanford, CA: Stanford University Press, 1995), 180.

5. Bruce Haley, *The Healthy Body and Victorian Culture* (Cambridge, MA: Harvard University Press, 1978), 253.

6. Sheila Rothman, *Living in the Shadow of Death: Tuberculosis and the Social Experience of Illness in American History* (New York: Basic Books, 1994), 4.

7. See, for example, R. A. Proctor, "Bodily Illness as a Mental Stimulant," *Cornhill Magazine,* April 1870, 412–26.

8. Rita Charon, "Medical Interpretation: Implications of Literary Theory of Narrative for Clinical Work," *Journal of Narrative and Life History* 3, no. 1 (1993): 91.

9. Harriet Martineau, *Life in the Sickroom: Essays. By an Invalid* (Boston: Leonard C. Bowles, and William Crosby, 1844). All references are to this edition and will subsequently be cited parenthetically in the text.

10. Michel Foucault, *The Birth of the Clinic: An Archaeology of Medical Perception,* trans. A. M. Sheridan Smith (New York: Pantheon Books, 1973). References are to this edition and will be cited parenthetically in the text.

11. M. Jeanne Peterson, *The Medical Profession in Mid-Victorian London* (Berkeley, CA: University of California Press, 1978), 37.

12. For a good analysis of these movements, see Logie Barrow, "Why Were Most Medical Heretics at Their Most Confident around the 1840s? (The Other Side of mid-Victorian Medicine)," in *British Medicine in an Age of Reform,* ed. Roger French and Andrew Wear (New York: Routledge, 1991), 165–85.

13. Alison Winter, "Harriet Martineau and the Reform of the Invalid in Victorian England," *Historical Journal* 38, no. 3 (1995): 604. All references to this insightful article will subsequently be cited parenthetically within the text.

14. Alison Winter argues that Martineau constructed a sickroom "directly engaged in the world of public affairs" (613). I prefer to see Martineau's representation of the sickroom as epitomizing the hazy boundaries between the ostensibly separate public and private spheres of Victorian England.

15. Roy Porter and Dorothy Porter, *Patient's Progress: Doctors and Doctoring in Eighteenth-Century England* (Stanford, CA: Stanford University Press, 1989), 13.

16. Martineau's biographers suggest that her illness was at least in part psychosomatic. In *Harriet Martineau on Women* (New Brunswick, NJ: Rutgers University Press, 1985), Gayle Graham Yates notes that Martineau was found after she died to have suffered from an ovarian tumor but writes that "Her exhaustion and her volatile behavior in the publication of the mesmerism letters suggest that emotional distress was at least a part of her illness" (13).

17. Diana Postlethwaite, "Mothering and Mesmerism in the Life of Harriet Martineau," *Signs: Journal of Women in Culture and Society* 14, no. 3 (1989): 588.

18. Alexander Shand, "The Pleasures of Sickness," *Blackwood's Edinburgh Magazine,* April 1889, 546.

19. For an interesting take on the relationship between the duration of an illness and the constitution of invalidism, see G. Whyte-Melville, "A Week in Bed," *Fraser's Magazine for Town and Country,* March 1864, 327–35.

20. George Eliot, *Middlemarch* (1871–72; reprint, Harmondsworth, England: Penguin, 1965), 546. References are to this edition and will be cited parenthetically in the text.

21. For an excellent study of the context of hysteria informing Martineau's work as well as of Martineau's attitudes toward mesmerism, see Postlethwaite, "Mothering and Mesmerism," 588. Postlethwaite argues that Martineau "used mesmerism to explore the interactions of passivity and power through the inwardly directed, emotional self-exploration that characterized her illness" (604).

22. Gillian Thomas, "Harriet Martineau," in *Dictionary of Literary Biography: Victorian Prose Writers before 1867,* ed. William B. Thesing (Detroit, MI: Gale Research Co., 1987), 173.

23. For an elaboration of this compelling argument, see Deirdre David, *Intellectual Woman and Victorian Patriarchy: Harriet Martineau, Elizabeth Barrett Browning, George Eliot* (Ithaca, NY: Cornell University Press, 1982).

24. In this sense, Martineau's study is like the American writer Charlotte Perkins Gilman's story "The Yellow Wallpaper," which has now become a cornerstone of feminist literary criticism. I am grateful to a reader for the University of Michigan Press for calling my attention to how Gilman's story might also be read as a "Life in the Sickroom."

25. For a good study of Martineau's understanding of issues of self-reliance, see Ann Hobart, "Harriet Martineau's Political Economy of Everyday Life," *Victorian Studies* 37, no. 2 (1994): 223–51.

26. Samuel Smiles, "Harriet Martineau," in *Brief Biographies* (Chicago, IL: Belford, Clarke and Co., 1883), 499.

"It Is More than Lame" ► Female Disability, Sexuality, and the Maternal in the Nineteenth-Century Novel

Cindy LaCom

At the June 1994 Society for Disability Studies meeting, a lively discussion followed papers on representations of disability in literature and, specifically, on disability as metaphor. One member of the audience resented having her disability reduced to a mere metaphor and asked what it would take to escape such reductionism. It is a good question, one being confronted more and more often by people working both in disability studies and in literary criticism. In *Pride against Prejudice: Transforming Attitudes to Disability,* Jenny Morris discusses the use of physical disability as a marker of evil and abnormality in film and literature and concludes, "[t]he more disability is used as a metaphor for evil, or just to induce a sense of unease, the more the cultural stereotype is confirmed."[1]

Though I agree with Morris that disability has for too long been exploited as a metaphor and appreciate the concerns voiced at the conference, the fact remains that disability has historically been used as a signifier to construct cultural standards of "normalcy" in everything from human sexuality to criminal behavior. As Diane Price Herndl puts it, "Ideology makes its appearance in representations," and one such "representation" is the body.[2]

The absence of disabled bodies in literary texts has been noted (and lamented) by many. Certain theorists and critics do explore the meanings of the body (and to an extent, or by implication, disability) in literature and art (Luce Irigaray, Susan Bordo, Rosemarie Garland Thompson, Paul C. Higgins, Judith Butler, Thomas Laqueur, to name a few). But most texts that examine how disability makes meaning are political or medical in nature, aimed at creating and nurturing a new civil rights movement or at disrupting an old medical model of disability.[3]

But if ideology makes its appearance in representations, it also makes its appearance in the absence of representation, as Judith Butler notes in *Bodies That Matter: On the Discursive Limits of "Sex":*

> it will be as important to think about how and to what end bodies are constructed as it will be to think about how and to what end bodies are not constructed and, further, to ask after how bodies which fail to materialize provide the necessary "outside," if not the necessary support, for the bodies which, in materializing the norm, qualify as bodies that matter.[4]

Disabled bodies have not been entirely erased from fiction; they are there in textual margins, and as David Mitchell and Sharon Snyder have suggested, "physical deformity—in its omnipresent service to the engine of the narrative—ironically enjoys an endlessly textualized existence."[5] This is especially true in the nineteenth-century British novel, where disabled bodies begin to appear—and to be constructed (often in opposition to "healthy" bodies)—with some regularity.

That most of these bodies are female is no accident, for the appearance of fictional female characters with physical disabilities in the nineteenth-century novel signaled very real cultural fears about women, female sexuality, and the maternal. I want to suggest that writers inscribed changing ideologies about female sexuality and the maternal on women's bodies and that this inscription occurred in and on disabled female bodies as well as on "healthy" female bodies.

Deborah Kent, an activist in the disability rights movement, has pointed out that far too many female characters with physical disabilities make "indifferent heroines." Prejudice, fear, and literary tropes traditionally either make monstrous the woman with physical disabilities or else banish her entirely to fictional borders. But this is not always the case, and I want further to explore the ideological work of literature in the nineteenth century by focusing on the figure of the indifferent heroine.[6] Though many authors included representations of female characters with physical disabilities in their novels, I want to focus on two novels—Anthony Trollope's *Barchester Towers* (1857), and Charlotte Yonge's *The Clever Woman of the Family* (1865)—which offer very different depictions of disability and, in doing so, offer antithetical depictions of woman's "nature" and her proper role in life.

During the nineteenth century, a patriarchal society increasingly confined woman to the home, valorized her maternal functions, and cherished her beauty. Thus, physical disabilities that "disfigured" women and kept them from becoming mothers were literally and symbolically crippling, and writers like Trollope (re)inscribed a negative attitude by associating female disability with diseased female sexuality and suspect morality. Medical and religious assumptions that connected a "whole" body with a "wholesome" soul further exiled women with physical disabilities from the materialized "norm" that Judith Butler examines. Consequently, women incapable of overseeing the domestic sphere and bearing children faced pity, suspicion, and/or hostility.

The increasing inscription of women as mothers was caused, in large part, by political and economic changes that fostered the growth of a middle class during the eighteenth and nineteenth centuries.[7] Cultural attitudes toward women underwent extensive revision, and the female body became a primary site for much of that revision. Medical men began to focus almost obsessively on female flesh, bone, and sexual organs as explanations of woman's "nature," and a proliferation of medical texts valorized woman's womb and her reproductive capacities. Prior to the eighteenth century, male and female bodies were viewed hierarchically, as different but comparable. In fact, up until the beginning of the eighteenth century, there was no word for "vagina" in European medical vernacular, for female sexual organs were considered inverted male sexual organs.[8] Legal and political distinctions between men and women existed, but they were based on gender, not sex. Well past the Renaissance, medical men believed that "there was but one sex whose more perfect exemplars were easily deemed male at birth and whose decidedly less perfect ones were labeled female."[9]

During the eighteenth century, however, the reproductive organs in men and women came to be seen as absolutely different, and these differences had political, legal, and economic ramifications. In "Orgasm, Generation, and the Politics of Reproductive Biology," Thomas Laqueur suggests that changing political views during the Enlightenment focused on women's bodies to justify a patriarchal hierarchy.

In striking contrast to the old teleology of the body as male, liberal theory begins with a neuter body, sexed but without gender, and of no consequence to cultural discourse. The body is regarded simply as the bearer of a rational subject, which itself constitutes the person. The problem for this theory then is how to derive the real world of male dominion of women . . . The dilemma, at least for theorists interested in the insubordination of women, is resolved by grounding the social and cultural differentiation of the sexes in a biology of incommensurability that liberal theory itself helped bring into being.[10]

Thus, the political and philosophical trends of two centuries were articulated next to an increasingly dichotomous view of male and female bodies used to justify oppression of women.

Medical discourses lent themselves to such justification. During the eighteenth century, the female skeleton, which had not been sketched before and was not referred to in medical training, became a popular means by which to illustrate "essential" differences between the sexes. The first drawings of women's skeletons revealed smaller heads and larger hips (emphasizing her reduced brain size and her inborn capacity for childbearing). As Linda Schiebinger notes, "If sex differences could be found in the skeleton, then sexual identity would no longer be a matter of sex organs appended to a neutral body . . . but would penetrate every muscle, vein and organ attached to and molded by the skeleton."[11]

Eighteenth-century medical texts also included heated debates about breast-feeding, but as the ideology of the domestic sphere gained power, more and more medical men urged women to stay home to breast-feed their children.[12] The intrusion into and revision of women's bodies (and therefore woman's nature) continued in nineteenth-century texts that focused on menstruation, pregnancy, and menopause, and the importance of a woman's uterus in her biological economy gained a position of central importance.[13] The reduction of woman to womb taught that woman's nature was primarily maternal, and a celebration of woman as the "angel in the house," articulated in John Ruskin's *Sesame and Lilies,* became commonplace in middle class and upper class England.

If woman's maternal capacities came to signify her moral strengths, her body was nonetheless seen as hovering on the edges of hysteria since pregnancy and menses in Victorian England "came to be considered pathological conditions."[14] As a result, the nineteenth century witnessed the articulation of conflicting views of the female body: women's bodies were seen both as vessels of morality and as inherently diseased and unclean. In order to valorize women's moral superiority, her body could not be both at once. So women were increasingly placed in one of two camps: good women and bad. Good women were obedient daughters, submissive wives, and moral mothers. Reflecting the belief that "[U]ncleanliness of mind and body act and react . . . and the perfect health of one is incompatible with an unhealthy state of the other," good women were, above all, whole/some.[15] Their physical bodies reflected and were reflected in their moral strengths and their maternal capacities.

Thus, as the female body came to function as a representation of feminine morality, the disabled body was increasingly read as a sign of either sexlessness or sexual deviance. Each was accompanied by specific characteristics in most fictional representations of female disability. The sexless invalid was typically ethereal, generous, and generally removed from society. She moved into one of the few subject positions available to her (which, it is worth noting, continue to constrain women with physical disabilities today), outlined by Susan Browne, Debra Connors, and Nanci Stern: she is "the happy, humble woman who has 'accepted her handicap' and is endlessly grateful for the help of others."[16] Mrs. Smith of Jane Austen's *Persuasion* (1818), disabled and poverty stricken after her husband's death, gratefully accepts help from the heroine, Anne Elliot, who is awed by Mrs. Smith's "cheerfulness and mental alacrity."[17] Lavvie Blythe, in Wilkie Collins's novel *Hide and Seek* (1854) is a physically disabled (and childless) woman whose husband brings home a young circus girl (deaf and dumb) based on his belief that Lavvie will be a good adoptive mother because she has learned to cope with—even welcome—suffering and pain. Another female character, Harriet Martineau's *Maria Young of Deerbrook* (1839), acknowledges the drawbacks of her disability but accepts that she will never marry and positions herself entirely outside the realm of sexuality: "I am out of the game . . . Women who have what I am not to have, a home, an intimate, a perpetual call out of themselves, may go on more safely."[18]

On other occasions, the sexless invalid is "a good woman who [has] been

cruelly wronged and whose illness only reveal[s] her piety," though this pattern—
zealous piety to cope with cruelty—is more common in nineteenth-century
American sentimental novels than in English novels.[19]

The other representation of female characters with disabilities is that which
emphasizes sexual deviance, which plays up the connection between "deformed"
body and deformed principles. This character, bitter, angry, and manipulative,
might display blatantly erotic behavior, a "perversion" exacerbated by her remaining childless, since her "crippled" body is considered incapable of bearing
life. In the same way that England's "odd women" (also called surplus spinsters)
were exiled in the last forty years of the nineteenth century—to Australia and
America, primarily—the sexually deviant disabled female character is also often
banished from fictive texts. This is the case with Madeline Neroni, the dark
temptress of Anthony Trollope's *Barchester Towers*, who, after disrupting the
town of Barchester, departs for her Italian villa at the novel's close to allow the
restoration of communal harmony.

Why, though, does a happy ending require her absence? She has served a
narrative purpose in drawing together the hero and heroine, but beyond that, her
ability to sexually interest all men—from the local bishop to the novel's hero—
constitutes a threat to those institutions that regulate order in Barchester. Neroni
represents what D. A. Miller calls the "narratable": she creates "instances of
disequilibrium [and] suspense"[20] and, like the "foreign body" that Miller likens
to the narratable, must be "assimilated or expelled."[21] Since the former remains
impossible, and since "traditional novelists typically desire worlds of greater
stability and wholeness," Neroni is expelled.[22] Trollope's eradication of Madame
Neroni constitutes an attempt, I will argue, to diminish and dismiss cultural
anxiety around illness and, more specifically, around female sexuality.

Though Madame Neroni is generally cataloged among the "bad" women who
function didactically in Trollope's fiction, recent interpretations seek a more
subversive meaning in her character. The authors of *Corrupt Relations* argue that
Neroni undermines the traditional morality of the story and the heroine's rather
insipid goodness "[t]hrough her unconventional past, her sexuality, and her cyn-
icism about Barchester pieties."[23] In their discussion of Dickens, Thackeray,
Trollope, and Collins, the authors argue that each challenges one of the most
fundamental creeds of Victorian sexual orthodoxy:

> that the virtuous woman has a nearly sacred social power. By placing 'bad' or
> even criminal characters like . . . Madeline Neroni . . . in positions of power,
> they imply—however circumspectly—the radical idea that the 'good' woman
> has little real independence or power. And by representing the 'bad' woman as
> a victim of a cruelly oppressive sexual system, they undermine the orthodox
> position even further.[24]

The question of whether or not Madeline Neroni is a subversive character embodying a challenge to Victorian ideals of good womanhood cannot be addressed, however, without an explanation of "what she is." And too many discussions of her character marginalize or overlook entirely her physical disability.

Trollope himself does not, and that may be the best place to start. Our introduction to Neroni tells us two things: she is beautiful, and "her person for many years had been disfigured by an accident."[25] This paradox is worth considering in detail. Her personhood, apparently constituted by her physical body, is deformed, but despite this (or because of it) she is beautiful. Her beauty, which is overtly sexual, represents itself as a "disfigured" body. Though Trollope may appear to challenge cultural norms by making Neroni sexual, he also condemns female sexuality by implying that it is inherently deformed. And by collapsing the boundaries between her "person" and her disfigurement, Trollope takes the first step toward making female sexuality a kind of dis-ease.

Neroni's beauty receives detailed and thorough attention. Because she cannot move, her face and especially her eyes assume great significance.

> They were dreadful eyes to look at . . . Cruelty was there . . . and a desire of masterhood, cunning, and a wish for mischief. And yet, as eyes they were very beautiful. (185)

Thus a tendency toward mischief, masterhood, and cunning is added to disfigurement to constitute her beauty and personhood. Madeline Neroni's beauty, residing in an unwholesome physical frame, embodies traits that differentiate her from the Victorian "good woman" like Eleanor Bold, the novel's heroine, who, despite her name, is appropriately modest and chaste. Neroni's face and eyes initially constitute the bait with which she attracts her prey, and we are invited to agree that "with such charms still glowing in her face, and with such deformity destroying her figure, she should resolve to be seen, but only to be seen reclining on a sofa" (185).

The charms of her face are meant to solicit our gaze, which then remains fixed on Madame Neroni's whole "physical person." Though Madeline's resolution to be seen contradicts and undermines the concealment of her maimed limbs with a large shawl, Trollope's management of her disability also irrevocably directs our attention to it; though he appears to cover her disfigurement, he in fact returns our gaze to it again and again, prompting our (potentially uncomfortable) desire to uncover and really see her.

For instance, the flurry of activity that precedes her safe deposit on the sofa calls attention to her disability. Her placement requires a cortege to carry her in, "head foremost, her head being the care of her brother and an Italian manservant [and] her feet . . . in the care of the lady's maid and the lady's Italian page" (196). The theatricality of it all is made explicit when we are told that

Neroni's sister "followed to see that all was done with grace and decorum" (196). Being carted about is hardly graceful, however, and the aesthetic awkwardness attendant upon her transport and placement echoes the awkwardness of her "person," which "she could only drag . . . painfully along with protruded hip and extended foot, in a manner less graceful than that of a hunchback" (185).

Like Duessa of Spenser's *Fairie Queene,* who conceals a deformed and hideous body beneath glorious robes, Geraldine in Coleridge's "Christabel," and Miss Havisham in Dickens' *Great Expectations,* Madame Neroni tries to disguise her deformity under rich and beautiful clothing. We never see beneath her robes, however, for she, unlike Duessa, Geraldine, and Miss Havisham, never disrobes (or is disrobed). She is thus able, again unlike her deformed (and divested) fictional sisters, to retain her sexual allure throughout the novel and also to retain her physical/moral ambiguity.

But if the men of Barchester clamor about her, we are reminded that their awareness of her disability ultimately repulses as much as it attracts her admirers. Different from the Eastern veiled woman Elaine Showalter discusses in *Sexual Anarchy,* Madeline nonetheless embodies a mysterious sexuality that both attracts and terrifies men: "The male gaze . . . is both self-empowering and self-endangering, for what lies behind the veil is the specter of female sexuality, a silent and terrible mouth that may wound or devour the male spectator."[26] Though obscured by a satin shawl, the mouth, those terrible lips that can potentially devour men, resides in each man's consciousness. An exemplification of such attraction/repulsion, the character Mr. Slope is infatuated with Madeline's beauty but resists her, aware that she is "from misfortune unfitted to be chosen as the wife of any man who wanted a useful mate . . . that she was a helpless, hopeless cripple" (283).

And though she attracts men like Mr. Slope and even Arabin, she is aware that she can neither "eat them matrimonially" nor "devour them by any escapade of a less legitimate description" (283). Too, though she recoils from the thought of marriage and is asexual, she nonetheless ultimately mourns her exclusion from those roles so important to good women in Victorian England: wifedom and motherhood.

The unsightliness and demarcation that represent her disability and constrain and order her sexuality find their penultimate expression toward the novel's conclusion where, in a conversation with Eleanor Bold about Arabin, Neroni laments, "What I would not give to be loved . . . by such a man—that is, if I were an object fit for any man to love!" (391). In that single and singular sentence, Madeline for the only time in the course of the novel refers simultaneously to her disability, to sexuality, and to a desire for love. She sacrifices Arabin because she recognizes that he would never want her, despite his fascination with her. The final verdict on her situation, on her "person" and the realities it produces, are that she will never have what the typical, whole/some Victorian woman—and

Neroni at heart—wants: union with a good man and a body/object that can nurture such a union and produce the children so important to her role in the domestic sphere. In finally enunciating her "punishment," that exclusion from what she really wants, Madeline Neroni simultaneously defines and erases herself, thus becoming one of those "outside" bodies that help materialize the "norm" Butler refers to. Recognizing her drawbacks, diagnosing correctly her (non)place in Victorian society, she removes herself from Barchester and from "real" womanhood in the same moment. Thus is Neroni banished from Barchester, whose social health and soundness are only then reconstituted.

Charlotte Yonge's novel, *The Clever Woman of the Family*, is also about a community whose health grows infirm before it is healed. Her novel, like Trollope's, includes a female character who is disabled, unable to walk. Yet her treatment of and portrayal of Ermine Williams is vastly different from the portrayal of Madeline Neroni.

Yonge, like Trollope, was one of the most prolific and popular writers of her day. Like Trollope, she is considered a conservative novelist. But if, like Trollope, she enforces a belief that the good woman ought to submit to male authority and remain in the home, her depiction of Ermine Williams raises questions about Yonge's actual response to cultural attitudes toward women, infirmity, and disability.

In one of the very few book-length studies of Yonge, Catherine Sandbach-Dahlstrom argues that Yonge subverts patriarchal values by revealing the cost to women of "adjusting to the conservative ideology."[27] Sandbach-Dahlstrom further contends that Yonge's use of a Christian paradigm allows her to subvert conventional ideology by "elevating the women characters, and endorsing the value system that women represent"—in short, by showing how piety imbues women with power. I agree with Mary Jean Corbett that religion "enabled [women] . . . to write in ways that those who sought access to literary authority on secular grounds could not," and certainly, this kind of authority informs Yonge's fiction.[28]

But I am uncomfortable reducing Ermine Williams to a Christian female martyr whose moral character "elevates" her. Because it overlooks the meanings written into Yonge's construction of female disability in *Clever Woman*, this argument is incomplete. Ermine Williams's disability becomes a signifier for the potentialities of a woman in Victorian society, which move her well beyond martyrdom.

Like Madeline Neroni, Ermine Williams becomes disabled in young adulthood. She, like Madeline, has had the opportunity to fall in love, though her suitor's family boycotts their marriage, and the accident that causes Ermine's disability effectively ends her relationship with Colin Keith.

In the first half of the novel, Ermine is referred to as a "great invalid, quite a cripple;"[29] in relation to her sister Alison she is labeled "the sick sister" (17); and

Alison describes her as "poor patient Ermine" (41). Ermine refers to herself as an "old cinder" (44)—she is disabled in an explosion that burns her legs—but she responds with irony and resistance to her community's pity, unwilling to be so easily categorized. To disrupt such categorization, Yonge includes descriptions of Ermine as outspoken, one whose ability to make friends with all also makes her a mediator in quarrels, and one whose anonymous publications as the Invalid in literary quarterlies "have much influence over people's minds" (52). If Ermine Williams is "crippled," she is also popular and powerful.

Nonetheless, living with her disability entails, for Ermine as for Madeline, what Carol Gill calls "a different social identity."[30] The disabilities of each are regarded as signs that alienate them from the traditional roles of wife and mother. As with Madeline Neroni, whose "unfortunate affliction precluded her from all hope of levanting with a lover" (283) (and I can only assume that a very bad pun is intended here by Trollope), Ermine's disability is automatically assumed to bar her from the possibility of a sexual union. Her sister worries that Colin's kindness "only rendered Ermine's condition more pitiable" (69). Ermine's "condition" (consisting of both her disability and her single status) is such an essential aspect of her identity that her sister wonders how she can contemplate a romantic relationship.

In keeping with cultural codes, Ermine initially rejects Colin's marriage proposal on the grounds of her disability. But by the novel's end, she and Colin Keith have married and have adopted two children. Though Yonge does not "allow" Ermine to bear her own children, her adopted son's exclamation, "You are mother!" (365) nonetheless disrupts the cultural expectation that categorically consigned nonambulatory and infirm women to nonmaternal space.

In addition to successfully becoming wife and mother, Ermine also does work that replaces those two very traditional "jobs" for women: she writes. Though she retains her anonymity and explains the publication of her articles to Colin by noting that "One must live" (62), her reasons for writing extend beyond economic need. Her claim that "what began as . . . a need to say out one's mind has become a resource for which we are thankful" (62) complicates Ermine's motives for writing: she must support herself, but she must also speak her mind. Like Yonge herself, Ermine writes because she enjoys it and takes pride in her vocation. And though she uses a pseudonym for publication (as did many real-life women writers in the nineteenth century), she arguably names herself by publishing as the Invalid and simultaneously revises traditional connotations attached to invalidism by writing articles that are regarded as astute and influential.

Though her writing does not define her in the eyes of her community, it defines her in our eyes, in the eyes of her lover, and in her own. Her writing is what ultimately distinguishes her from Rachel Curtis, the not-so-clever heroine of the novel's title, who, after a shot at independence, confesses that "a woman's tone of thought is commonly moulded by the masculine intellect, which, under one form or another, becomes the master of her soul" (337). However, Ermine has had little such masculine guidance; her father died, and her brother left before she began writing and publishing. She tells Colin that Rachel is "just what I should have been without Papa and Edward to keep me down" (95), but it is only after Papa and Edward are gone, when she is no longer "kept down," that Ermine becomes truly independent.

Ermine, unlike Madeline Neroni, need not be "put outside the boundaries of the community, outside its middling 'marches.'"[31] Her continued presence in the community indicates that Ermine, unlike Madeline, has become a marker not of dis-ease but of a kind of health and wholeness. Yonge's enunciation of an ideology that values a woman's independence and celebrates a wholeness based not solely on corporeal parts but also on intellectual and emotional facilities revises Trollope's world, where disability and its diseased sexuality is exiled and replaced by the whole body and wholesome/nonsexual beauty of Eleanor Bold.

Resolution of communal anxiety about Ermine's disability occurs when she assumes the acceptable roles of wife and mother. Though her new titles reinforce conservative Victorian ideology that consigned woman to home and defined her in terms of husband and children, Yonge nevertheless revises cultural assumptions about the disabled woman and collapses Trollope's equation of female sexuality and female "deformity." Yonge refuses to reduce Ermine to either a spiritualized being whose self-effacing behavior apparently explains a lack of sexual desire or to a monstrous creature whose body, being all, transforms her into a kind of sexual black widow. Instead, Yonge begins to confront social anxiety around women's infirmity and female sexuality by uniting both in Ermine Williams while celebrating her continued vocation as a writer. Refusing to reduce woman to mere legs and limb, Yonge ultimately challenges us to see more than just the "person" of Ermine Williams.

Ermine's move into the realm of sexuality and her inclusion as an integral part of her community constitute signs of hope and a deconstruction of cultural norms. It is fair to say that Yonge uses Ermine's disability as metaphor and that I choose to read it as such. Writing about the "realities" of her disability—the daily tasks of getting out of bed, bathing herself, preparing meals, confronting discrimination (which for the most part occurs offscreen)—is difficult, if not impossible, because of Victorian taboos against detailed descriptions of any bodily act not public and "appropriate." Sexual scenes are always coded (this is true even in seduction novels, though works like *My Secret Life*, pornographic memoirs published anonymously at the end of the nineteenth century, were very explicit about sexual acts),[32] and details about childbearing, breast-feeding, even dressing are vague, if they are included at all. I have never read a Victorian novel where a character urinates, brushes her teeth, or clips her toenails.

Given that descriptions of such acts are censored, it is impossible to get the "true" story of female disability in nineteenth-century England (or of women's lives in general, perhaps). It is possible, however, to explore the intersections between disability, female sexuality, and the maternal and to read disability both literally and as a metaphor that makes meaning. A metaphoric reading of female disability may reinforce sexual and social myths. But it also offers critical insights into how woman's "nature" and her "person" have been historically constructed and, in so doing, allows us to reread literature's "indifferent heroines" and to reassess the very important stories they tell.

NOTES

1. Jenny Morris, *Pride against Prejudice: Transforming Attitudes to Disability* (Philadelphia, PA: New Society Publishers, 1991), 93.

2. Diane Price Herndl, *Invalid Women: Figuring Feminine Illness in American Fiction and Culture, 1840–1940* (Chapel Hill, NC: University of North Carolina Press 1993), 8–9.

3. For discussions of this absence of disability in literature, see Morris, *Pride against Prejudice*; Editorial, Elspeth Morrison, *Feminist Arts News* 2, no. 10 and Deborah Kent, "In Search of a Heroine: Images of Women with Disabilities in Fiction and Drama," in *Women with Disabilities* (Philadelphia, PA: Temple University Press, 1988) for further discussion of the depiction (or lack thereof) of disabled women in literature.

A sampling of texts that discuss disability from more political or medical positions include Mary Jo Deegan and Nancy A. Brooks, *Women and Disability: The Double Handicap* (New Brunswick, NJ: Transaction Books, 1985); Claire H. Liachowitz, *Disability as Social Construct: Legislative Roots* (Philadelphia, PA: Pennsylvania University Press, 1988); Martha Minow, *Making All the Difference: Inclusion, Exclusion and American Law* (Ithaca, NY: Cornell University Press, 1990); and Joseph Shapiro, *No Pity: People with Disabilities Forging a New Civil Rights Movement* (New York: Times Books/Random House, 1993).

4. Judith Butler, *Bodies That Matter: On the Discursive Limits of "Sex"* (New York: Routledge, 1993), 16.

5. David Mitchell and Sharon Snyder, "Narrative Prosthetics: Postmodern Discourses of Disability in Film, Theory, and the Arts," in *End Results and Starting Points: Expanding the Field of Disability Studies,* ed. Elaine Makas and Lynn Schlesinger (Portland, ME: The Society for Disability Studies and the Edmund S. Muskie Institute of Public Affairs 1996), 211–13.

6. Deborah Kent, "In Search of a Heroine: Images of Women with Disabilities in Fiction and Drama," in *Women with Disabilities: Essays in Psychology, Culture and Politics,* ed. Adrienne Asch and Michelle Fine (Philadelphia, PA: Temple University Press, 1988).

7. In *Desire and Domestic Fiction: A Political History of the Novel* (New York: Oxford University Press, 1987), Nancy Armstrong discusses the intersections between novels, conduct literature, and the growth of the middle class. She argues that prior to the eighteenth century, England's rural economy had allotted women's traditional work some

value. Their labor—making butter, selling eggs, weaving, tending livestock—contributed to a household's economic stability. But in the eighteenth and nineteenth centuries, numerous factors occasioned a decreasing valuation of women's work. Two contributed most significantly to the change: the population shift from the country to rapidly growing cities due to the advent of the industrial revolution, and the rise of the middle class.

The woman who remained at home became a symbol of middle class status, and her sole "employment" became that of domestic management. Where conduct books for women had previously included "advice for the care of livestock or the concoction of medicinal cures" (67), in the eighteenth century they increasingly focused on the proper care of husband and children.

8. See Thomas Laqueur, *Making Sex: Body and Gender from the Greeks to Freud* (Cambridge, MA: Harvard University Press, 1990), especially chapters two and three.

9. Ibid., 134–42.

10. Thomas Laqueur, "Orgasm, Generation, and the Politics of Reproductive Biology," in *The Making of the Modern Body: Sexuality and Society in the Nineteenth Century,* ed. Catherine Gallagher and Thomas Laqueur (Cambridge, MA: Harvard University Press, 1987), 19.

11. Linda Schiebinger, "Skeletons in the Closet: The First Illustrations of the Female Skeleton in Eighteenth-Century Anatomy," in *The Making of the Modern Body: Sexuality and Society in the Nineteenth Century,* ed. Catherine Gallagher and Thomas Laqueur (Cambridge, MA: Harvard University Press, 1987), 53.

12. See Elizabeth Kowaleski-Wallace, *Their Mother's Daughters: Hannah More, Maria Edgeworth, and Patriarchal Complicity* (Oxford: Oxford University Press, 1991); and, for information on the controversy over breast-feeding versus wet nursing in America during the nineteenth century, see Barbara Ehrenreich and Deirdre English, *For Her Own Good: 150 Years of the Experts' Advice to Women* (New York: Doubleday, 1978). Ehrenreich and English discuss the increased control of male doctors in the realm of childbirth in the nineteenth century in "Witches, Midwives, and Nurses." Attempts to eradicate midwifery, historically practiced by women, were largely successful, and by the beginning of the twentieth century, the delivery of infants was practiced almost solely by licensed medical men.

13. Sally Shuttleworth discusses at length the place of menstruation in nineteenth-century medical discourses in her excellent article, "Female circulation: Medical Discourse and Popular Advertising in the mid-Victorian Era," in *Body/Politics: Women and the Discourses of Science,* ed. Mary Jacobus et al. (New York: Routledge, 1990). See also Mary Poovey, "'Scenes of an Indelicate Character': The Medical 'Treatment' of Victorian Women," in *The Making of the Modern Body,* ed. Catherine Gallagher and Thomas Laqueur (Berkeley, CA: University of California Press, 1987); and Elaine Showalter, *The Female Malady: Women, Madness, and English Culture* (New York: Penguin, 1985).

14. Diane Price Herndl focuses on images of the invalid woman in Victorian and modern American literature in *Invalid Women,* 26.

15. Quoted in Bruce Haley, *The Healthy Body and Victorian Culture* (Cambridge, MA: Harvard University Press, 1978), 23.

16. Susan Browne, Debra Connors, and Nanci Stern, eds., *With the Power of Each Breath* (San Francisco, CA: Cleis Press, 1985), 77.

17. Jane Austen, *Persuasion* (1818; reprint, New York: New American, 1980), 239.

18. Harriet Martineau, *Deerbrook* (1839; reprint, New York: Dial Press, 1984), 35.

19. Herndl, *Invalid Women*, 50.

20. D. A. Miller, *Narrative and Its Discontents: Problems of Closure in the Traditional Novel* (Princeton, NJ: Princeton University Press, 1981), 17.

21. Ibid., 117.

22. Ibid., 265.

23. Richard Barikman, Susan McDonald, and Myra Stark, eds., *Corrupt Relations: Dickens, Thackeray, Trollope, Collins, and the Victorian Social System* (New York: Columbia University Press, 1982), 204.

24. Ibid., 9.

25. Anthony Trollope, *The Warden and Barchester Towers* (1857; reprint, New York: Book League, 1942), 184. All future references will be cited parenthetically in the text.

26. Elaine Showalter, *Sexual Anarchy: Gender and Culture at the Fin de Siècle* (New York: Viking, 1990), 146.

27. Catherine Sandbach-Dahlstrom, *Be Good Sweet Maid: Charlotte Yonge's Fiction* (Stockholm: Almquist, 1984), 106.

28. Mary Jean Corbett, *Representing Femininity: Middle-Class Subjectivity in Victorian and Edwardian Women's Autobiographies* (Oxford: Oxford University Press, 1992), 75.

29. Charlotte Yonge, *The Clever Woman of the Family* (1865; reprint, New York: Virago, 1985), 31. All future references will be cited parenthetically in the text.

30. Carol Gill, "What Doctors Didn't Want to Know," in *The Disability Rag* (May/ June 1992): 12.

31. Miller, *Narrative and Its Discontents*, 115.

32. In *The Other Victorians: A Study of Sexuality and Pornography in Mid-Nineteenth-Century England* (New York: Bantam Books, 1967), Steven Marcus examines Victorian views of sexuality through a reading of a variety of sexual discourses to argue that Victorian pornography "had a historical meaning and even a historical function" (288). For further information on the proliferation of pornography in Victorian England, see also Ronald Pearsall, *The Worm in the Bud: The World of Victorian Sexuality* (New York: Penguin Books, 1969); and Kellow Chesney, "Prostitution," chap. 10 in *The Victorian Underworld* (New York: Schocken Books, 1972).

The "Talking Cure" (Again) ▶ Gossip and the Paralyzed Patriarchy

Jan Gordon

Lawrence's most startling variation of the Sleeping Beauty theme deals with the archetypal modern woman whose husband practices two professions Lawrence despised: industrialism and intellectualism. Regrettably for the story, Sir Clifford Chatterley is also a cripple . . . That it was a war wound that paralyzed Clifford deepens the symbol, yet in itself it is a poor one, for Lawrence's fable. It would have been a stronger story if Lawrence had made Clifford's lack of sex the result of overintellectualism: there was a suggestion of this early in the book, in the character of Michaelis, with whom Connie had a love affair before she met the gamekeeper.[1]

Harry T. Moore, an influential early critic of D. H. Lawrence's work, would locate the thematic weakness of *Lady Chatterley's Lover* in Sir Clifford's *disability.* Whereas the physically localized and historically determined handicap might evoke the sensitive reader's genuine sympathy for the "betrayed" heir, the mental impairment of overintellectualism would displace any literal disability in the "cultural body" of late empire. In allegorizing the physical dysfunction as in reality a cultural malaise, Moore himself would be numbered among those Lawrence would have condemned as substituting the head for the body. Once the dysfunction was so allegorized, however, readers would cease to think of the *disability* save as an appendage of history. The critic here, as is so often the case, acts as a coconspirator in the repression of the physical.

This critical strategy is all too familiar to students of British romanticism. During the late 1960s and early 1970s, several leading critics identified the operations of the natural world with a special kind of romantic imagination. In commentary, they often overlooked the price paid for such an easy allegorization of natural processes: once a cloud becomes a synecdoche for mutability or a River Duddon in Wordsworth's sonnets for a specific representation of temporality, clouds and rivers cease to exist as merely natural phenomena but are experienced only under some emotional erasure. This strategically "denatured nature" participates in the very crisis to which it testifies. For, once made a product of the transforming poetic imagination, the experience of any spontaneous joy of first exposures is forever foreclosed in much romantic poetry. The natural world, once subjected to the romantic tendency to allegorize this exposure as therapeutic, must come to function in a secondary capacity, like Wordsworth's "foster mother," entrusted only with mollifying an imprisoning amnesia.[2]

As the British romantic poets often denatured nature in the process of endowing her with "extranatural" meanings—thereby conspiring with the very practices of the industrial revolution that they otherwise sought to condemn—so critics of the novel often fold corporeal dysfunction within some larger historical crisis *under which* it comes to be read. This tendency may well represent a sophisticated denial of both the specific dysfunction and any consideration of the comparative benefits of specific therapies that a belief in historical or social determinism might not countenance. It may also account for the relative immunity to disciplined study that narratives of disability seem to enjoy in our critical culture. Weakness or dysfunction in the cultural or critical body is, after all, traditionally resistant to all save the most invasive of therapies: revolution or some alternative redistribution of the currents of lifeblood of power.[3]

Our initial response to disability all too often alternates between two related reflexes, each of which would deny it a functional, continuing, narrative presence. The ocular stare would "fix" handicapped individuals as discontinuities. As with the close reading of any text, we presume to look *behind* the specific disability to a recuperable cause or moment of instantiation: how did one get that way? The handicapped individual thereby becomes the repository of some secret that can only be re-covered as a special, "readerly" interpretation that privileges the metaphorical as opposed to the metonymic syntagmatic order.[4] Or, alternatively, the dysfunctional body is experienced as a reflexive "turning away," the averted gaze that renders the presence of the disabled visually, rather than historically, discontinuous. Both the stare and the averted gaze deny the narrative of disability a place alongside other narratives that it would complement, illuminate, or even deconstruct.

Were Sir Clifford Chatterley's wound a symbolic manifestation of the twentieth-century penchant for overintellectualism, an affliction of the head, then some variant of the Rousseau Treatment, like that which the gamekeeper Mellors administers to the equally self-conscious Lady Chatterley, might be therapeutically indicated. And yet, in the novel Lawrence wrote, as opposed to the one the author of *The Intelligent Heart* would have had him write, Sir Clifford's therapy assumes an altogether different, even oppositional, course from hers. A little less self-consciousness and conversation *about* sexual "matters" and more attention to "acts" may in fact have been an effective prescription for marital ennui among the members of the Chatterley's social class accustomed to brisk walks, country air, and the odd vacation in Biarritz.[5] But neither forgetting the head nor exercising the body is viable therapy for Sir Clifford's more focused complaint, nor its easy accommodation by more traditional images of a paralyzed patriarchy.

And yet, Sir Clifford Chatterley too is helped by a therapy as radical in its own way as that which Mellors brings to Lady Chatterley. Traditionally, however, this therapeutic intervention in his physically impaired condition has been overlooked by generations of Lawrence's literary critics who have customarily found Lady Chatterley's being "out of touch" more accessible to narratives of liberation than that of Sir Clifford, the gentleman confined to a wheelchair. Disabilities of the heart and head are apparently more amenable to both critical and therapeutic intervention. Perhaps it is for this very reason that some "conversion" of physical disability to either a moral impairment or a defect of consciousness occurs so often in nineteenth-century British fiction. This tendency *becomes* a discipline of course in Freud's *Studies on Hysteria,* whose fin de siècle composition places it in a chronological cusp between say, Dickens or George Eliot and Lawrence's achievement in *Lady Chatterley's Lover.* When the traumatic agent thought to be responsible for corporeal pain is miraculously converted to, first, an agent provocateur and then to a double agent that transforms bodily pain into a historically misplaced symbolization, the "talking cure," by which psychoanalysis emerges as a distinctive discipline, becomes a potential intervention.[6]

Because the radical Protestantism that informs so much of the history of British fiction dictates that physical disabilities or dysfunctions represent an inherited share in some spiritually originary deformity or disobedience—that "turning away from God's grace" that was, even etymologically, the per*version* of Adam and Eve—we might logically enough expect narratives of disability and their prescribed therapies to have a shared instrumental function within some larger, totalizing narrative. If a specific handicap thus functions as a mark of the distance separating full divine or social acceptance (sanction), therapeutic narratives, insofar as they address moral or spiritual dysfunction as collateral to the physical complaint, might guide (or misguide) our reading. Often, as we shall see, some obscure voice, previously denied or repressed, is crucial to these therapeutic narratives. If some inner voice, often indistinguishable from a dialogic encounter with the divine in Protestant theology, often ministers to the spiritually downtrodden or morally infirm, so some attendant voice, ministering to the disabled but frequently indistinguishable from its repressed self-interest, comes to be allied with narratives of disability.

A model text may be Charlotte Bronte's *Jane Eyre,* wherein Rochester's history of spiritual and material self-indulgence is punished by a fire that leaves his body disabled and his estate in ruins. This doubly deformed patriarchy paradoxically enables him to marry his former governess turned heiress by making his moral-physical incapacitation equivalent to her (previous) incapacity of social rank. The emergent marital economy of compensation is signaled by the mysterious call of a voice in the night, by which the lovers summon each other. This inner voice is nothing less than the symbolic release of the repressed screams of hidden madness in the attic on the one hand and Jane Eyre's missionary zeal on the other, each of which as an alternative "calling" had threatened to render the partners ineligible for a legal marriage. Rochester needs her voice as a therapeutic eye, given his partial spiritual and physical blindness. And a marriage with one's therapeutic attendant cum guide civilizes what had been either a socially threatening relationship or no relationship at all as a Florence Nightingale marriage.

A similar kind of conversational attentiveness will become instrumental in converting the paralyzed Sir Clifford Chatterley. Ivy Bolton, the woman from Tevershall initially brought in by Lady Chatterley to assist her in the care of a disabled husband, at the outset appears as one more of Lawrence's highly self-conscious modern women, not unlike Constance Chatterley in fact.

> Mrs. Bolton was admirable in many ways. But she had that queer sort of bossiness, endless assertion of her own will, which is one of the signs of insanity in modern woman.[7]

Before the reader encounters Mellors, quite laconic by comparison, Mrs. Bolton is nonetheless the only life at Wragby Hall. Before her arrival as a hands-on health care professional (she has a qualification as a nurse and has previously attended the ill miners in Sir Clifford's employ), the ancestral Chatterley estate, denuded of its large oaks for trench timber during the Great War, has become the "weary warren" (VI, 65) of a now discontinuous succession. Encompassing both literally and figuratively bleak prospects of ever more marginally productive Midland coal pits, the familial seat has long since ceased to be a place of either contemplation or vision.

At virtually every turn, Lawrence suggests that the inmates of Wragby Hall and their frequent weekend guests do not suffer from overintellectualism but from its antipode: the confines of a newly "narrow 'great world'" (I, 44), a wonderful euphemism for the confined vistas of what had formerly constituted the nation's landed patriarchy. With rents no longer sufficient to cover their elegant lifestyle, Sir Clifford has turned to writing amateur stories and light journalism for the "illustrated papers," the forerunners of contemporary British tabloids, through which he supplements the Wragby living. Private theatricals and Lady Chatterley's nightly readings from the classics complete what passes for intellectual activity, which mirrors the confinements of Sir Clifford's physical existence.

The lack of stimulation to both head and body is what initially leads Lady Chatterley to engage Mrs. Bolton to minister to Sir Clifford's physical and, after she learns how to type, intellectual needs. Lawrence makes it quite clear that in fact Mrs. Bolton and Lady Chatterley effectively change places. For not only has Mrs. Bolton been enamored of Mellors in his youth but she literally, as Lady Chatterley has done metaphorically, has *lost* her husband to the mines as a result of an industrial accident. Lady Chatterley takes Sir Clifford's hired man, as it were, and Sir Clifford commences an affair with her amanuensis—at the outset symbolically equivalent infidelities among the gentry with those committed to its rehabilitation.

> Clifford, however, inside himself, never quite forgave Connie for giving up her personal care of him to a strange hired woman. It killed, he said to himself, the real flower of the intimacy between him and her. But Connie didn't mind that. The fine flower of their intimacy was to her rather like an orchid, a bulb stuck parasite on her tree of life. (86)

Though readers, literary critics, and the judiciary have all taken a keen interest in the details of Lady Chatterley's sexual awakening from the sterility of Wragby Hall and her own frigidity (and Lawrence to his credit keeps them thematically separate but equal), no critic discusses her husband's renewed capacity for human intimacy in the absence of Lady Chatterley, a transformation explicitly detailed in the novel. Is this oversight a consequence of our inability to imagine a story line for Clifford Chatterley beyond or outside his physical incapacitation? If such were indeed the case, then Sir Clifford's disability not only prevents authentic sexual and intellectual engagement but any critical encounter as well. The reader would be absolved, as D. H. Lawrence clearly was not, from judging or even caring about his rehabilitation. The paralyzed knight-errant from the Great War would remain, as has been his historical fate, a kind of shut-in from whom we avert our critical eyes.

Yet, the example of Lady Chatterley would suggest that this need not be the case at all. For, were the particular disability to be internalized so that the shattered body we see is symbolic of some larger, perhaps collective, social dysfunction (such as overintellectualism perhaps) that could be revealed, then that very revelation would come to be identified with a therapeutic procedure and not seen merely as an act of discovery. The complaint that renders the individual dysfunctional must be *seen to be hidden*. This anomaly is certainly applicable to Lady Chatterley's situation. Her vague longing for a genuine wider world, suggested in increasingly long walks through the ancestral estate and the sickly pallor that alarms her friends, would seem to indicate not an identifiable illness or disability but a *syndrome*. By contrast, the cause of Sir Clifford's paralysis is so transparent and his dependencies so obvious as to leave virtually no room for critical interpretation. He is altogether too *marked* by his disability. Or is he?

Because the disabled individual so often suffers from pain that is visible to himself and others either directly or indirectly—in the obvious limitations to free movement, the burden of prosthetic devices or continuous medication, or self-consciousness at the way these restrictions are perceived by others—the disabled body is more *open* to at least the illusion of continuous surveillance that is often masked as care or concern but that may be prurient. And it is surely this very *openness,* the *publicité* of dysfunction, that would seem to conspire against the secret, interior life or self that, as Charles Taylor has reminded us, has been the traditional fount of freedom in the Western liberal imagination.[8] The release of Clifford Chatterley's interiority, as a consequence of Mrs. Bolton's dialogic ministrations, is a task no less difficult than that by which Mellors touches Lady Chatterley's "interior space," equally hidden behind the demands of social existence and its assorted crutches, which have made her too into a glossy text, all surface, for the illustrated papers.

The gossip's access to a celebrity she would otherwise never come to know and Sir Clifford's access to a village life from which his estate has kept him forever distant create a *relationship* as radical as that of Connie and her gamekeeper. It should, by all odds, evoke a similar interest in the reader, and yet the critical silence regarding it would suggest otherwise. Although they do not bedeck each other's bodies with flowers, the thrill is there once gossip is perceived as defining an erogenous zone.

> She was thrilled to a weird passion. And his "educating" her roused in her a passion of excitement and response much deeper than any love affair could have done. In truth the very fact that there could be no love affair left her free to thrill her very marrow with this other passion, the peculiar passion for knowing, *knowing* as he knew. There was no mistake that the woman was in some way in love with him: whatever force we give to the word love. (104)

If *Lady Chatterley's Lover* is indeed the hymn in praise of the liberated body unfettered by psychological disabilities, what are we to make of this other passion between Sir Clifford and his hired nurse, which transcends class and educational barriers as surely as the more conventional passion of Connie and Mellors? If the very impossibility of conventional sexual intercourse is itself erotic, then the social revolution symbolized by Lady Chatterley's flight is thematically unnecessary. Lawrence's novel would then appear less *necessarily* revolutionary and perhaps more the forerunner of a novel like Nicholson Baker's *Vox,* where "talking about it" so completely displaces the sexual act that intercourse remains the only nonerotic activity left in the modern world. In other words, the political and sexual revolution that Lawrence's achievement would seem to advocate is mediated by another interest: the possibility of alternative therapies that mime some of the symptoms of the disability—just as immunization is often effected by administering a measured dose of the illness to the patient. If the love affair of Lady Chatterley and the gamekeeper has its memorably "kinky" moments (appending flowers to sexual organs as part of foreplay), the parallel relationship of the clingy Ivy Bolton and Sir Clifford Chatterley constitutes, at least in Lawrence's narrative, an "intimacy of perversity" (303) which begs the reader's comparison of respective therapeutic regimens for the differentially disabled.

After all, from her initial delight in "having his body in her charge" (103), Mrs. Bolton advances to genuine conversational intimacies of the very sort with which Constance Chatterley has always felt insecure, avoiding as she does the compulsory after-dinner chats at Wragby Hall with the excuse of chronic headaches. Gossip has succeeded where conventional lovemaking techniques are either irrelevant or not applicable, given Sir Clifford's war injury. Gossip is as much a *transaction* as traditional sexual intercourse, and, if we critics admit Mellors's reticence and working class verbal ellipses as instrumental to Lady Chatterley's transformation, then we must tolerate Mrs. Bolton's excessive talkativeness as having a potentially similar appeal for Lady Chatterley's husband. And though Sir Clifford's appetite for the consumption of village gossip from his nurse/caretaker may seem narcissistic or at least self-reflexive given the fact that he readily consumes the same genre of which he has been a primary producer, Lady Chatterley's sexual awakening also requires heightened self-esteem. There could be no better expression of the extent to which the British landed aristocracy, though in love with itself, was deficient in the knowledge of how to love itself *differently* in the light of reduced public demand for its services.

The same gossip that would condemn Lady Chatterley's behavior—for her affair will become "Tevershall talk" by the end of *Lady Chatterley's Lover* — would function as an agent of therapeutic liberation for the disabled patriarch, freeing him from the narrow space into which history, as both family fortune and the catastrophic effects of war, has plunged his body and spirit. In contradistinction to the geographically centered noble estate or the historically continuous noble family name, gossip testifies to the impossibility of recovering an antecedent narrative appropriate to other representations of sterility in *Lady Chatterley's Lover*. Approximately contemporaneous with Lawrence's novel, Martin Heidegger was to condemn the operational dynamics of gossip under the word *Gerede:* the uprooted idle talk that floats homelessly about modern culture, much as the orphan or uprooted gentry does in nineteenth-century British fiction.[9] This discourse is possessed without really making it one's own, as it is perpetually passed on.

If gossip were simultaneously the cure for a paralysis that chronically afflicts the British patriarchy, and also the public response that would condemn an equally radical therapy, then this discursive attention would leave nothing outside itself. The cure, if not worse than the illness, would be indistinguishable from it, insofar as it *marks* or otherwise identifies its presence. And, because gossip is one possible representation of what we designate as *public* opinion, its therapeutic application comes to be virtually indistinguishable from some communal pain suffered not merely by a single privileged class but by everyone. The disability would have gone public in some double sense: it is simultaneously a social reproduction of the Other's pain—at least metaphorically the agent by which it is spread as a contagion—and yet, crucial to the pain's management, if not its containment.

The tendency to attribute the physical or emotional disabilities of the privileged to overintellectualism has a long tradition in European literature. And just as frequently, the "small talk"—a wonderful euphemism for gossip—that would otherwise disgust and devalue the participants as intrusive or otherwise demeaning comes to be enlisted as a therapy of choice. This is perhaps nowhere better illustrated than in that other "talking cure" applied in various incarnations to that most exquisite of patriarchal disabilities, gout, in British fiction preceding that of Lawrence.

If—to slightly amend Susan Sontag—it is not the specific nature of an illness but rather the way in which its "legible disabilities" come to be read that endows it with a unique periodicity, then the paralyses of gout would appear to qualify as the patriarchal infirmity par excellence of the eighteenth and nineteenth centuries.[10] Its victims included Dr. Johnson and Dean Swift and later, to judge from his diet, Emma Woodhouse's father, Charles Darwin, and the expatriate Joseph Conrad, who was particularly vulnerable to its attacks when J. M. Dent's deadline for manuscript submissions was not met. Medically, gout is a metabolic disorder characterized by hyperuricemia due to the excessive production or decreased excretion of uric acid, which is deposited as sharp crystals in the soft tissues. About twenty percent of gout patients report that an immediate male ancestor was also afflicted, an incidence that, though not really higher than that occurring with other metabolic disorders (say diabetes), is sufficient to have lent the illness the dimensions of an inheritable property.[11] A hobbled Sir Leicester Dedlock of Dickens' *Bleak House,* married to a much younger, elusive woman, can keep up with neither her shadowy movements nor her fears, gripped as he is by what Dickens terms the "demon of the patrician order."

> Other men's fathers may have died of the rheumatism, or may have taken contagion from the tainted blood of the sick vulgar, but the Dedlock family have communicated something exclusive, even to the levelling process of dying, by dying of their own family gout.[12]

Sir Leicester Dedlock's illness is all the more significant since *Bleak House* is a novel wherein the "tainted blood of the sick vulgar," embodied in the contagion of smallpox that passes from Jo the Crossing Sweeper to the narrator, Esther Summerson, threatens to make no social distinctions among those it would inscribe. Sir Leicester Dedlock's odd gait, then, like that other gate to Chesney Wold, barred to the prospective easements of the ill rabble, would signify a quasi-incestuous familial narrative. Consanguineous marriages arranged among descendants of the same family tree in an attempt to preserve wealth have perpetuated gout so that it is passed along in successive generations. Like the family plate and the portraits of successive Lady Dedlocks that grace the mantelpiece at Chesney Wold, the disability serves as an heirloom. In the imagination of the eighteenth and nineteenth centuries, gout was only internally communicable, maybe even a "countersyphilis." If that particular social disease (syphilis) was contracted by figuratively straying too far from one's own family (or its internalized social preferences and values), so gout was a similar judgment upon economically and socially incestuous investment practices: the pain attendant upon liking too much of the identical good things. Social recuperation, financial accumulation, overintellectualism, and fluid retention were thereby thematically aligned.

Hence, in British literature and visual art, gout has characteristically been an accompaniment to luxuriant consumption and self-indulgence. In Hogarth the complaint assumes a moral dimension as a corpulent companion to Sloth, and in Rowlandson's 1799 engraving *The Gout*, the painful immobility is represented by a red, swollen toe (doubly so, since it rests upon an equally oversized Georgian settee) being invaded by a fiery Satan with long, lean talons. Gout then is, to be sure, a moral visitation of the same sort that Harry T. Moore would have preferred to have Sir Clifford Chatterley suffer rather than the more bathetic war wound that preserves for Sir Clifford a modicum of reader sympathy. For only if the narrative of disability is converted to or otherwise imagined to be a retribution for some identifiable moral transgression can it *justify* an unhappy wife's sexual redemption. Moral transgressions are deserved (and hence redeemable) only when the individual bears some responsibility for his disability, a responsibility difficult to represent in the arbitrary forces of history or their corollary, military attack.

In both *Lady Chatterley's Lover* and the various "gout wards" that figuratively (and occasionally literally) recur in British novels of the eighteenth and nineteenth centuries, narratives of *physical disability* come to be partially attributable to some noncirculating *surplus*. Though clinically what one inherits is the *susceptibility* to an adverse response to an excess of urates, the cultural representations of the complaint often displace the course of the malady onto its effective *cause*; it is as if diabetes were defined as the consequence of an excessive desire for sugar! One suspects that the Renaissance model of the human body (as a repository of circulating humors that must be kept in proper balance in order to preserve health) had a continuing life beyond those diagnoses that attributed melancholy to an excess of spleen and that overintellectualism might have its home there, as well.

Tobias Smollett's Matthew Bramble hopes to "discharge the over-flowings of his spleen"[13] upon his correspondent, Dr. Lewis, in the subtext of *The Expedition of Humphry Clinker,* entitled "The Lamentations of Matthew Bramble," by taking part in that seasonal *discharge* at the therapeutic watering hole of Bath. In the process of his therapy, the hypochondriacal Bramble comes to believe that illnesses share a binary system according to the body's fluid balance; gout is a complaint of obstruction, whereas he imagines himself to dwell among those seeking relief from diarrhea, that deflux of unobstructed physiological (and social) fluidity.

> If these waters, from a small degree of astringency, are of some service in the *diabetes, diarrhoea,* and *night sweats,* when the secretions are too much increased, must not they so harm in the same proportion when the humours are obstructed, as in the *asthma, scurvy, gout,* and *dropsy?*[14]

Bramble's nephew, James Melford, as it turns out, is much closer to the mark in his diagnosis, which, like that of so many of Lawrence's critics, is more literary than pathological.

> Those follies that move my uncle's spleen, excite my laughter. He is as tender as a man without skin; who cannot bear the slightest touch without flinching. What tickles another would give him torment; and yet he has what may be called lucid intervals, when he is remarkably facetious—Indeed I never knew a hypochondriac so apt to be infected with good humour . . . but when his spirits are not exerted *externally,* they seem to recoil and prey upon himself.[15] (emphasis added)

In Melford's astute reading of his uncle's disability, it is neither "high *goût*"[16] nor the overcrowding and stench of Bath that awakens Matthew's paralytic paroxysms but rather the obstruction of some natural benevolence that afflicts the student of Henry MacKenzie's popular *Man of Feeling.* In the context of Smollett's novel, gout has become a synecdoche for Bramble's hypochondria—metaphysically, the inability to organize his symptoms into a coherent whole that can be consistently and univocally *denominated.* As part of his hypochondria, gout is the quasi-periodic assertion that there *is,* in fact, what so many eighteenth-century historicists would deny—a secret consciousness that constitutes something left over, a pain that has escaped the enabling of the vast impersonal systems and forces that served as the era's organizational machinery and diagnostic key.

Throughout *The Expedition of Humphry Clinker,* the constitution of the body is regarded as a function of some circulation that is designated under the rubric *oeconomy,* and that behaves as if the flow of energy were in fact directed by an organ of the body. Hence, hypochondria, gout, and any attendant physical and social paralysis are part of a system of inflation (inflammation) as it were, which multiplies symptoms by obscuring the distances between them. Bramble's problem is a failure of integration, defined as a circuit that would transact an exchange involving the excess of feeling and some object. Bramble is unable to vent his sensibility; gout is a consequence of some self-reflexive consumption, the tendency of the body to feed too much upon itself. Only later in his journey does Bramble finally succeed in an act of practical benevolence by voluntarily reorganizing the financial bankruptcy of his childhood friend, Baynard, heretofore unable to avoid a life of wanton luxury.

Bramble's gout-induced paralysis is cured when the body comes to be defined as an instrument of sympathetic *work* in the world rather than a passive receptor. What had previously been regarded as the ineffective water therapy at Bath is imagined to become effective when it represents the possibility of a metaphoric immunity.

> We should sometimes increase the motion of the machine, to *unclog the wheels of life*; and now and then take a plunge into the waters of excess in order to case-harden the constitution.[17]

A minuscule dose of luxury that immunizes ("case-hardens") the constitution against further indulgence serves to convert what had been a self-reflexive consumption into a therapy that promotes renewed physical vehicularity. What is intriguing here is the unstated analogy by which the restoration of economic balance in another's financial account invisibly (as with Adam Smith's "invisible hand" in the 1776 *Wealth of Nations*) restores the fluid balance, so as to break the cycles of hypersensitivity, gout, and depression, all of which had characterized Bramble's disability. There is a relationship between the general economy and the individual corporeal economy. If the paralysis of gout is marked by an accumulation of insoluble deposits in the soft tissues of the body where they impede locomotion and real work, so the paralysis of the political body of eighteenth-century England is a result of the sedentary, noncirculating wealth that is luxury.

The overflow of goodwill known as benevolence, which ultimately mobilizes the disabled, is nonetheless antithetical to another privileged patriarchal practice: inscription. For in the same letter in which Bramble announces to his epistolary correspondent, Dr. Lewis, that he no longer needs the latter's medical counsel, the now recovering paralytic belatedly recognizes that his compulsive writing is a symptom of that very disability. Tobias Smollett, who had apprenticed and later practiced (unsuccessfully) as a surgeon, allows his novel to self-destruct, putting an end to the privileged closure of the "letter" (and by implication his indulgence in the disciplined study of letters) as an adjunct to his gouty hero's reabsorption into an economy in which excess is redistributed. Epistolarity itself, at the conclusion of one of the century's most popular epistolary novels, is imagined as yet one more luxurious self-indulgence, not unlike Sir Clifford's repetitive essays for popular tabloids. Genuine transactive exchange, an economic and discursive deployment of the dialogic, must supplant the private indulgence of the solitary writing machine with its tendency to subsidize iteration, intransitive accumulation, and social (as well as formal) enclosure.

Narratives of disability are thus often, if not dependent *upon*, at least allied *with*, other narratives with which they might share ontologies of paralysis, restricted mobility, or the presence of sedentary deposits that must be cleared in order to restore systemic balance. As a result of the probable exaggeration of the role of inheritance in subsidizing its genealogical reiterations, gout came to be associated with maintaining the family line: hence the ease with which the disorder was elided with writing, the leisure of the book and library, and other "entitlements" of the historically privileged. History itself thus comes to be perceived of as a burden, a surplus—be it in overintellectualism, an excess of leisure time, or too heavy a familial lineage—that induces a psychological disability. Any therapy would, logically enough, involve the lifting of this burden of history by substituting an alternative, lighter narrative that might restore mobility by enabling the handicapped body to imagine a-filiative families whose blood lines and wealth it might be excused from maintaining.

Any narrative of recovery in a life line of the handicapped patriarchy often comes to depend upon excising the story line of the "letter" (and the narratives it would presume to authorize) and replacing it with an altogether different, and occasionally radically different, narrative. In Sir Walter Scott's *Waverley*, the heir's education until his seventeenth year consists mostly of desultory hours spent in "insignificant and trifling" studies of Scottish tradition and genealogical history at the hands of his uncle, Sir Everard Waverley, a man obsessed not only with his own pedigree as patriarch of Waverley-Honour but also with his vision of its political negation, represented in the disability of the Hanoverian succession. Edward is dispatched from one arena of "suppressed vexation" to another, the domain of the baron of Bradwardine, a fellow Jacobite, who holds ancient title to the living of Tully-Veolan, a near ruin symbolic of decadent lowland gentry. Bradwardine exemplifies what passes for overintellectualism, a pedant whose library is filled with obscure Scottish poets of little artistic value, now reduced to ciphers by which genealogical descent is established and authentic family crests are separated from usurpers and counterfeiters.

And, like so many pedants, the baron of Bradwardine is afflicted with paralyzing gout attacks that render him immobilized for days on end, a paralysis that Scott would have us read politically. The attempt to repetition a dead genealogical past (there is no male heir and, given the geographic enclosure and isolation of Tully-Veolan, no real prospects for the forlorn Rose Bradwardine) is part and parcel of the crisis of familial as well as political, succession.

> But although Edward and he differed *toto coelo*, as the Baron would have said, upon this subject, yet they met upon history, as on a neutral ground, in which each claimed an interest. The Baron, indeed only cumbered his memory with

matters of fact—the cold, dry, hard outlines which history delineates. Edward, on the contrary, loved to fill up and round out the sketch with the colouring of a warm and vivid imagination which gives light and life to the actors and speakers in the drama of past ages.[18]

There could be no better deconstruction of the putative neutrality of history. For the baron of Bradwardine, the past is to be recovered *as is* in the various rituals that govern his life in the present; whereas, for his ward, Edward Waverley, history is more akin to fancy, merely one more imaginative narrative among others.

Hence, the luxurious clarets and game and offal-laden banquets that Bradwardine enjoys to excess with his similarly debauched neighbors (similar to the heavy, late dinners at the Chatterleys' Wragby) are but a reminder of some larger paralysis, in this instance marked by the onset of gout. Mock jousts, drinking contests that function to bond a community of aging males, and empty pledges of loyalty to class or family honor, now reduced to paying tribute money to an assortment of Highland banditti, comprise the decadent life of Tully-Veolan. To conceive of history as a recoverable commodity is to be paralyzed by the very agents that are emblematic of a decadence, the resistance to recovery *as is,* in favor of progressive dissimulation.

Typically, the therapy of choice in British fiction involves a flight into the primitive, which offers an alternative narrative for which inscription provides no preparation. Edward Waverley's escape into the Highlands and his temporary adoption by Chief Fergus Mac-Ivor introduces him to a culture where "hospitality . . . had yet its line of economy."[19] The entertainment is "uncommonly vocalic,"[20] mingling the feats of heroes, the complaints of lovers, and the wars of contending tribes, none of which can be translated into the highly codified lines of familial descent and noble prerogative to which his earlier education had been given over. The cure lies in a forced exposure to the prehistory of the nation with its oral as opposed to written culture. During his flight from overintellectualism and into the communal society of Glennaluoich, Edward Waverley encounters genuine martial voracity in support of honor rather than a voracity displaced onto culinary appetite and mock rituals of male bonding. Though wounded in an ankle—a common site of gout—the future heir is quickly restored to full mobility by the folk pharmacopia and oral invocations of a tribal medicine man, Ivy Bolton's antecedent.

In each instance, the Highlands as a sanatorium of civilized disability embodies values antithetical to those espoused by a landed patriarchy beneath the clouds whose self-image is foundational. The overreliance upon memory is replaced by communal participation: the past is narrated in successive "lays," spontaneously supplemented in each recitative so as to constitute a continuous, ongoing epic that obliterates class differences as well as the distinction between past and present—not unlike Mrs. Bolton's gossip. The Highland "family" is neither biologically determined nor defined by arcane baronial crests but is rather an a-filiative convention into which Edward Waverley is absorbed as a son, despite his linguistic and cultural estrangement. Decisions are arrived at consensually, rather than directed by arbitrary historical precedent.

And yet, no matter how different and refreshing this exposure to the Highlands is for Edward Waverley, the politics of Scott's novel demands that it be identified in some sense with what he authentically *is*. Just as Ivy Bolton's importance to Clifford Chatterley depends upon her being *read* as what the life of the gentry has *become* in the twentieth century (gossip), so the oral, primitive culture of the impoverished tribes, as they eke out an increasingly marginal existence within greatly reduced mountain enclaves in the Highlands, is really not that remote from the life of the confined gentry from which Edward has descended. But, retrospectively, the Highlands, like Bath for Smollett's Matthew Bramble, figuratively restores a mobility by introducing an alternative narrative. Edward Waverley can no more conventionally marry Flora Mac-Ivor (who, given the misplaced alliances of the tribes, is ultimately condemned to live out her days in a continental convent) than Sir Clifford can wed Ivy Bolton. But the oral exchange, like nurse Bolton's share in Sir Clifford's rehabilitation, must be narrated as the revelation of an heretofore denied or repressed interest that, as foundational—as foundational as the Highland tribes to the history of Scotland—must "out" if genuine political renewal is to occur. Once exposed to what he is, as opposed to what he has learned of the basis for his expectations, Edward Waverley, like the hypochondriacal Bramble, is "case-hardened." His blood permanently purified by the vocalic liquidity of an oral culture from the inherited tendency to launch painful precipitates into the joints of his lower extremities, Edward Waverley is free to marry Rose Bradwardine and to renew an interrupted succession. This interruption had been narrated as the prospect of sterility and paralysis attendant upon a culture devoted to historical recovery and highly endogamous marital settlements.

Similarly, Sir Leicester Dedlock's vulnerability to gout in *Bleak House* belongs to the order of social enclosure and privatization: lists of the peerage; family libraries; lawyers; and the endless array of private correspondence that creates and is created by the enhanced status of the letter. In Dickens's novel, a paralyzed Chancery itself is an institution dedicated to the incessant repetition of the antecedent, a place where all deliberations are invariably referred back until time (and the contested proceeds of wills and testaments) is exhausted. The paralysis shared by writing, an heirless patriarchy, an overcrowded court docket that never produces a verdict, and gout is threatened by another illness that, like gossip, promises to trickle up as the pustule of the extrafamilial and that spreads not like letters (with a specific addressivity) but rather like gossip, which touches all while appearing to lack any recuperable originating author(ity). If the paralysis of gout is associated with the closure of writing in *Bleak House*, smallpox behaves analogously to gossip in its random circulation. Of course, it is none other than Inspector Bucket, who takes pride in an ear keenly attuned to nuance, French accents, and local gossip, who cuts through the paralysis of the Chancery suit to discover an a-filiative "relationship" that is no part of the historically inscripted "inking" that so stains characters and surfaces in *Bleak House*.

Like Ivy Bolton at Wragby, Bucket comes to dominate a privatizing employer's time and space. Though descendant from a working class family "in service," the inspector is so socially mobile and uninhibited as to be equally at home in Tulkinghorn's secret chambers, in Tom-all-Alone's, in Chesney Wold's library and its dripping, rheumatic grounds, as a midnight traveling companion to Esther Summerson, and at police stations, where he is known to everyone. Orality and those with an enhanced sensitivity to it work to bring an elite, though increasingly immobile, patriarchy into contact with a local channel. In the process, gossip is internalized, brought into the libraries, texts, and exclusive codes that had traditionally defined a historically mandated patriarchy. From one perspective, this immersion in an alternative informational channel represents, in its exposure, the triumph of surveillance. In its resistance to precise reproduction (Bucket prides himself upon never carrying a pen!) or repetition *as is,* gossip as a narrative suggests the possibility of a *differential reproduction,* a wonderful synecdoche for a fertility that would not be consanguineous—an idea to which strong patriarchies are traditionally resistant. But, both discursively and genealogically, this is the form that any renewal at Wragby will assume.

This convention is perhaps nowhere better illustrated than in the plight of Casaubon in George Eliot's *Middlemarch*. When we first encounter him, the scholar appears as a lingering relic of the eighteenth century, looking for an elusive Key to All Mythologies, writing the odd, arcane, clerical tract, *accumulating* documents meticulously arranged in his highly compartmentalized library, not unlike an Encyclopedist born a shade late. Collector of minute facts and parergae, Edward Casaubon is only a slightly less eccentric version of the disabled patriarchy exposed in *Waverley* or *Lady Chatterley's Lover*. None of his research bears any *issue* in worthy publication, a sterility not at all lost upon Dorothea Brooke, his wife, committed as she is to pragmatic projects for the improvement of daily life.

In her epigraph to the fifth chapter of *Middlemarch*, on the occasion of Casaubon's painfully circuitous, quasi-incestuous marriage proposal to a woman less than half his age—the same gesture toward historical recovery that defines his work—George Eliot cites Robert Burton's *Anatomy of Melancholy* (1621) in order to construct a narrative tradition wherein both his physical and intellectual disabilities find a common home.

Hard students are commonly troubled with gouts, catarrhs, rheums, cachexia, bradypepsia, bad eyes, stone, and collick, crudities, appellations, vertigo, winds, consumptions, and all such diseases as come from over-much sitting: they are most part lean, dry, and ill-coloured . . . and all through immoderate pains and extraordinary studies.[21]

Casaubon's hobbled gait and ghostly pallor are made over into that familiar syndrome of (overintellectual) complaints in which lifestyle ailments are mixed with occupational hazards. The pain of scholarship is translated into physical disability in a conversion process that owes little to any physiological bond. The now familiar gout is a quickly precipitated deposit from an accumulated retention that *drops* (hence the Latin *gutta*) into the soft tissues and joints, entirely in harmony with the scholar's "banked" stock of research and even his conversational style, always "in reserve."[22] Casaubon is unable to vent his stream of feeling—either for research or genuine affection for his wife—and so it accumulates in depositions of enclosure, those reservoirs of dammed up emotion that form, collectively, the infamous metaphoric basin of Dorothea's life without prospects during their Roman honeymoon.

Yet, in what must surely be the most notorious instance of medical misdiagnosis in nineteenth-century British fiction, Casaubon's life-threatening disability, as it turns out, is not our familiar gout syndrome but a defective heart whose arrhythmia has been detected by the new Dr. Lydgate's new instrument, the stethoscope. In a novel where an intellectual premium is placed upon either the recuperation of ancient, univocal narrative origins or the construction of futuristic plans, George Eliot is suggesting that in fact medical progress is characterized by the displacement of narratives of disability. Dr. Lydgate's instrument "opens" the disabled body in such a way as to identify an alternative center for the production of meaning. In this instance, the futility of traditional therapy, recommended by the scholar's equally arrogant friend, Brooke, should not go unremarked, if for no other reason than its comparative effectiveness when administered by Ivy Bolton in the rehabilitation of Sir Clifford.

> Why you might take to some light study: conchology, now: I always think that must be a light study. Or get Dorothea to read you light things.[23]

A light discourse administered by Dorothea Brooke is neither imaginable given the seriousness of her projects nor likely to be effective in Casaubon's terminal case, yet it continues to remain a viable therapeutic narrative, even after the assumptions that grounded the original narrative of disability are no longer adequate, a fate shared with other imaginative models in *Middlemarch*. Yet Casaubon's clear resistance to what he cannot hoard and classify is betrayed by the codicil to his will, in which he would *foreclose* the possibility of a marriage raised by the community's gossip. *Public opinion* is a collective narrative for which Casaubon has exhibited profound contempt, which surely partially explains his delay in publishing his work, but not so distant from his concerns as to escape his futile attempt to enclose it within that ultimate nineteenth-century narrative of disability: the last will by which he would structure the lives of others in absentia. Casaubon's resistance to oral speculation is, then, nothing less than the repressed truth of a life dedicated to historical recuperation. No wonder it is that truth that will come to comprise the therapy, that immersion in a wider public life, to which Dorothea will convert her energies in the novel's penultimate chapters.

Nineteenth-century narratives of disability, because they are often so easily associated with a diminished, if not handicapped, patriarchy and its public role, are often read as abstractions—like the overintellectualism that Harry T. Moore thought to be Sir Clifford's real disability. And sure enough, that disability, too, would render the victim out of touch with everyday life, for which benevolence, light reading, a more fluid discursive or real economy, even gossip itself might provide a useful therapy. These home remedies would presumably put the disabled in touch with that *publicité* so easily allegorized as the "real" or transactive world. But, it would only give him a symbolic rehabilitation, which would continue, even maintain the paralysis.

In this regard, Naumann, the "Nazarene" painter encountered in Rome by the newly married Casaubon and his wife, has it aesthetically right when he comments that the scholar's "starchy" face is "too abstract to be represented"[24] in any portrait. Once allied with metaphysical conditions or pathological syndromes that blur distinctions between and among representations or symptoms, artists and critics often substitute imaginary "representations" like that of the "deformed line" (both graphically and historically). Unable to represent the negation of representation,[25] we fill the absence. In Conrad's *The Secret Agent*, the actual ideology of a cell of anarchists is difficult to represent, save as a negation that would destroy all social and legal conventions (including those that arbitrarily enable a civilization to mark time). The interest in ideological deformation can only be represented as corporeal deformations: Verloc's chronic narcolepsy, which turns night into day for him; Michaelis's obesity, which renders him immobile without the physical assistance that renders him vulnerable to police surveillance; and Karly Yundt's gouty knees, which have deformed his walk and appearance.

If Conrad converts a shaky belief in ideological deformation into genuine physical disability, Freud's *Studies on Hysteria*—the Freud who often initially tested his well-heeled patients for excessive urates at the commencement of therapy—would appear to have reversed Conrad's trajectory.[26] The analyst would presume to convert a genuine paralysis (like the extreme facial neuralgia that afflicts "Frau Cacilie") into a narrative disability, attendant upon errors in symbolization. The majority of these errors have their origins for Freud in substitutions in which family members displace lovers and vice versa. Neurosis was once defined by Freud as "an abnormal attachment to the past," but retrospectively, it seems of a piece with other instances of the excess of history that paralyzes so many patriarchs in British fiction. His "talking cure," as with Ivy Bolton's, is one more attempt to "make the past really past."

If indeed narratives of disability define a field of interdisciplinary interests, those engaged in its study would be required to define how and why these narratives are different from other narratives. A tentative prolegomenon of the *relationship* between narratives of disability and conventional discursive practice might include the following observations.

1. Physical disability may or may not *inscribe* the individual, but once the disability is narrated, the body often behaves *as if* it were a text.
2. Even though a particular disability may appear as an arbitrary or discontinuous opening in the life of a subject, the narrative of that disability can usually be accommodated by a historical tradition that it may supplement, be indistinguishable from, or even deconstruct.
3. Because the narrative of disability has a different "life" from either the forces that occasioned it or the narratives by and in which it is socially reproduced, any study of disability narratives might operate in a gap between the disability and its representations.
4. Traditional literary criticism often *symbolically converts* a genuine physical or mental disability into a narrative that may enable intellectual or emotional access to the disability while occluding its unique or individuating characteristics. The corporeal body is easily appropriated by other "bodies" (social, political, ancestral).
5. Because narratives of disability are inextricably bound to identity formation and self-image, the public consumption of disability narratives over time partially determines the integrative (social) acceptance of the subject.
6. Although disabilities may be similar, the narratives of the respective disabilities might diverge to such an extent as to call forth differential therapeutic narratives.

Back to Sir Clifford and Lady Chatterley and their respective narratives of disability. The narratives that would presume to constitute their respective therapies assume apparently dissimilar courses. Hers seems a logical extension of that dubious nature cure prescribed by so many nineteenth-century medical practitioners: brisk walks, mountain air, sea bathing, and a measured dose of that other *petite mort*, the sublime exposure to a noncontinuous "prospect." In practice, her therapy consists of limiting extended conversational exchange. A literal bounce is restored to Sir Clifford's wheelchair by its apparent antipode, the noisy, incessant small talk with the village gossip that opens a dead patriarchal space to the same extent that Mellors's syntactic ellipses create a new sensitivity in Lady Chatterley's maternal space. Both are brought to a new knowledge—sociopolitical on the one hand, physical on the other—that had previously been denied. Not any overintellectualism, but its opposite, the refusal to ac*knowledge* experience exogamous to their class interests, is at the heart of the Chatterleys' *shared* disabilities and, I would argue, their *differentially related* therapeutic narratives.[27]

In this instance, the history of literary criticism displays a tendency to convert a disability into a surplus. If, for Harry T. Moore, Lady Chatterley's recovery bears a resemblance to the Sleeping Beauty legend, why should not the narrative of Sir Clifford's disability recall the infamous Sultan Shahriar, the captive of that most persecuted of gossips, the Scheherazade of the *Arabian Nights*? These analogies make sense of course only if the pair's handicaps are read metaphorically, as part of a larger paralysis impacting the British ruling class at a specific juncture. Sir Clifford's oral cohabitation with Ivy Bolton could have no conceivable therapeutic value in relieving the emotional and physical pain of a shattered body, which must remain, as one suspects must be true of Lady Chatterley's orgasms, beyond discourse. Ivy Bolton's equally radical treatment would thus represent one more way in which Sir Clifford cannot choose but to remain a passive listener to a better storyteller. And that is surely a definition of what it means to be disabled, rather than the cure with which it comes to be identified.

NOTES

1. Harry T. Moore, *The Intelligent Heart: The Story of D. H. Lawrence* (London and Toronto: Heinemann, 1955), 359–60.

2. The essays in Meyer Abrams, *The Correspondent Breeze: Essays in English Romanticism* (New York: Norton, 1984), are in so many ways antithetical to the strategies and assumption of Paul De Man in *The Rhetoric of Romanticism* (New York: Columbia, 1986), insofar as they assume some self-consciousness of a direct correspondence between natural and imaginative states informing British romanticism. The progressive "denaturing" of nature in nineteenth-century models of mentalism is one of the subjects of J. H. Van den Berg, *The Changing Nature of Man: Introduction to Historical Psychology* (New York: Norton, 1983), a book less well known than it should be.

3. The comparative diagnoses of the afflictions of corporeal and political bodies in the nineteenth century—and the misreadings that often arise as a consequence—are the subject of a collection of marvelous essays by Mary Poovey, *Making a Social Body: British Cultural Formation 1830–1864* (Chicago, IL, and London: University of Chicago Press, 1995).

4. For a detailed theoretical discussion of these oppositional modes of reading inscription—readerly (metonymic) and recuperative (metaphoric)—see Mieke Bal, "De-

Disciplining the Eye," *Critical Inquiry* 16 (spring 1990): 506–31. The disabled body as a "marked text" is treated in Elaine Scarry, *The Body in Pain* (Oxford: Oxford University Press, 1985), though the author is less suggestive in distinguishing between the reading of the disabled body and the ways in which we read the uniquely or especially abled body and the different sorts of pain experienced by the objects of these differential readings.

5. H. M. Daleski, *The Forked Flame: A Study of D. H. Lawrence* (1968; reprint, Madison, WI: University of Wisconsin Press, 1987) has remarked upon the thematic importance of anal intercourse in *Lady Chatterley's Lover* as initiating an alternative paradigm of pleasure from, at least physiologically, the "nether" world. This "indelicate therapy," if not a birth control technique, would parallel the pleasure that Sir Clifford obtains from a source regarded as socially and discursively "beneath" him.

6. For a discussion of the ways in which Freud "writes down" the corporeal bodies of his patients and replaces them with "talking" or "hysterogenic" bodies more accessible to verbal analysis, see my "Freud's 'Secret Agent' and the *Fin du Corps*," in *Fin de Siècle/Fin du Globe: Fears and Fantasies of the Late Nineteenth Century,* ed. John Stokes (London: Macmillan, 1992), 117–38.

7. D. H. Lawrence, *Lady Chatterley's Lover,* ed. Richard Hoggart (Harmondsworth: Penguin, 1961), 101. All references to Lawrence's novel in the text are indicated by the appropriate page number in the Hoggart edition.

8. Charles Taylor, *The Ethics of Authenticity* (Cambridge, MA, and London: Harvard University Press, 1991), esp. 24–36.

9. Martin Heidegger, *Being and Time,* trans. John Macquarrie and Edward Robinson (Oxford: Basil Blackwell, 1980), 212. Heidegger's discussion would contrast the idleness of gossip with the work—"hard struggle"—necessary to attain what he would classify as authentic knowledge, like Clifford Chatterley's knowledge of German mining technology. Gossip thus, in Heidegger's critical model, comes to define a dispossessive relationship with an object of potential comprehension, not unlike that which Mellors would implicitly advocate for him and Lady Chatterley.

Patricia Meyer Spacks, *Gossip* (New York: Alfred Knopf, 1985), is an attempt to define the role of "small talk" as an agent in the empowerment of women. For a critique of those ideas, see my review of Spacks's work in *Modern Language Notes,* 101, no. 5 (1986): 1273–79 or my *Gossip and Subversion in Nineteenth Century British Fiction: Echo's Economies* (Basingstoke 2d London: Macmillan, 1996). Neither Spacks nor I, however, deal with the therapeutic dimensions of gossip in narratives of disability.

10. Susan Sontag, *AIDS and Its Metaphors* (New York: Farrar Straus and Giroux, 1988), esp. 24–30. Sontag sees particular disabilities as having a periodicity that cannot be explained by anything we know of their "organic" progress: leprosy in the middle ages and tuberculosis among the "wasted" romantics would be two cases in point. For a more complete attempt to give gout a metaphoric meaning, see my " 'The Key to Dedlock's Gait': Gout as Resistance," in *Literature and Sickness,* ed. David Bevan (Amsterdam and Atlanta, GA: Rodopi, 1992), 25–52.

11. Tsa'ai-Fan Yu and Lawrence Berger, eds. *The Kidney in Gout and Hyperuricemia* (Mt. Kisco, NY: Futura, 1982), 155.

12. Charles Dickens, *Bleak House,* ed. Norman Page (Harmondsworth: Penguin, 1971), 271.

13. Tobias Smollett, *The Expedition of Humphry Clinker,* ed. Angus Ross (Harmondsworth: Penguin, 1983), 63.

14. Ibid., 52.

15. Ibid., 79.

16. Ibid., 85. The pun involving the French word for "taste" and the medical complaint recurs in Smollett's novel, as it often does, later, among Balzac's misers. The fact that the illness can be represented as one of a material hoarding that is genetically transferable endows it with unique deconstructive possibilities among literature's greedy.

17. Ibid., 381.

18. Sir Walter Scott, *Waverley,* ed. Andrew Hook (Harmondsworth: Penguin, 1972), 59.

19. Ibid., 163.

20. Ibid., 173.

21. George Eliot, *Middlemarch,* ed. W. H. Harvey (Harmondsworth: Penguin, 1972), 66.

22. Ibid., 73. The initial diagnosis of Casaubon's illness is partially dependent upon a substitution of academic interests for the excessive protein consumption believed to be a contributing factor to his gout. The "feed/ing/ too much on the inward sources" (4), since it is also applicable to his "contained" marriage proposal, comprises that typical resistance to *renewal* that became a common mode of representing totally unrelated physical disabilities.

23. Ibid., 320.

24. Ibid., 249.

25. If the romantic sublime in its topographical discontinuities (ragged peaks, deep ravines, broken "prospects") was hypostasized as a natural disability that nonetheless constituted a therapy for certain physiological disabilities, then the role of the sublime is filled with irony. One "disability" would constitute the potential therapy for another: "broken" nature for a "broken" or "jaded" heart. As an often interrupted or half-understood wisdom, gossip would have a function similar to that of the sublime. For a theory of "sublime ironies," see Thomas Weiskel, *The Romantic Sublime: Studies in the Structure and Psychology of Transcendence* (Baltimore, MD, and London: Johns Hopkins University Press, 1986).

26. Freud's habit of initially discounting "gouty diathesis" in his patients as a first stage in any treatment is the subject of his lengthy footnote to "Frau Emmy Von N." See *The Standard Edition of the Complete Works of Sigmund Freud in Twenty-Four Volumes,* vol. 2, ed. James Strachey (London: Hogarth Press, 1953–66), 71.

27. The Chatterley's quasi-incestuous obsession with what they (already) are might be suggested in the ironic twist that Lawrence gives the so-called *Blutbrüderschaft* theme. Sir Clifford's adaptation of the latest in German technology to his mines seems part of a larger interest in Saxon origins shared by the Lady Chatterley, who had lost her virginity as a bohemian music student in Dresden. Given the German origins of the handicap sustained in the Great War, Sir Clifford's devotion to their technology is another example of being in love with that which is killing, familiar to gout-afflicted patriarchs of eighteenth- and nineteenth-century British novels but also to the familial politics of World War I, fought between cousins.

From Social Welfare to Civil Rights ▶ The Representation of Disability in Twentieth-Century German Literature

Elizabeth C. Hamilton

Any definition of disability is always a product of its historical context. The movement of disability discourse within and among antagonistic paradigms in twentieth-century Germany warrants special attention, for German social models of the past hundred years have profoundly shaped present-day understanding of what disability is, both in Germany and throughout the world. People working in the seemingly disparate fields of medicine, law, and art have continuously vied for the authority to pronounce a final judgment—and indeed, prescribe appropriate treatment—and have hence configured disability in the very attempt to define it. While disability has long been present in the German arena as a "public problem," it has only recently entered into public debate as an issue of individual experience. Because the political, social, and economic value of the disabled individual to society has historically been measured in Germany in terms of a person's diminished ability to perform work, a disabled individual's claim to the rights of full citizenship has frequently stood in direct conflict with the interests of the social totality. This study traces the many and often contradictory articulations of disability that have arisen in a century-long political contest of social welfare and individual civil rights.[1]

Four twentieth-century German prose works predict and confront this tension, albeit by different literary means and to different ends: Leonhard Frank's 1918 collection of novellas, *Der Mensch ist gut* (The human being is good)[2] criticizes the Imperial German government's engagement in World War I and depicts the early organization of the Communist Party in Germany. The disabled soldiers portrayed in the novellas are upheld as reminders of the meaningless destruction wrought by the war and thus serve the work's ultimately hopeful orientation toward the future. Günter Grass's 1959 novel, *Die Blechtrommel* (The tin Drum), confronts National Socialist rule and World War II and asks how citizens of the new Federal Republic might come to terms with the legacy of the murderous Nazi society. One of the disabilities portrayed in this novel, the stunted growth of the figure Oskar Mazareth, is commonly understood to symbolize the "dwarfish" or "stunted" ethics of National Socialism, the hold that German fascism had on the middle classes, and the consequently troubled framework in which to situate a new German nation. Recent testimonial literature by people with disabilities eschews the symbolic approach and details personal accounts of discrimination and ostracism that result from having a disability. Two recent works (Andrea Buch, ed., *An den Rand gedrängt* [Pushed to the Margins] (Reinbek: Rowohlt, 1980), and Sigrid Arnade, ed., *Weder Küsse noch Karriere* [Neither kisses nor Careers] (Frankfurt: Fisher, 1992), problematize traditional literary and social metaphors that present disability as a burden or liability to a social whole and in an attempt to set the record straight invite discussion of disability in terms of subjective experience and individual civil rights. Analyzing the portrayals of disability within these texts, I hope to demonstrate that disability resists ahistorical characterization because the experience of disability is not historically constant.

Consider first *Der Mensch ist gut*. Author Frank introduces the character Robert as he receives the news that his son has died on the "field of honor" (8). Throughout the narration, Robert questions this and other metaphors such as "the altar of the Fatherland" that are, in the narrative, part of the German prowar propaganda used during World War I (22). Robert finds that these metaphors neither comfort grieving parents nor provide the general public sound justification for continuing the war.

Das Feld der Ehre war nicht sichtbar, nicht vorstellbar, war Robert nicht begreifbar. Das war kein Feld, kein Acker, war keine Fläche, war nicht Nebel und nicht Luft. Es war das absolute Nichts. Und daran sollte er sich halten.

[The field of honor was not visible, was not imaginable, was not conceivable to Robert. It was not a field, not land, not a surface, not mist, not air. It was absolute nothingness. And he was supposed to cling to it.] (Leonhard Frank, *Der Mensch ist gut* [Zürich: Max Rascher Verlag, 1918; München: Nymphenburger Verlagshandlung, 1964], 9)

For Robert, the "field of honor" and the "altar of the Fatherland" are metaphors that serve the German government's projection of itself as an institution worthy of its citizens' lives. *Der Mensch ist gut* goes on to criticize the German government that elevates its own image over its citizens and their needs.

Der Mensch ist gut depicts the attitudes behind the early organization of the Communist Party in Germany and argues that pacifism can efficiently and effectively defeat the real enemy, the "absence of love" (12).[3] To a great extent, Frank laments the circumstances facing newly disabled soldiers and writes on behalf of those who might yet be disabled in war. Frank devotes an entire chapter to the *Kriegskrüppel,* or, literally, "war cripple,"[4] portraying the harsh realities that soldiers wounded in war and those who underwent amputation will face.[5] The surgeon who has performed countless amputations bitterly anticipates the widespread unemployment likely facing the war cripple.

> Hunderttausende werden mit ähnlichen Gründen abgefertigt von den Unternehmern. Hundertausende—Schlosser, Schreiner, Spengler, Maurer, Schmiede, Bergleute, Handlanger, Taglöhner, Erdarbeiter, Bauarbeiter—verlassen als Abgewiesene, stillgeworden und hoffnungslos, die Fabriken, die Werkstätten, die Baubüros. In den Arbeitsnachweisen hängen Tafeln, auf denen steht: "Für diese Arbeiten kommen nur kräftige, unbeschädigte Leute in Frage." "Kräftige, unbeschädigte Leute haben den Vorzug." "Für diese Stellen kommen . . ."

> [Hundreds of thousands of them will, for the same reasons, be given the once-over and sent on their way by their employers. Hundreds of thousands—metalworkers, carpenters, plumbers, bricklayers, smiths, miners, handymen, day laborers, construction workers—rejected, silenced, and hopeless, they'll leave the factories, the workshops, the bosses' offices. The employment agencies will hang signs that read: "For these jobs, only strong, undamaged people will be considered." "Strong, undamaged people preferred." "For the following positions . . ."] (159)

Elaborating upon the distressing realities that these soldiers disabled in war will face, Frank exposes the metaphors designed to entice young men into military service as rhetorical devices that validate existing political and social structures. In his portrayal of the war cripple, Frank criticizes a political program that does not meet the needs of individuals who fall outside of the norm, which in this case is "undamaged." In this progressive criticism, however, lies his adherence to conventional notions, for Frank in effect reifies able bodiedness as an essential and indisputable norm. Although Frank speaks ostensibly on behalf of people with disabilities, he, if unwittingly, attributes value to certain disabilities based on their origin, elevating those disabilities that result from war wounds above disabilities that are congenital or acquired through accidents or debilitating disease.[6] *Der Mensch ist gut* cannot be understood to support the rights of disabled people per se but instead those of a select group of people. The compassion Frank shows is great, and his advocacy on the war cripple's behalf is sincere and unselfish. Indeed, he presents the war cripples as victims of deceit, for the obstacles they will face in getting jobs, walking, dancing, or having sex have been imposed upon them by the very people who promised them "honor" and the sanctity of an "altar." Frank seeks to reconcile these disabled individuals to their rights and sees as a source of reconciliation a changed political system that will not inflict disability upon its citizens. Put more simply, Frank seeks to prevent war-incurred disability.

Despite his well-intentioned efforts, however, Frank in many ways reproduces the oppressive thought patterns that he overtly challenges. When Frank mourns the war cripple's lost limbs in order to criticize the government policies that caused disability, Frank upholds not only a normative and overly simple standard of able bodiedness but also the notion that able bodiedness is a right.[7] He faults the government for turning able-bodied men into war cripples, because he knows that war cripples will be treated as though they were ordinary people with disabilities, and surely, these soldiers deserve better. Arguing their blamelessness, Frank, if inadvertently, suggests that some people "deserve" their disabilities and thus upholds the mythology of punishment and blame as components of disability.[8] Depicting disability as a product of damage, Frank upholds the notion that disability is derived from able bodiedness and is not to be considered an experience in its own right. When able bodiedness is validated in this manner, it is impossible to speak of disability as anything but a problem or a flaw whose solution lies in its prevention or cure. Thus, while *Der Mensch ist gut* gives evidence of the movement of disability-related discourse into political spheres, it also exhibits remnants of the mythological and moralistic thinking that surrounded disability in earlier centuries.

The development of scientific professions and the application of scientific methods to human subjects marks a comprehensive discursive shift at the end of the nineteenth and beginning of the twentieth centuries.[9] One result of this development was an increase in public attention to people with disabilities. Some aspects of this attention were quite liberating, in particular the debate over the most appropriate language with which to discuss disability. Carl von Kügelgen's essay, "Nicht Krüppel—Sieger!" [Not cripple—Victor!] was published in 1919, one year after Frank's *Der Mensch ist gut.* In his essay, von Kügelgen describes the punishing and ostracizing term *cripple* and calls for widespread use of a less degrading term. Note in particular his anger at being measured against the norm.

Der Einzelne wird am Bilde der Volksmassen gemessen und, wenn Wesentliches fehlt, mit dem Ausdruck "Krüppel" gestraft, der hier ganz im alten Sinn des Minderwertigen gebraucht wird.

[The individual is measured against the image of the masses, and, if some essential part is missing, is punished with the expression "cripple," that only conveys the old sense of inferiority.] (Carl von Kügelgen, "Nicht Krüppel— Sieger!" in *Gedanken und Erfahrungen eines Einarmigen.* (Langensalze: Beyer and Söhne, 1919), quoted in Helmut Bernsmeier, *Krüppel oder Körperbehinderter?* In *Der Sprachdienst* 24n. 12 (1980): 177–79)

Hans Würtz, a leading specialist in disability education and administrative director of the Oskar-Helene-Heim in Berlin, offered a somewhat contradictory assessment of the quality and conditions of life that the disabled person could expect. He concluded in his 1921 study, "Das Seelenleben des Krüppels" (The inner life of the Cripple):

> Der Krüppel steht in innerer Spannung gegen die Gesunden. Er geht nicht gern aus sich heraus . . . Die Möglichkeiten unbefangenen Gemeinschaftsbewußt-seins sind in dem Krüppel ganz verschüttet . . . Alles Auffällige schaft eine Sonderstellung. Sonderstellungen verknüpfen sich mit besonderen Gefühlen und Wissensregungen. Ein besonderes Seelenleben grenzt gegen das gemein-sam Seelische der Gemeinschaft ab.

> [The cripple exists in an inner tension with the healthy. He does not like to be drawn out . . . The possibilities of unrestrained social awareness are threat-ened or completely buried . . . Any conspicuous difference creates an unusual status. Unusual statuses are accompanied by unusual feelings and intellectual inclinations. A unusual inner life creates a barrier to the collective spirit of the society.] (Hans Würtz, "Das Seelenben des Krüppels," in *Krüppelkundliche Erziehung und das Gesetz betr. öffent-liche Krüppelfürsorge* [Leipzig: Voß, 1921], quoted in Joachin S. Hohmann, *Schon auf den ersten Blick. Lesebuch zur Geschichte Unserer Feindbilder* [Darmstadt: Luchterhand, 1981].)

Würtz maintained that a "cripple" was as socially ill as he was emotionally ill. He wrote that "sofern daher der Krüppel seelisch leidet, ist er durchweg ge-meinschaftskrank" [insofar as the cripple suffers spiritually, he is without excep-tion socially sick]. Würtz concluded that this social illness dictated social treat-ment: "Der Krüppel ist daher gemeinschaftsfähig zu machen. Das ist der Sinn der Krüppelpädagogik" [The cripple is to be made socially acceptable. That is the objective of cripple pedagogy] (Wurtz, "Das Seelenben," quoted in Hohmann, *Auf den ersten Blick*, 199). Although many of Würtz's initial assessments recall deeply rooted stereotypes of people with disabilities, his programs were in fact quite progressive in their emphasis on social integration. Only a few years later, official policy would mandate the extermination of people with disabilities.

Despite the attempts of a few educators and doctors to apply the findings of social science in the service of people with disabilities, extremists versed in the language of social Darwinism began to find a foothold in conservative circles eager to "strengthen" the German *Volk*. A number of *Rassenhygieniker*, or theo-rists espousing a notion of "racial hygiene," proclaimed the concept of the "sur-vival of the fittest" to be an imperative, that is, that those who are physically stronger *should* survive those who are weaker. The science of racial eugenics became the overarching authority for medical and political policy that mandated the eradication of disability. The pronounced differentness of a disabled person with respect to his or her nondisabled peers received great attention from scientists, whose studies "proved" to government policymakers that people with disabilities have a degenerative effect on the societies in which they live. From the late nineteenth century to the period of National Socialist rule, theories of racial hygiene called for restrictions on intermarriage between the disabled and the able bodied and mandatory abortions and sterilization in the event that a child was likely to be born with a disability. Karl Binding and Alfred Hoche's 1920 study, "Die Freigabe der Vernichtung lebensunwerten Lebens. Ihr Maß und Form" [Permission to exterminate life unworthy of Life: Its extent and Form], concluded that the lives of disabled people were "absolut zwecklos . . . Für ihre Angehörigen wie für die Gesellschaft bilden sie eine furchtbare schwere Belastung" [absolutely purposeless . . . They create for their relatives as well as for society a terribly heavy burden] (Karl Binding and Alfred Hoche, *Die Friegabe der Vernichtung lebensunwerten Lebens. Ihr Maß und Form* [Leipzig meiner, 1920], quoted in Helmut Bernsmeier, *Arbeitstext* [Stuttgart: Reclam, 1983], 71).

Binding and Hoche's work provided the rationale for the Nazi campaign to rid the German population of the "burdensome" disabled and so protect the *Volk* from this degenerative element. Plans for the removal of the "life unworthy of life" were embraced and executed with nationalistic fervor.[10] Klaus Dörner's 1967 study, "Nationalsozialismus und Lebensvernichtung" [National Socialism and the Extermination of Life] (Klaus Dörner, "Nationalsozialismus und Lebensvernichtung," in *Vierteljahresschrift für Zeitgeschichte* (1967): 121–52) estimates that Nazi doctors killed between 100,000 and 125,000 people with physical and mental disabilities (146). Poore (Carol Poore, "Disability as Disobedience? An Essay on Germany in the Aftermath of the United Nations Year for People with Disabilities," in *New German Critique* 27 (fall 1982): 161–95) points out that the Nazi regime's conception of health was predicated on an unmitigated parallel between the body and the mind and describes how this simple relationship was projected intact onto the concept of the body politic.

[It is clear] that the ideological short-circuit of drawing direct parallels between body and mind fit into a larger opposition being set up between health and sickness. And, indeed, this was not viewed merely as the health or sickness of the individual patient, but in a much more encompassing sense as the health or sickness of the Volk and the nation. (176)

After the end of the war, the Nazi policies of eugenics ended, and virtually no public discussion or even simple acknowledgment of these practices took place. In the abrupt turnabout from National Socialism toward a consumer-driven, achievement- and performance-oriented society, or *Leistungsgesellschaft*, political attention to disability focused primarily on war veterans. In the early years of the Federal Republic, the emphasis was on providing health care and social benefits and on developing and extensive program of work-oriented rehabilitation. Nursing homes and sheltered workshops for people with disabilities adhered to the widespread belief in the therapeutic value of work and operated on the notion of "Arbeit als—und statt—Therapie" [work as—and instead of—therapy] (Udo Sierck, *Arbeit ist die beste Medizin. Zur Geschichte der Rehabilitationspolitik* [Hamburg: Konkret, 1992], 9). Sierck points out that work was not conceived as an enjoyable activity that might lead to self-fulfillment or pride, but instead work was viewed as a method of controlling behavior. Once again, then, people with disabilities were viewed in terms of deviance and dangerousness that put society, that is, "normal" people, at risk, and it was reasoned that work-oriented therapy would minimize this risk. Sierck writes:

> Die Idee von Tätigkeit als Selbstverwirklichung spielt keine Rolle. Der Aspekt der Produktivität stand einseitig im Vordergrund. Die Arbeit wurde für die Erziehung zu Ordnung, Sauberkeit, Disziplin, zur Gewöhnung an Leistungsfähigkeit und -bereitschaft genutzt. Sie ging einher mit dem Versuch, abweichendes Verhalten zu unterdrücken und an die geltenden sozialen, moralischen und politischen Werte anzupassen.

> [The idea of work as self-development never played a role. The issue of productivity alone was foregrounded. Work was used to educate [a person] to be orderly, clean, disciplined, and trained in competitiveness and efficiency. It went hand in hand with the attempt to suppress deviant behavior and to [ensure the] conform[ation] to prevailing social, moral, and political values.] (9)

Noteworthy are the ways in which the goals of postwar rehabilitation parallel the ideals of National Socialism: the suppression of deviant behavior; education toward orderliness, cleanliness, and discipline; and the measurement of a person's perceived usefulness to the larger society.[11] To be sure, the actual physical liquidation of people with disabilities was no longer sanctioned after the war and the language of degeneration had softened, but the drive toward normalization had survived intact.

Oskar Mazerath, the narrator and main character of Günter Grass's *Die Blechtrommel*, exhibits all of the abnormal characteristics that, under National Socialism, would logically mandate his death; in a notably similar fashion, Oskar also offends the self-image of the newly developing Federal Republic. Narrating the novel in both first and third person voices, Oskar chronicles and reflects upon twentieth-century German politics and culture as they are played out in the lives of three generations. The narrative's pivotal question asks how citizens of the newly established Federal Republic might comprehend the atrocities of National Socialism and the widespread acceptance of Hitler's murderous policies.

The figure of Oskar Mazerath is most often understood as a metaphor, and this metaphoric quality is most evident in the characteristics that mark Oskar as "disabled." Only three feet high and, later in his life, hunchbacked, Oskar can indeed be partly understood in symbolic terms. Oskar Mazerath is obnoxious and loud, misshapen and uncontrollable. Supremely annoying and unattractive, Oskar is in every respect burdensome to those around him. He drums incessantly and screams so that he shatters glass. These traits, drawn from a stockpile of stereotypes that are highly specific to the disabled, have an important function in the novel, for they symbolize Oskar's resistance to the ideology of fascism and the activities of his own family members that ultimately advance National Socialism. Oskar first resisted his father's goals at the age of three, when he willfully stopped growing so that he might not be forced to follow in his father's footsteps and that "his shadows" might not be measured against those of his parents' generation.

> Um nicht mit einer Kasse klappern zu müssen, hielt ich mich an die Trommel und wuchs seit meinem dritten Geburtstag keinen Fingerbreit mehr, blieg der Dreijährige, aber auch Dreimalkluge, den die Erwachsenen alle überragten, der den Erwachsenen so überlegen sein sollte, der seinen Schatten nicht mit ihrem Schatten messen wollte.

> [To avoid playing the cash register I clung to my drum and from my third birthday on refused to grow by so much a finger's breadth. I remained the precocious three-year-old, towered over by grownups but superior to all grownups, who refused to measure his shadow with theirs.] (Günter Grass, *The Tin Drum*, trans. Ralph Manheim [New York: Random House, 1964], 60)

Here it becomes evident that the figure of Oskar Mazerath is more than a symbol. It is important to note that Oskar does not merely embody resistance to National Socialism, he enacts resistance with his body and in the ways in which he expresses himself. His drumming and shattering glass reveal themselves to be modes of both expression and perception. Werner Schwann notes that "trommelnd versetzt er sich in die Gedanken anderer Menschen und durchschaut sie" [drumming, he transports himself into the thoughts of other people and sees through them] and that the breaking of glass "gestattet gelegentlich (z.B. beim Zersingen von Brillengläsern) eine neue Optik" [facilitates now and then (e.g., when singing so that he shatters eyeglasses) a new visual perspective] (Werner Schwann, *Ich bin doch Kein Unmensch. Kriegs-und Nachkriegszert im deutschen Roman* [Freiburg: Rombach, 1990], 21). Here, Oskar deliberately disrupts narrative conventions. Oskar's drumming and glass-shattering songs are not held up as an alternative to more conventional speech; they are instead an attempt to problematize the very way that meaning is produced in language and in society. His is a critical voice that demands to be heard.

It must be pointed out, however, that the figure of Oskar Mazerath does not only embody and enact resistance to fascism; the symbolic quality of his character also signals Oskar's complicity with the Nazi offense. Hildegard Emmel emphasizes the metaphoric quality of Oskar's portrayal: "The life story of *Die Blechtrommeler* that seems to emerge is for the artist Grass only a means to an end, that of expressing what is unnarratable in narrative form" (Hildegard Emmel, *History of the German Novel,* trans. Ellen Summerfield [Detroit: Wayne State University Press, 1984], 341). The self-imposed nature of Oskar's disability provides, as I have discussed, a compelling argument that Oskar enacts resistance to German fascism. It can nonetheless be argued that Oskar has allied himself with the Nazi goals. Hanspeter Brode writes: "Das permanente Trommeln verweist sicherlich auf die gesamte Zeitsituation prägende Aggressivität; es signalisiert martialisches Tun und militärische Disziplinierung" [The permanent drumming clearly refers to the aggressivity that marked the entire period; it signals martial conduct and military discipline] (Hanspeter Brode, "Die Zeitgeschichte in der 'Blechtrommel' von Günker Grass. Entwurf eines Textinternen Kommunikations modells," in Rolf Geißler, ed., *Günter Grass Materialienbuch* [Darmstadt: Luchterhand, 1976], 86–114). Oskar's family members treat even the adult Oskar like a child, and Oskar uses this to his advantage and escapes accountability for his role in the deaths of Alfred Mazerath, Jan Bronski, and his own mother. Emmel points out the ambiguity surrounding Oskar and his dwarfed body, writing that *Die Blechtrommel* "shows how the seemingly childish Oskar is drawn into the events, does not resist, and finally, whether intentionally or not, commits deeds which harm others" (Emmel, *German Novel,* 343). In this sense, Oskar's body does indeed have representational quality, symbolizing the stunted ethics of middle class Germans during National Socialism. Noel Thomas writes: "Oskar gives shape to the amorality of the age in which he lives. He reflects in fractured manner the extent to which truth, morality, and religion have been eroded under the impact of bourgeois attitudes and politics" (Noel L. Thomas, *Grass: Die Blechtrommel. Critical Guides to German Texts,* ed. Martin Swales [London: Grant and Cutler Ltd., 1985], 85).

The symbolic quality of his portrayal does not lessen the impact of the resistance to fascism that Oskar enacts. The power of his resistance is a product of the confidence Oskar has in himself and the authority he claims to tell his own story. Schwann writes:

> Hier besteht ein Erzähler mit bemerkenswerter Klarheit auf der Erkennbarkeit seiner Individualität und indirekt auch auf der Erzählbarkeit seiner Geschichte, denn ein Held ist er nicht im Sinne eines Heros, sondern in dem, daß er sich als veritable Hauptperson einer berichtenswerten Handlung vorstellt.

[This narrator is remarkably clear about the recognizability of his individuality and also, indirectly, about the narratability of his story, because he is not a hero in the [conventional sense], but instead in the sense that he presents himself as the veritable main character of a plot worth telling.] (Schwann, *Unmensch*, 15)

Yet within Grass's depiction of both the Nazi period and the emerging Federal Republic, it is clearly the nonconforming and uncontrollable Oskar who has the most to lose: "Oskar bleibt den Widersprüchen der Welt in einem viel intensiveren Maße ausgeliefert als seine Mitmenschen, die sich auf eine bequeme Art in der Alltäglichkeit einzurücken verstehen" [Oskar remains subjected to the contradictions of the world to a much more intensive degree than his fellow human beings who only know how to move in daily life in a comfortable manner] (Schwann, *Unmensch*, 48). The ambiguity of narrative agency, then, is both the overarching form and theme of Grass's critique of twentieth-century Germany.

The picaresque structure of the narrative deserves attention here, for the *Schelmenroman* genre is an important facet of this novel's ability to engage in this critique. The *Schelmenroman*, as opposed to the teleological *Bildungsroman*, is likely necessary after the end of the war, when literary and intellectual foundations were shattered. There is little hope of linear development here. Even Oskar's decision to grow again proves futile: he only grows a few centimeters and develops a humpback in the process. Oskar is an outsider, and like any good picaresque novel hero, he satirizes society from his view from below (or without). His disability plays an important role in affecting this satire. Schwann writes: "Da man ihn auch geistig für zurückgeblieben hält, benimmt man sich in seiner Nähe so ungeschickt, wie man in Wahrheit ist" [Since people around Oskar consider him to be mentally retarded as well, they are as careless in his presence as in they are in truth] (Schwann, *Unmensch*, 22). For these reasons, *Die Blechtrommel* marks a turning point in twentieth-century prose representations of the disabled outsider. The narrative problematizes Oskar's relationship to the social whole and demonstrates the contribution he makes to shaping that society. The novel reminds readers that not only the educated Bildungsbürger is involved in building this German nation. To be sure, Oskar's stunted growth functions as a metaphor for the stunted ethics of the German middle classes. Yet Grass must be credited for creating a "dynamic metaphor," one that is supremely active and capable of affecting change. Oskar is not merely acted upon or even held up for his didactic qualities. Grass puts tired stereotypes of disability to work by constantly repositioning them within a dynamic framework. Through this repositioning, *Die Blechtrommel* accentuates the tension between social welfare, that is, what is good for the emerging German nation, and Oskar Mazerath's claim to acknowledgment as a full citizen. Oskar demands to be recognized as an active member of his society. He is not only shaped by, he also shapes, the German nation in which he lives.

The German social network provides a model of rehabilitation and care that many nations emulate. Disability policy nonetheless operates on the notion that disability is a social problem and not an issue of individual civil rights. Although Germany does not have a strong tradition of civil rights, the first article of the constitution of the Federal Republic does make an unequivocal claim to promote universal human rights: "Die Würde des Menschen ist unantastbar" [The dignity of the human being is inviolable] (Art. 1 Abs. 1 Satz 2 GG). The claim to protect the "dignity of the human being," however, is not sufficient to guarantee self-determination to people with disabilities. Increasingly subject to cost-benefit analysis, disability policy frequently elevates the welfare of the many above the welfare of the few. This tendency subordinates people with disabilities and precludes their full integration into the activities of daily living, thus putting their claim to the rights of full citizenship at risk. Clear discrepancies exist in the contemporary German social welfare state with regard to people with disabilities: on one hand, the often-praised "social network," the federally run and state-run system of insurances that is the primary marker of the German social welfare state, provides high-quality, comprehensive health care; on the other hand, this very system defines disability by measuring the reduction of a person's capacity to work against a standard or a norm, thus perpetuating the notion that disabled people are less than whole. Since 1974, West German law has defined disability using the normative instrument "MdE," or "Minderung der Erwerbsfähigkeit" factor: the factor indicating the degree to which the capacity of the individual to work is diminished (Georg Schmidt, *Schwerbehinderte und ihr Recht* [Köln: Bund-Verlag, 1994], 15). This factor was renamed as "Grad der Behinderung" ("GdB"), or "degree of disability," in 1986, yet the resulting designation is still one that measures the reduction of one's capacity to work. Thus a person might be designated "50%" or "75%" and would receive corresponding benefits.[12] While the law itself has not changed since German unification, the effects of unification on the lives of people with disabilities living in the former East Germany warrant a fuller investigation that is beyond the scope of this study.

It remains remarkably unclear, however, exactly how "work" is defined so as to arrive at the GdB factor. Carol Poore draws attention to the overwhelming deference to the German market economy and highlights the "contradictions associated with the whole complex of work, employment, and performance, connected as they are to certain deeply-rooted ideas about the "value" of the individual to a society based on profit" (Carol Poore, "Disability as Disobedience," 188). Poore further identifies an area in which tension exists between an individual's responsibility to his or her society and that individual's opportunity for personal development.

The central problem underlying this practice of defining disability as decreased work potential is that work or performance is not perceived as being a possibly creative or fulfilling activity. Rather, it is viewed primarily from the point of view of economic gain and social control. (190)

This formulaic approach to defining disability gives rise to tension between an individual's claim to the rights of full citizenship and the well-being of a social totality, for such a definition of disability quite literally renders a disabled person burdensome to the social whole. This person's claim to full civil rights thus stands in clear conflict with the interests of the social totality.

Recent testimonial works previously cited (Andrea Buch, ed., *Ann den Rand gedrängt* [Pushed to the Margins]; and Sigrid Arnade, ed., *Weder Küsse nach Karriere* [Neither Kisses nor Careers]) provide varied and differentiated accounts of many of the physical and mental conditions that, despite their seeming unrelatedness, fall under the medical and political designation "disability." A broad range of physical and mental conditions is covered in each of these works, including blindness, spinal cord injury, cerebral palsy, thalidomide syndrome, and others. The people interviewed cite little more than the social responses to disability as "qualities" they share with other people designated disabled: limited interaction with their nondisabled peers; a paternalistic health care system; severely reduced access to education and employment; lack of involvement in decision-making processes that affect their daily lives; and the nondisabled community's pervasive though erroneous perception that sexuality simply does not exist in the lives of people with disabilities. These testimonies question a model of disability that is based on an ostensibly ahistorical notion of "wholeness" and in doing so call for new analysis of the very term *disability* and its impact on human lives.

Marking a significant discursive shift, these works explore the many and varied manifestations of disability itself. The authors and editors examine disability as a topic, and, relinquishing all traces of mythology and metaphor, use language that describes disability as an experience. Their writing introduces a disability-centered perspective and offers insightful critique of the merits of disability as a literary device. The interview and personal narrative forms introduce a new voice into disability discourse: the voice of the individual who lives with a disability. This newer voice operates in the tradition of social critique undertaken by Leonhard Frank and Günter Grass, yet the individuals who speak in *An den Rand gedrängt* and *Weder Küsse noch Karriere* reconfigure the terms of disability discourse by claiming a central voice. In other words, the people interviewed do not view themselves as symptoms of a larger social problem or a burden to German society; instead they view any unreflected deference to German society to be a burden to *them*. While this type of inversion is an important first step toward emancipation, the writers of these collections do not adhere to the notion that a social whole is necessarily the antagonistic opposite of an individual. Instead, the writers of these narratives insist upon recognition as an integral part of the German society. Their texts give evidence of the writers' developing consciousness as members of a particular social group. Most evident is their call for new evaluation of the role and history of people with disabilities in Germany. Finally, it is important to note that the voices in these testimonial collections are predominantly the voices of women. Expanding upon the efforts of the German women's movement of the 1970s and similarly concluding that "the personal is political,"[13] which was a popular slogan of the German women's movement of the 1970s, Buch and Arnade seek expressly to elevate the subjectivity of the women interviewed and acknowledge their authority. Buch writes that the interviews "spiegeln die subjektiven Erfahrungshorizonte der einzelnen Verfasserinnen wider" [reflect the subjective range of experiences of the individual writers] (10).

An den Rand gedrängt features interviews with people who have disabilities as well as their family members, friends, therapists, social workers, teachers, and primary caretakers. Common to the entries are the critique of "therapeutic" efforts to integrate people with disabilities into the *Leistungsgesellschaft* and the conviction that unreasonable demands are placed on individuals to achieve. Buch is doubtful that these demands can afford anyone a fulfilling life, arguing that the typical strategies of this rigorous pursuit are particularly inappropriate to many people with disabilities. The writers of *An den Rand gedrängt* argue that the rewards are elusive and ask why people with disabilities should be "therapeutically" trained toward these ends. They ask instead to be recognized as individuals and treated with dignity. One young woman, Regina Schier, contemplates the potential effects of the interview and writes:

Ich hoffe und wünsche mir, daß aus diesem Bericht über mein Leben ersichtlich wird, daß ein behinderter Mensch in erster Linie "Mensch" ist und erst in zweiter Linie "Behinderter."

[I hope and wish that it will be evident from this report of my life that a disabled person is first and foremost a "person" and only after that, "disabled."] (42)

Sigrid Arnade's collection of interviews, *Weder Küsse noch Karriere*, documents the experiences of twelve women who have disabilities. Arnade's work posits their double discriminatory treatment, first as women and then as women with disabilities. The latter type of discrimination ironically works to neutralize the former. Women with disabilities, Arnade argues, are in effect stripped of all gender: "Behinderte Frauen werden kaum als Frauen wahrgenommen" [Disabled women are hardly perceived as women] (202). All of the women interviewed describe the social obstacles that hinder and in many cases prevent meaningful interpersonal relationships. The exploration and expression of sexuality were rendered for these women virtually impossible by the general public's widespread unwillingness to engage with them on any meaningful level. Such isolation was further complicated by the fact that even parents, family members, teachers, and doctors refused to acknowledge, and thus discounted, sexuality as an aspect of their lives.

> Herzschmerzen hat [Else] vor allem in der Jugend gehabt als ihre Schwestern heirateten und es für sie klar war, daß sie nie heiraten würde. "Eine behinderte Frau heiratet nicht. Mit diesem Satz meiner Eltern bin ich aufgewachsen und habe ihn als junger Mensch nie angezweifelt."

> [Else was above all heartsick in her youth when her sisters married and it was clear to her that she would never marry. "A disabled woman does not marry. With this, my parents' statement, I grew up, and as a young person, never doubted it]." (82)

This expressly political book asks the important theoretical question: what is a woman? In an attempt to answer, Arnade's work reminds readers that human beings are always members of more than one social group. Her protocols examine the lives of women with disabilities in order to study the ways in which they negotiate belonging to two historically oppressed groups. This testimonial work illuminates the conflicting impulses that raise the question of how identity categories are defined and prioritized. Consider the following brief example: the right to abortion, when gained, is frequently assumed to empower women. Yet, in a position stemming directly from Nazi ideology, German women who have disabilities are more often than not counseled to terminate pregnancy. Further, the topic of abortion sparks heated debate among disabled women who oppose abortion that is primarily undertaken to prevent the birth of a disabled child. Indeed, in this situation, women with disabilities have expressed a distinct sense of disempowerment. Arnade writes:

> Nichtbehinderte Frauen kämpfen seit Jahren für das Selbstbestimmungsrecht in bezug auf einen Schwangerschaftsabbruch und die Sterilisation. Da haben es Frauen mit Behinderung leichter: Von ihnen wird geradezu erwartet, daß sie ein Kind abtreiben lassen, wenn sie schwanger geworden sind. Auch dem Sterilisationswunsch einer behinderten Frau wird problemlos entsprochen.

> [Nondisabled women have been fighting for years for the right to make their own decisions about abortion and sterilization. Here, women with disabilities have it easier: it is virtually expected that they have abortions if they become pregnant. Even a disabled woman's desire to be sterilized will be accommodated without problems.] (203)[14]

Arnade also addresses the incidence of rape among women with disabilities in Germany. Significantly, she was in 1992 not able to find reliable statistics documenting the frequency of rape of women with disabilities, but she nonetheless judged the number of rapes to be high, writing that

[behinderte Frauen] sind dem Täter sogar noch hilfloser ausgeliefert, da sie sich oftmals nicht wehren können. Die Vergewaltigung behinderter Frauen wird tabuisiert und taucht folglich in keiner Statistik auf. [(women with disabilities) are even more helpless against a perpetrator, since they are often not able to defend themselves. The rape of disabled women is made taboo and does not show up in any statistics.] (202)

The women interviewed in *Weder Küsse noch Karriere* also describe their frustrated attempts to find meaningful work. Those women who did find work reported regular encounters with condescending employers and coworkers, and they felt that they were required to perform at a higher level of expertise simply to be regarded as adequate. They were often required to perform menial tasks and were discouraged from having contact with other workers or clients: "Bei dieser Tätigkeit sitzt sie den ganzen Tag an der Schreibmaschine und tippt, hat also keinen Kontakt zu Kunden oder Geschäftspartnern. Dafür wollte man sie haben, aber das wollte Rose nicht" [In this job she sits at her typewriter all day and types, without any contact with customers or business associates. They wanted her to do that, but that is not what Rose wanted] (42).

Testimonial literature such as Andrea Buch's *An den Rand gedrängt* and Sigrid Arnade's *Weder Küsse noch Karriere* advances disability discourse significantly by chronicling the actual experiences of individuals who live with disabilities. It is important to note that neither Buch nor Arnade places much emphasis on curing or preventing disability. They take pains to recognize disability as an experience in its own right and do not subscribe to long-standing notions of derivation from a standard of able bodiedness or of the socially degenerative effects of disability. The terminology they use is not bound to mythological or other narrative systems that engage in explaining or ascribing larger meaning to disability, and the authors discredit overly simplified, universalized symbols of disability. Instead, they advocate self-representation and the exchange of practical information in the effort to gain social and political strength. In this vein, such testimonial literature enriches both the representation of disability in writing and the very real lives of people with disabilities.

People with disabilities today make up a significant portion of the German population. It is estimated that six million people out of 80 million, or around 7.5 percent, have some sort of disability. Although this is currently more people than comprise several major German political parties,[15] people with disabilities in Germany enjoy astonishingly little political power. As more people with disabilities organize themselves and mobilize their energies in attaining political strength, they will not simply remove the "liability" of disability, they will reshape the contours that define the human experience.

NOTES

1. I undertake this study with the intention to subject my own use of the term *disability* to scrutiny. I acknowledge from the outset that my operative definition of disability is informed by the Americans with Disabilities Act of 1990 and designates a physical or mental condition that interferes with a major life function such as walking, hearing, breathing, or learning; or being perceived as having such a condition. (See Public Law 101–336, 102 Cong., 2nd sess. (23 January 1990), Americans with Disabilities Act of 1990, sec. 2a(7).) I rely heavily on this definition because it places disability squarely within the context of individual civil rights and provides a clear contrast to the more normative and society-oriented German definition. Further, in the spirit of the interdisciplinary approach that I take in this analysis, I make use of the American definition in an attempt to "exploit the hermeneutic potential of intersecting borders between the world of ethnographer and native" (Jeffrey M. Peck "Going Native: Establishing Authority in German Studies," in Frank Trommler, Michael Geyer, Jeffrey Peck, eds. "Germany as the Other: Towards an American Agenda for German Studies. A Colloquium," in *German Studies Review* 13 (1990): 129). Official political borders have already been opened, as policymakers in both Germany and the United States have frequently considered social structures in each state as models for their own projects; an example pertinent to this study of disability is the United States' recent interest in the German health care system. By including an American definition of disability in this study of German literature, I hope to chip away at the notion that political boundaries form closed histories and cultures.

2. All translations from the German are mine unless otherwise noted.

3. The original phrase is "Nichtvorhandensein der Liebe."

4. I shall retain the term *war cripple* in my translations of quotations from the novellas. Although the degrading tenor of the term is apparent today, *war cripple* best conveys the social stature of soldiers disabled in war at the time of the novellas' appearance. Further, as I shall argue in this essay, it is this very social position with which Frank takes issue.

5. I have deliberately avoided terms such as *amputee* and tried to minimize my use of *the disabled* because these terms reduce an individual to that which makes him or her different from the "norm."

6. I do not wish to imply that those people injured in war are in any way undeserving of the rights or the respect that Frank seeks for them. I wish instead to point out that Frank cannot be understood to speak for "the disabled" as a group, as disabilities have many origins.

7. Frank seems to suggest that "able bodiedness" is the natural consequence of simply having a requisite number of body parts.

8. See Hans-Jörg Uther's discussion of disability as punishment in his study of Ger-

man popular narratives, *Behinderte in populären Erzählungen. Studien zur historischen und vergleichenden Erzählforschung* (Berlin: Walter de Gruyter, 1981).

9. Along with disability, other social issues such as the role of race or sexual orientation moved in similar fashion among discursive realms. James Jones notes, for example, that "homosexuality moved slowly from the strictly moral and legal realm, which encompassed social attitudes, to the realm of science, which dealt with reason and ratio" (James W. Jones *"We of the Third Sex": Literary Representations of Homosexuality in Wilhelmine Germany,* German Life and Civilization [New York: Lang, 1990], 46). Jones points out that while the topic of homosexuality did not lose its moral stigma, medicine did radically alter its view by the end of the nineteenth century. Clearly, the professions of social sciences engaged in classification of human activity on an ever-growing scale. Thus the interrogation of norms such as Frank undertakes in *Der Mensch ist gut* is certainly in keeping with the early twentieth century's efforts to classify, quantify, and name aspects of human life.

10. A number of book-length studies document the treatment of people with disabilities under National Socialism. See in particular Ernst Klee, *"Euthanasie" im NS-Staat. Die Vernichtung lebensunwerten Lebens* (Frankfurt: Fischer, 1983); and Götz Aly, "Medicine against the Useless," chap. 2 in Götz Aly, Peter Chroust, and Christian Pross, *Cleansing the Fatherland. Nazi Medicine and Racial Hygiene,* trans. Belinda Cooper (Baltimore, MD: Johns Hopkins University Press, 1994). Two particularly important sources of information on the role of doctors under National Socialism are Robert N. Proctor, *Racial Hygiene. Medicine under the Nazis* (Cambridge, MA: Harvard University Press, 1988); and Robert Jay Lifton, *The Nazi Doctors. Medical Killing and the Psychology of Genocide* (New York: HarperCollins, 1986).

11. While National Socialists carried these notions to their most heinous extreme, these strategies of social control are by no means unique to the Nazi period.

12. See as well the discussion of abortion in C. Ewinkel and G. Hermes, eds., *Geschlecht: behindert. Besonderes Merkmal: Frau* (München: AG SPAK, 1992), 69–87.

13. "The personal is political" was a popular slogan of the German women's movement of the 1970s.

14. See as well the discussion of abortion in C. Ewinkel and G. Hermes, eds. *Geschlecht: behindert. Besonderes Merkmal: Frau.* (Munich: AG SPAK, 1992), 69–87.

15. Membership in Bündnis 90/Die Grünen in January 1993 numbered 40,700; the Freie Demokratische Partei (FDP) 92,475; the Sozialdemokratische Partei Deutschlands (SPD) 886,000; and the Christlich-Demokratische Union (CDU) 684,300 (Petra Zwickert, ed. *Harenberg Lexikon der Gegenwart 95* [Dortmund: Harenberg, 1994]). I do not wish to imply that it is possible to group all people with disabilities in Germany into one political party, for as I have indicated earlier, disability is by no means an exclusive or overriding aspect of human identity; as such, it defies reason to suggest that all disabled people would choose membership in the same political party. Indeed, disabled people's lack of strength as a unified political power would seem to illustrate this fact.

Disabled Women as Powerful Women in Petry, Morrison, and Lorde ▶ Revising Black Female Subjectivity

Rosemarie Garland Thomson

Perhaps the fundamental aim of African American women's writing is to construct a black female subject that displaces the negative cultural images generated by America's aggregate history of racism and sexism. Such a collective project of cultural revision challenges the African American woman writer to produce a narrative of self that authenticates black women's oppressive history yet offers a model for transcending that history's limitations. In other words, the writer must recast the dominant representations of black womanhood without violating the elements that have been shaped by the experience of being a black woman in America. Her task is thus to render oppression without reinscribing it: to build a figure of black female selfhood on the narrow space between victimization and assimilation, so that she neither repudiates her history nor embraces the conventional scripts of womanhood that have excluded her.

In Audre Lorde's explicitly revisionist narrative of self, *Zami: A New Spelling of My Name*, the narrator Audre/Zami at once poses this problem and implies a solution.

> My mother was a very powerful woman. This was so in a time when that word-combination of *woman* and *powerful* was almost unexpressible in the white american [sic] common tongue, except or unless it was accompanied by some aberrant explaining adjective like blind, or hunchback, or crazy, or Black. Therefore when I was growing up, *powerful woman* equaled something else quite different from ordinary woman, from simply "woman." It certainly did not, on the other hand equal "man." What then? What was the third designation?[1]

Acknowledging that the dominant definition of "woman" excludes personal power, Lorde searches here for language to express her experience of the oxymoronic "powerful woman." Rejecting both "woman" and "man," she imagines this iconoclastic black female as occupying a "third designation" distinct from the only two available normative options. This woman thus falls outside standard categories and necessarily into the realm of the "aberrant," intelligible only if inflected by "explaining adjective[s]" invoking that which is outside what counts as normal. For Lorde, the designations "blind," "hunchback," "crazy," and "Black" become the only available semantic vehicles into the ontological safe space of the extraordinary, where alternative ways of being can be articulated and validated. Using these adjectives, Lorde equates the body's form with subjective identity. Indeed, Lorde uses the devalued bodily characteristics associated with race and disability to represent any state or feeling that differs from the privileged norm. The material experience of always being extraordinary, of never coinciding with the normative requirements of womanhood or manhood, is the fact of existence that shapes the identity Lorde creates in her "biomythography." The body is the source of both the freedom and the condemnation from which Lorde's mythic self, her own third designation, emerges.

What is clear in this passage and throughout Lorde's biomythography is that difference, not sameness, is her principle of identity. Being outside the ordinary is both essential and emancipatory in her self-definition: she is a lesbian as well as "fat, Black, nearly blind, and ambidextrous," a cluster of attributions at once excluding and affirming (*Zami* 240). By claiming her extraordinary body as the ground of identity, she repudiates the norms of "woman" and "man." Assimilation to the norm would be for her an act of self-effacement in which she would be a deviant pretender. Instead, Lorde figures herself as inassimilable, so unique in body, birth, history, and behavior that distinction becomes the principle of her identity and her power.

Lorde's third designation is one manifestation of a figure sprinkled through African American women's writings, a figure whose body bears the marks we think of as "disabilities." This figure's extraordinary body disqualifies her from the restrictions and benefits of conventional womanhood, freeing her to create an identity that incorporates a body distinguished by the markings—some painfully inflicted, some congenital—of her individual and cultural history. These disabled figures present a version of black female subjectivity that insists upon and celebrates physical difference. By flaunting rather than obscuring these figures' physical differences, the authors establish the extraordinary body as a site of historical inscription rather than physical deviance and simultaneously repudiate such cultural master narratives as normalcy, wholeness, and the feminine ideal.

I trace here a genealogy of this disabled figure—who might be more precisely called extraordinary—from its inception as Mrs. Hedges in Ann Petry's 1946 novel *The Street;* through more fully developed manifestations in Toni Morrison's first five novels, *The Bluest Eye* (1970), *Sula* (1973), *Song of Solomon* (1977), *Tar Baby* (1981), and *Beloved* (1987);[2] and finally to Audre/Zami in Audre Lorde's 1982 biomythography, *Zami: A New Spelling of My Name.* Together, these disabled female figures gesture toward an antiassimilationist, politicized rhetoric of difference born of the civil rights and the Black Arts movements of the 1960s. Characters such as Morrison's Eva Peace, Baby Suggs, and Pilate Dead and Lorde's Zami offer an African American female self grounded in the singular body that bears the etchings of history and whose validation, power, and identity derive from physical difference and resistance to cultural norms. These women enable their authors to represent a particularized self who both embodies and transcends cultural subjugation, claiming physical difference as exceptional rather than inferior. Beginning with Petry's Mrs. Hedges, an ambiguous precursor in the modernist grotesque tradition, I examine here eleven figures and their rhetorical roles. Following Mrs. Hedges are Morrison's disabled women, Eva Peace, Marie Thérèse Foucault, Baby Suggs, Nan, and Pauline Breedlove; the physically marked figures of Pilate Dead, Sula, Sethe, and her mother; and, finally, the multiply distinctive central figure of Audre in Lorde's *Zami*. In varying degrees, these figures each occupy the radical subject position Lorde terms the *third designation*. In these revisionist narratives of black womanhood, the body as a site of history and identity is at once burden and means of redemption.[3]

Physically disabled characters appear with some frequency, but usually peripherally, in African American literature.[4] I focus here on the figures created by Petry, Morrison, and Lorde to reveal the shift in African American literary representation from a modernist to a postmodernist mode, a change that parallels the ideological move of minority groups from assimilation to affirmation of cultural and ethnic differences.[5]

The representation of disability I find in Morrison and Lorde—and to a degree in Petry—reflects a shift in the meaning attached to bodily difference that is consonant with the positive identity politics characteristic of the post–civil rights era, in which racial and gender variations are reinterpreted as differences to be accommodated or celebrated rather than erased. This change in perspective on bodily difference can be traced historically in early legislation that compensated for disability in the workplace and the military and later in the legislation exemplified by the 1990 Americans with Disabilities Act requiring that disabilities be accommodated.[6] With their disabled figures, Petry begins and Morrison and Lorde develop a postmodern perspective of particularity in which physical differences—racial, gender, cultural, or sexual—are seen as politicized marks of variation that must be recognized and accommodated within a democratic society. The rhetorical framing of bodily difference thus moves from a politics of sympathetic advocacy to a politics of affirmative identity.

The Extraordinary Woman as Powerful Woman: Ann Petry's *The Street*

The conventions of naturalism structure *The Street*'s primary narrative, creating a modernist rendering of alienation and desperation.[7] Petry's "street" is a neutral—even hostile—world, bereft of transcendental signifiers, without the traditional ideologies of unity and meaning that could provide adequate tools for living. Rooted in racism and sexism, the novel's rhetoric of despair renders all characters except the heroine, Lutie, as modernist grotesques, of which Mrs. Hedges is the paradigm. Focusing on Lutie's unswerving journey toward disaster, *The Street* traces the failure of the dominant versions of True or New Womanhood to come to terms with modern, institutionalized racism and sexism.[8]

A subdued counternarrative can be extracted from this novel, however, by imaginatively reading Petry's physically disabled antiheroine, Mrs. Hedges. This character anticipates the positive identity politics that African American women's writing articulates after the 1960s and tentatively begins forging a new, specifically black, figure of womanhood. The model of black female subjectivity that Mrs. Hedges inaugurates refuses the derivative cultural script of the patriarchal woman and instead acknowledges the violations and exclusions of the oppressed body. Defining themselves apart from the conventional model of white femininity from which they have forever been excluded, Mrs. Hedges and her heiresses extravagantly claim the authority of their bodies as well as their individual and collective histories as the basis of their identities. This version of black womanhood is fully developed in the physically disabled figures created forty years later by Morrison and Lorde. As their prototype, Mrs. Hedges embodies not the rule but the exception, testifying to the dialectical relationship between the subjugation and the realization of the black female self in modern American culture.

Mrs. Hedges functions as a foreboding and forbidding element of the deterministic environment that defeats Petry's spunky and earnest protagonist, Lutie Johnson. A "very black" woman of "enormous bulk," Mrs. Hedges is "so huge that the people [in her hometown] never really got used to the sight of her" (*Street* 5, 242). A frightening precursor to Lorde's "powerful woman," she is "a mountain of a woman" with "powerful hands," whose strength and size violate the diminutive and delicate stereotype of womanhood and defy categorization. Mrs. Hedges is an inexplicable monster who seems to Lutie like "a creature that had strayed from another planet" (*Street* 237, 236). If Mrs. Hedges's hugeness precludes the femininity of which Lutie is the black type, it is her physical disability that definitely renders Mrs. Hedges Lutie's grotesque opposite. The reader knows from the outset that Mrs. Hedges has some mysterious, awful bodily condition that she hides by wearing a bandanna and staying at home, sitting at her window above the rest of humanity in the street. She operates as an ominous quasi monster who evokes the Gothic and embodies the grotesque conventions that create the sense of impending, menacing, impersonal fate characteristic of both naturalist and modernist narrative.

Not until halfway through the novel does Petry humanize Mrs. Hedges by revealing the story of her disability, the "mass of scars—terrible scars" covering most of her body after she escaped from a tenement fire by squeezing herself through a tiny basement window (*Street* 237). When Petry briefly shifts the omniscient narration typical of naturalism to Mrs. Hedges's perspective to explain her disability, the novel allows the reader some empathy and understanding but refuses Mrs. Hedges any pity. Recounting the incident that has determined Mrs. Hedges's life and identity, the novel conceals her interior, just as Mrs. Hedges hides her scars from public view. We learn what she does to survive but not how she feels about it. She appears chiefly through a normative perspective.

> When she walked into [employment agencies], there was an uncontrollable revulsion in the faces of the white people who looked at her. They stared in amazement at her enormous size, at the blackness of her skin. They glanced at each other, tried in vain to control their faces or didn't bother to try at all, simply let her see what a monstrosity they thought she was. (*Street* 241)

Mrs. Hedges remains throughout the novel resolutely other, apparently unmoved, and finally inscrutable. As the grotesque, toughened embodiment of the brutal life dictated by the street, she inspires mainly "dismay" or "horror," leading Lutie to conclude that "It would never be possible to develop any real liking for her" (*Street* 247, 239).

Nevertheless, a striking ambiguity in Mrs. Hedges's figuration suggests a possible oppositional subtext in which she is the literary foremother of the postmodern black heroines. Narrative comments such as "all those years [Lutie had] been heading straight as an arrow for that street" indicate that *The Street* is primarily intended as a narrative of social determinism in which the "walled enclosure" of racism and its institutions finally surrounds the heroine (*Street* 426, 430). Such generic constraints demand that Mrs. Hedges function as the disturbingly grotesque product of racism and poverty. Representing the unacceptable fate that the hapless heroine must endure if she is to thrive on the street, Mrs. Hedges—who offers Lutie the alternative of prostitution—is part of Lutie's oppressive social environment. She is both the street's victim and its threat. Nevertheless, Mrs. Hedges remains unrescued and survives the street; indeed, she becomes its queen—precisely because she is the antithesis of the conventional Lutie.[9] Juxtaposing Lutie and Mrs. Hedges makes *The Street* not simply a fatalistic vision of racist, sexist society but a feminist critique of conventional womanhood inflected by race issues. Moreover, viewed from this perspective, Mrs. Hedges allows us to explore her potential as a radically revised heroine.

Lutie is precisely what Mrs. Hedges is not: the perfect lady, a version of the nineteenth-century domestic heroine, cast out of the patriarchal home for which she was fashioned and abandoned in Harlem during World War II. Motherless and fortuneless, Lutie must make her way in the world, in the tradition of the heroines of nineteenth-century women's fiction.[10] Armed with beauty, morality, a spunky industriousness, self-reliance, faith in the American success narrative, and what Nancy Cott has called "passionlessness," Lutie is a granddaughter of the True Woman, the traditional feminine version of the self-made man.[11] Her only available cultural model for life is Ben Franklin, whom she undauntedly invokes in a paradoxical mantra of self-blame and self-encouragement.[12] Ready to sacrifice herself for the manhood of her son and her husband, Lutie is republican motherhood incarnate. She can never triumph, however, in Petry's realm of implacable racism and sexism, inflected by the universalized impotence and alienation so characteristic of the modernist aesthetic.

Each of Lutie's conventional feminine assets turns out to be a disastrous liability in the twentieth-century context of "the Street." Rather than evoking respect and admiration, Lutie's beauty compels the lust of every man she meets, inciting men to fight for ownership of her as if she were a piece of meat. Her idealized passionlessness makes their desire for and power over her a greater threat than necessary. For example, Boots, whom she bludgeons to death in a self-destructive moment of released rage, might have made a suitable lover if Lutie had been able to somehow accept his sexuality and avoid his coercion. Her Emersonian self-reliance and fear of moral contamination of herself and her son prevent her from bonding with women such as Mrs. Hedges's "girls" or anyone else who might help her negotiate life on the street. Lutie's adopted mode of femininity is so ineffective in a world shaped by racism and sexism that she literally and metaphorically cannot even read the signs in Petry's wind-whipped opening scene. Every act, every decision comes from the individualist sensibility that seems to Lutie the only coherent narrative of self but that leads her inexorably toward ruin.

Whereas the street and its dangers are illegible to Lutie, Mrs. Hedges is almost omniscient. Instead of retreating because of her disability, she actively engages the world on her own terms from her window, refusing to "expose herself to the curious, prying eyes of the world" (*Street* 247). The opposite of sexually objectified Lutie, Mrs. Hedges has the gaze, a voice, and agency—the personally empowering elements that culture has persistently denied women. With her "rich" and "sweet voice," she gently but authoritatively advises, manages, and connects with the folks on the street (*Street* 5, 8). Her "unwinking," "eager-eyed stare" clearly apprehends and comprehends both the street's squalor and its potential (*Street* 245, 68). Displaying no emotion but much generosity, she is the powerful "lady with the snake's eyes" that seem to penetrate people, reading their thoughts (*Street* 8). Both malevolent and benevolent, Mrs. Hedges uses her powerful body to rescue the defenseless Lutie from her predatory landlord and to regulate his sexual aggression thereafter.

Seeing without being seen, knowing without being known, staging without being staged, acting without being acted upon, the figure of Mrs. Hedges inverts the cultural choreography of gender so concisely described by John Berger: "men act and women appear."[13] In contrast, the guileless and exposed Lutie is ceaselessly the victim of both her inadvertent and deliberate attempts to capture the male gaze—for example, when she heads to Junto's bar for relaxation or auditions for singing jobs. Mrs. Hedges's body may be violated and shaped by her history of enduring racist and sexist institutions, but it is also the instrument with which she is able to define herself apart from the cultural script of womanhood that destroys Lutie. By juxtaposing these two women, *The Street* effectively dislodges the gender system's myth of the power and advantage of feminine beauty and the rewards of male devotion, suggesting alternative forms of female empowerment.

Anticipating Lorde's call for a third designation, Mrs. Hedges repudiates the dominant script of femininity without falling into a masculinized mode. Instead, she establishes a woman-centered life and maintains a truce of sorts with the coercive male power that controls the street. In the brutal environment of racism, sexism, and poverty, Mrs. Hedges forges a community of women that figuratively and literally nourishes its members even while it is circumscribed by an inescapable power hierarchy that would grant her nothing but scorn. Outside of the sexual economy herself, Mrs. Hedges has set up a household of "girls" who manipulate the sexual exchange system to satisfy their own material needs. Above all, the figure of Mrs. Hedges insists upon the demands, restrictions, and obligations of the body. Because, as she notes wryly, "Mary and me don't live here on air," she begins to charge the young men who come around for sex (*Street* 250). Nevertheless, her relations to this prostitution and to Junto, the omnipotent white male who controls the street, are very ambiguous. Mrs. Hedges is in one sense utterly complicit with the dominant order that oppresses them all and is the ultimate threat to Lutie's freedom. Yet her actions are an adaptation to brutal adversity that allows her and the girls to make a life for themselves mostly on their own terms: choosing their customers, tending the sick, watching kids after school, and looking out for one another. Despite being—from Lutie's perspective—perversely compromising, threatening, and repellent, Mrs. Hedges nevertheless testifies with her indomitable corporeality to the grandeur and authority of "an absolutely incredible will to live" (*Street* 245). While Lutie's attempted inviolable self proves brittle and vulnerable, Mrs. Hedges refuses victimization, witnessing with her extraordinary body the abiding power of the violated self to endure injustice and yet prevail.

From the Grotesque to the Cyborg

Even though Petry's portrayal of Mrs. Hedges is one of qualified positive empowerment, *The Street*'s treatment of this character seems nevertheless to be dictated predominantly by the conventions of the modernist grotesque. Such a reading implies that the grotesque might be worth exploring as a problematic yet potentially suggestive way of representing physical disability. The problem occurs when we employ an aesthetic category such as the grotesque in an inherently politicized critical project. When the interpretive framework of the grotesque's visual fantasies and extravagances is translated into the predominantly realistic conventions of literary representation and criticism, the grotesque becomes equated with physically disabled characters. Therefore, using the grotesque as an analytic strategy invites both critics and readers to view representations of disability through an aesthetic rather than a political framework. Aestheticizing disability as the grotesque precludes analysis of how those representations support or challenge the sociopolitical relations that make disability a form of cultural otherness.

The grotesque as a mode of liminality that blurs accepted categories is nevertheless suggestive for my purposes. Geoffrey Galt Harpham defines the grotesque figure as "stand[ing] at the margin of consciousness between the known and the unknown, the perceived and the unperceived, calling into question the adequacy of our ways of organizing the world, of dividing the continuum of experience into knowable parts." Such a sense of the grotesque as "something illegitimately *in* something else" tends to neutralize alienation and repugnance and to highlight the potential for an iconoclastic liminality that can accommodate new forms of identity—precisely the project of the African American women writers I consider here. Anthropologist Victor Turner contends that liminal figures occupy "a realm of pure possibility whence novel configurations of ideas and relations may arise."[14]

By refusing with their very beings to conform to social rules and categories, the disabled women operate as physical alternatives to the status quo. Their opposition to the dominant order is not intellectual; rather, it is an immutable ontological state. The experience of bodily lack, difference, and marginalization is recast here as a radical, affirmative state of alternative physical configuration particularized by history.[15] When a figure that might ordinarily appear merely as grotesque—like Mrs. Hedges—is thus reformulated through liminality, a sociopolitical perspective begins to emerge.

Mrs. Hedges's figuration as an ambiguous modernist grotesque opens the way for a postmodern representation of disabled figures that more fully exploits the potential of third designations and liminal identities. The most fundamental aspect of postmodern thought for the purposes of this analysis is its willingness—perhaps its demand—to relinquish the principles of unity and sameness in interpreting self and world. What I am calling postmodern here are alternative, affirmative narratives that do not depend on a faith in oneness or a range of valued concepts such as wholeness, purity, autonomy, and boundedness—characteristics of the ideology of unity that both sanction the normative self and generate its opposite, the corporeal other. The disabled figures in these novels explore narratives of the body in a postnormal world, similar to the postgender world sometimes invoked by feminists, which upsets the traditional normal/abnormal dichotomy.[16]

The principle of unity undergirds the dominant discourse of abnormality, expressed in ideas such as social Darwinism and the statistical conception of the norm, both of which arose in the nineteenth century. The notion of a human norm that polices human physical variation both generates a unified community whose differences are effaced and defines an outside and inside. The concept of the norm that Foucault finds emerging in the eighteenth century thus characterizes bodies with the differences we call disabilities as deviant rather than distinctive. So while prodigious or "monstrous" bodies have always been a focus of human interest, the normal/abnormal dichotomy of the modern mind limits the explanation of differences to pathology. Although the idea of abnormality as an interpretive frame for physical disability displaced such rationales as divine punishment or moral corruption, the dichotomy of normal/abnormal nevertheless devalues disability rather than defining it on its own terms. Like "powerful woman," the term *disabled person* is oxymoronic because "disabled" nullifies the dominant version of personhood expressed in, for example, the Emersonian self-possessed individual.[17]

Whereas the notion of a hybrid self might act as a guiding metaphor for those who consider themselves nondisabled, for people with disabilities such hybridization is often consonant with actual experience. The disabled person always fuses the physically typical with the physically atypical. The disabled body is also often merged with prosthetics such as wheelchairs, hearing aids, or white canes.[18] Disability is also sometimes experienced as a transformation, or a violation, of self, creating classification dilemmas or ambiguous status. All persons with physical disabilities thus embody the "illegitimate fusion" of the cultural categories "normal," which qualifies a person for human status, and "abnormal," which disqualifies him or her. Within this liminal space the disabled person must constitute something akin to identity. According to the principle of unity, the disabled person becomes grotesque either in the sense of a gargoyle, breaching boundaries, or in the sense of a eunuch, one who is incomplete, not whole. But if unity is no longer the organizing principle of world and self—as the modernists lamented and the postmodernists celebrate—then the grotesque sheds its twisted, repugnant, and despair-laden implications and becomes a cyborg:[19] the affirmed survivor of cultural otherness, ready to engage the postmodern world on its own terms. The paradoxes of body, self, and world that positivism sought to untangle with taxonomies and that modernism bemoaned with grotesques have become the stuff with which a postmodern sensibility explains itself and—paradoxically—constructs its meaning.

The Extraordinary Body as the Historicized Body: Toni Morrison's Disabled Women

Such hybrid figures repeatedly appear in Toni Morrison's first five novels, published between 1970 and 1987. Among other things, each novel elaborates alternative modes of self for the African American woman. The successors of Petry's Mrs. Hedges, Morrison's disabled and marked women have changed, we might say, from grotesques to cyborgs. Each character discussed here functions as what Morrison has called "the pariah figure."

> There are several levels of the pariah figure working in my writing. The black community is a pariah community. Black people are pariahs. The civilization of black people that lives apart from but in juxtaposition to other civilizations is a pariah relationship . . . But a community contains pariahs within it that are very useful for the conscience of that community.[20]

Marginalized by the exclusionary hierarchy of appearance commonly known as "beauty" or "normalcy," Eva Peace, Marie Thérèse Foucault, Baby Suggs, Nan, Pilate Dead, Sula Peace, Sethe, and Sethe's mother are all pariah figures whose place in "the conscience of th[e] community" is to probe the interrelations of identity, history, and the body. Each woman is excluded from the cultural center because of her deviant bodily marks or configurations, as well as by being black, poor, female, and—in some cases—old. While some of these women are central and others peripheral characters, all of them possess a narrative power, often associated with the supernatural, that far outstrips the marginal social status accorded them by the dominant order. Their "deformities," "disabilities," and "abnormalities" are the bodily imprints and the judgments of social stigmatization—rejection, isolation, lowered expectations, poverty, exploitation, enslavement, murder, rape. Excluded because of their bodies from all privileged categories, Morrison's pariah figures explore the potential for being and agency outside culturally sanctioned spaces.[21]

These characters enable Morrison's novels to represent a narrative of self that simultaneously embraces and transcends the individual and collective history of oppression. Although Morrison's novels certainly celebrate black American culture, they also insist that its very shape and spirit have been informed by the institutions, injustices, and resonating, devastating consequences of racism. Nevertheless, Morrison's characters are not victimized or demoralized, nor do they lead diminished lives. A scene from *Beloved* succinctly illustrates how Morrison represents the tension between the need both to incorporate the experience of oppression and to surmount it. The young heroine, Sethe, just escaped from slavery, is able to look with full horror at the young black men hanging dead in the sycamore trees and, at precisely the same moment, to recognize the arresting beauty of those trees. Refraining from reconciling those images, and thus attenuating the contradiction's force, Sethe embeds the disharmony in her memory for a lifetime. Sethe's refusal to allow either spectacle to cancel out the other, her sharpening of this paradox that potentially threatens all meaning and coherence, exemplifies the mode of being and knowing that Morrison represents as fundamental to the African American self. This self affirms the human ability to survive pain, loss, and the denial of both self and culture without abridging experiences of passion, beauty, attachment, and joy. As physical witnesses to violations and oppression, the extraordinary bodies of these women act as a collective conscience by testifying to the power and dignity inherent in this specifically African American narrative of self.

The prototype for all eight women is Eva Peace, the matriarchal grandmother who pervades Morrison's 1973 novel, *Sula*. Eva's leg has been amputated, perhaps on her own initiative so that she can collect insurance money that will feed her children. Like Mrs. Hedges's forcing her imposing body through the basement window to escape the fire, Eva's act of tough desperation both reshapes her body and guarantees her survival. All of Morrison's protagonists are in similar situations: they literally constitute themselves with a free-ranging agency whose terms are tragically circumscribed by an adversarial social order. Self-violation, however, is no concession for Eva or for Mrs. Hedges; rather, it is an act of self-production that at once resists domination and witnesses oppression's virulence. Eva differs from her fellow amputee, Melville's Captain Ahab, in that Ahab's amputation enslaves him in an obsessive pursuit of Moby Dick, while Eva's amputation frees her from poverty. Ahab's transformation is wrought by wholly uncontrollable external forces, while Eva's is accomplished on her own terms. Indeed, physical disability neither diminishes nor corrupts Morrison's extraordinary women; rather, it affirms the self in context. Eva's disability augments her power and dignity, inspiring awe and becoming a mark of superiority.

Morrison represents Eva as a goddess/queen/creatrix character, rich with mythic allusions and proportions, even though she is by dominant standards just an old, black, one-legged woman who runs a boardinghouse. Eva is a rewritten, black Eve, striding the realms of the ordinary and the extraordinary, a female version of the African American trickster whose asymmetrical legs suggest presence in both the material and the supernatural worlds and signal empowerment rather than inadequacy. The trickster is ambivalence personified, violating behavioral norms with outrageous antics and reversing cultural categories that make sense of the social order.[22] As a trickster figure, Eva transgresses the existing social order, opening up the possibility for an alternative narrative of the embodied self as unique rather than normative. Revising as well the Biblical myth of Eve's original sin, Eva creates a mythic narrative of the maternal grounded in physical existence—eating, defecating, dying, and the material, mundane demands of earthly survival. Her power encompasses birth and nurturing as well as death: she severs her leg to sustain her "beloved baby boy," Plum, whom she later immolates when his heroin addiction blunts the life she once gave him (*Sula* 34). Morrison rewrites Eve's apple as the meager three red beets that remain for Eva to feed her children after her husband abandons her to poverty. In short, Eva is a goddess not of the Western spiritual order but of the flesh—flesh made extraordinary not by idealization but by history. Her enduring body is both her identity and her ultimate resource.

Eva's legacy to her world is sustenance. Not always benevolent and never sentimentalized, Eva provides food and shelter, the material needs of life. Eva is the "creator and sovereign" of a peculiar, rambling, incoherent boardinghouse, filled with living, singing, addiction, and casual lovemaking (*Sula* 29). This "woolly house" is replete with trees bearing womblike pears in the yard and "a pot of something always cooking on the stove" (*Sula* 29–30). Directing her children, as well as a continuous stream of friends, boarders, and adopted strays, Eva reigns—much like Mrs. Hedges—over an unorthodox communal household from her incongruous throne, a wagon in her third-floor bedroom where she reads dreams and distributes "goobers from deep inside her pockets" to gaggles of children (*Sula* 29). Naming her own children and renaming others with a mystical and determining vision, Eva possesses, like Adam, the power denied Eve: to name and thus to define. For example, she renames three very different abandoned boys she adopts as "Dewey King," apparently recognizing that the bond of a shared name would enable them to emerge from rejection and isolation and to survive (*Sula* 39). Thus, in the liminal space of what Michelle Fine and Adrienne Asch have called the social "rolelessness" of disabled women, Morrison erects a rich narrative countermythology around the pariah figure Eva, investing her with the power and authority that the dominant order would withhold.[23]

The quasi-supernatural character Marie Thérèse Foucault, from Morrison's 1981 novel *Tar Baby*, resembles Eva Peace. Thérèse's narrative role is essential, although she occupies little space in the novel. Known on Dominique for her "magic breasts," the now blind Thérèse is a former wet nurse for white babies and a washerwoman for the wealthy whites who control a nearby island (*TB* 92). Like Eva, Thérèse has mysterious powers; she is a caretaker, a trickster, and an Eve figure whom the narrator calls "a lying crone with a craving for apples" (*TB* 93). Like the blind seer Tiresias, Thérèse has the knowledge associated with the gaze, but without the sense of sight. With omniscience reminiscent of Mrs. Hedges's, Thérèse senses the stalking presence of Son, the novel's protagonist, weeks before any of the sighted characters become aware of him. Like both Eva and Mrs. Hedges, Thérèse unobtrusively manages the main characters from her position on the edge of society. She leaves Son food, enables him to pilfer the white people's provisions, and finally escorts him through the dark to his ambiguous destiny. A spiritual mentor as well, Thérèse coaxes both Son and her nephew to reconnect with their black culture, their "ancient properties," after they have been lured away by white culture (*TB* 263). Personifying the mythical, supernatural element in the novel, Thérèse is suspected of being "one of the blind race" who escaped slavery and currently roam the island freely on horseback, seeing with "the eye of the mind" (*TB* 130–31).

Thérèse vividly illustrates an essential aspect of all the mythical disabled women in these novels: her narrative prestige and power—both magical and material—are exactly the opposite of the position the real world accords such figures. Thérèse's extraordinary knowledge and authority within the mythic black culture contrast starkly with her powerless, inconsequential, and even invisible position within the dominant culture. To the whites, she is an intractable servant, poor, old, blind, uneducated, haughty, superstitious, ungrateful—and bad at English. Repeatedly fired, she is simply rehired by her employers, who do not even recognize her. However, being resolutely outside the dominant order gives Thérèse authority. She will not speak to the deferential black servants, or "acknowledge the presence of the white Americans in her world," or include them in her imaginative stories, or even simply look at them (*TB* 94). Such denials free her from the cultural perspective that would obliterate her. Blind and invisible to the privileged, Thérèse nevertheless senses the pulse and sets the stride for the black community that Morrison celebrates. By elevating the lowest figure on the dominant scale of human value to power and status, the novel inverts that hierarchy.

Beloved, the 1987 fictional exploration of the female self under slavery, features two disabled figures, limping Baby Suggs and one-armed Nan, whose bodies bear witness to racism's violations and to their own survival.[24] Baby Suggs and Nan—following Eva, Thérèse, and Mrs. Hedges—nurture, guide, and tend to the material needs of the black community from an effaced position of authority. After her son buys her out of slavery, "Baby Suggs, holy" establishes a kind of maternal ministry and community welfare center, similar to Eva's, in her intergenerational, female home, where "two pots simmered on the stove," "the lamp burned all night," and she "loved, cautioned, fed, chastised and soothed" every black man, woman, and child who passed through (*Beloved* 87). Until she is worn out by life, Baby Suggs is also a priestess of the flesh, leading the community in neopagan, outdoor ceremonies, rich with dancing, crying, and singing, in which she delivers potent, moving sermons imploring the people to deeply love their own flesh, their strong and worthy bodies that are broken, tormented, and despised by others. Afterward, she "dance[s] with her twisted hip the rest of what her heart ha[s] to say" (*Beloved* 89). Baby Suggs knows the significance of the body for black women: her flesh has been owned by someone else, her eight children have been stolen from her, and her disabled hip has quite literally reduced her value in the perverse economy of slavery.

Less developed than Baby Suggs, Nan, Sethe's early caretaker, also has the power to survive, nurture, and remember. Like Thérèse, Nan is a wet nurse; like

Eva, she is an amputee. Nan is also a preserver of culture and history, telling the young girl Sethe—*Beloved*'s protagonist—in their vanishing African language the story of Sethe's birth, revealing that she was the sole child whom her enslaved mother valued, the only one not born of a rape and thrown overboard. Although Sethe never acknowledges it explicitly, part of her mother's legacy is the certainly ambiguous moral capacity to commit infanticide, a paradoxical power shared with Eva Peace.

Morrison creates another group of women whose bodies are extraordinary not because of functional limitation but because of formal particularity.[25] The first is Pilate Dead, born without a navel, who is a priestess and the maverick aunt of Milkman Dead, *Song of Solomon*'s protagonist. Like Mrs. Hedges, Eva, and Baby Suggs, Pilate is the matriarch of an unorthodox household, "a collection of lunatics," where mysterious arts of the flesh such as wine making, potion making, and lovemaking are practiced. In Pilate's house, three generations of women reign like the three graces or Eumenides, black goddesses who sought vengeance for crimes against family members (*SS* 20). Self-named, Pilate ceremoniously hangs through her earlobe her Biblical name ensconced in a tiny brass box. Just as Thérèse lures Son back to his black roots, Pilate and her housewomen entice Milkman with their siren songs, but instead of destruction he finds a revitalizing connection with his history and ancestors.

Pilate's extraordinary body differentiates her from the other characters, marking her off in a liminal, often magical, space of possibility. Morrison describes this effect in an interview.

I was trying to draw the character of a sister to a man, a sister who was different, and part of my visualization of her included that she had no navel. Then it became an enormous thing for her. It also had to come at the beginning of the book so the reader would know to expect anything of her. It had to be a thing that was very powerful in its absence but of no consequence in its presence. It couldn't be anything grotesque, but something to set her apart, to make her literally invent herself.[26]

Morrison suggests here that a character's embodied difference enables her to "invent herself," to realize a distinctive identity apart from the canonical body that acts out conventional, white scripts. All these women literally embody a principle of identity formation predicated on the extraordinary rather than the ordinary. Assuming much narrative significance, these women's bodies resist assimilation into a narrow category of humanness and challenge all exclusionary physical standards in racial and gender systems. By seeing all offers of either assimilation or tolerance as condescension, they insist that there is nothing into which they wish to assimilate and that there is nothing in themselves that must be tolerated.

Similarly to Pilate Dead, Eva Peace's granddaughter, Sula, is set apart by a dark facial birthmark that gives "her otherwise plain face a broken excitement and blue-blade threat" (*Sula* 52). Sula's physical marking is both the cause and the manifestation of her otherness. Suggesting her ambiguous position within the community, Sula's birthmark is interpreted by others as a snake, a tadpole, her mother's ashes, or a rose, depending on each character's position. As a rose, the birthmark alludes to the blossoms on the skin that early Christians interpreted as stigmatic marks of grace and alludes to the African goddess of love, Erzulie, whose sign is a rose.[27] The serpent, of course, associates Sula with the biblical Eve and with her grandmother, the revised, black Eve. The way that Sula's birthmark becomes the anchor for someone else's narrative meaning captures the essence of how cultural otherness is produced. What the dominant order perceives as bodily differences act as depositories of meaning that serve the psychological and political perspectives of that group. The extraordinary aspect of her body makes her a spectacle among spectators, the point of reference for social boundaries. The body that acts and appears different becomes a marked pariah and disrupter of the social order. In such a role, Sula enables "others [to] define themselves" by offering up her differences so that the community can clarify itself (*Sula* 95). As with the other extraordinary women, her body serves as "the conscience of th[e] community."[28]

Both Sethe and her unnamed, enslaved, rebellious, hanged mother have markings that map their histories upon their bodies, at once imposing identity and differentiating them from the unmarked. Sethe's mother's slave status is literally integrated into her flesh, branded on her as on a steer or a Greek slave. Her mouth has also been permanently fixed in a ghastly, ironic "smile," fashioned by the master's punitive bit rather than by her own feelings (*Beloved* 203).[29] With the dignified, tough pride of a survivor, Sethe's mother, in her only direct encounter with her daughter, brandishes her stigmata before Sethe as a means of identification, prompting the innocent child to plead, "Mark the mark on me too," as a bond with her mother (*Beloved* 61). Answered with a slap from her outraged mother, Sethe finds eventually that the legacy of enslavement provides her with her own inscription, a deep intricate scar on her back from the brutal beating that was the price of her freedom.

Recalling Sula's differentiating birthmark, Sethe's scar is interpreted by others alternately as a chokecherry tree and a wrought-iron maze. Sethe herself must decipher this memory-charged inscription, borne on her back and hidden from her own view, in order to fathom her history and quiet her ghosts. This ambiguous badge, at once a curse and a gift from her mother, represents their bond as well as Sethe's redemption from her mother's fate. As with each marked female character, Sethe's bodily reconfiguration is paradoxical, embodying simultaneously the terrible price demanded and the extraordinary character produced by her history and identity. The communal role of the extraordinary women is to preserve otherness and its meanings with the very shapes of their bodies and to sustain the communal body by nurturing and care. Their marked bodies witness the communal bond created by slavery and the differentiation each individual history has wrought. These women's bodies *re-member*: they recall and reconstitute history and community.

Morrison's extraordinary women emerge most clearly when contrasted with a final physically disabled female character who serves quite a different rhetorical function from the others. Pauline Breedlove, mother and wife of the brutalized and brutal Breedlove family in Morrison's first novel, *The Bluest Eye*, bears the label of bodily deviance and the markings of history, just like her successors. But Pauline does not display the authority, dignity, or quasi-supernatural powers of figures like Eva, Thérèse, or Pilate. Although Pauline is a washerwoman and caretaker of white children like Thérèse, has a disabled foot and a limp like Baby Suggs, and has survived poverty, abuse, deprivation, and animosity, she is never a priestess or mythical goddess figure. Instead of enabling other members of her community, she devastates them. Indeed, Morrison strips Pauline of precisely what she endows the other disabled women with. While they are empowered, Pauline is diminished, for she has desecrated herself by her complicity with oppression. By internalizing the judgment of inferiority handed down to her, Pauline betrays her own flesh and consequently that of her children, husband, and racial community. The stigmata of being black in a white culture, being a woman in a man's world, being poor in a rich society, or even limping through a world that idealizes physical ability do not diminish Pauline and destroy her daughter, Pecola. Rather, the convergence of circumstances, character, and choice that makes Pauline embrace "ugly" and her role of "the ideal servant" with neither question nor defiance robs her of the dignity, grace, beauty, and love accorded the other extraordinary women (*BE* 34, 100).

Pauline is Morrison's sympathetic study of violations of the soul and perversions of potential perpetrated by racism's institutions. Her misplaced priorities estrange her from the sustaining community of other black women so that Pauline never hears sermons by the likes of Baby Suggs, eats in kitchens like Eva's, or even feels the validating solidarity of the whores who live upstairs. Bereft of such sustenance, she is tragically seduced into self-loathing, squandering her potential by finding her praise and satisfaction keeping a rich white family's house and loving their blue-eyed, blond-haired girl instead of her own daughter. With no sources of resistance, Pauline accedes to the destructive ideologies of female martyrdom, bourgeois respectability, denial of the flesh, and romantic love. Such beliefs lead her to accept disability as imperfection, to idealize white physical beauty as equal to virtue, and to embrace the role of the ideal, praise-lulled, black servant in a luxurious white household. Much like Petry's Lurie, Pauline has embraced the cultural scripts all the other marked women have rejected. Her faith in these ideological sins against blackness, femaleness, and self functions in the novel as an apostasy that nullifies her daughter, Pecola. For this violation, Morrison denies Pauline one of her chief rhetorical emblems of empowerment: the inclusive, woman-centered, black home where she might have reigned as a priestess of the flesh.

Pauline's experiences demonstrate that even while the novels authorize and validate the possibility of a more utopic world of alternative embodiment, they also surround the women's lives by a realist, adversarial social order that circumscribes both their actions and their relationships. Although few characters actually occupy the dominant subject position, it is nevertheless pervasive, a ubiquitous force that relentlessly disrupts and limits the black characters. The slave owner, Schoolteacher, for example, appears only briefly in *Beloved;* yet the dreadful consequences of his acts reverberate throughout the novel, rupturing and distorting relationships everywhere within the black community. Even the arguably benevolent white men such as Valerian in *Tar Baby,* Mr. Garner in *Beloved,* and Pauline's appreciative employer in *The Bluest Eye* unwittingly inflict damage because their dominant perspective and values are incompatible with the well-being of black people. The cruel paradox fundamental to Morrison's novels is that the destructive interlocking race/gender/class systems govern her characters even while the characters have power to act within those systems. We see this delimitation of agency, for example, in *Sula* when Eva severs her leg to save Plum from hunger and later burns him to save him from spiritual starvation, and—even more strongly—in *Beloved* when Sethe turns back the slave master by slashing her baby's throat.

By insisting that the historicized body informs identity, Morrison recalls Leonard Kriegel's "Survivor Cripple," whose principle is that "self-creation is limited by the very accidents that give it shape" and that agency lies in "the will to manipulate that which has manipulated him *[sic]*." The women's disabilities and marks are either material traces of racism or the congenital variations upon which cultural otherness is built. These physical traces are a discourse inscribed by history upon the flesh of human beings, what Paule Marshall calls "life-sores."[30] The disabilities, then, are not metaphors for lives twisted by oppression but the identifying, affirming, and valued manifestations of bodily uniqueness and personal history. The body is a text that the women insist upon interpreting themselves, even as they resist fantasies and fears others project on them. The women's histories are emblazoned upon their flesh, evidence of dignified endurance and profound vitality.

The Extraordinary Subject: Audre Lorde's *Zami: A New Spelling of My Name*

Whereas Petry's and Morrison's disabled women tend to occupy the margins of their fiction, Audre Lorde's 1982 "biomythography," *Zami: A New Spelling of*

My Name, places the marked woman and the claims of her body at its very center, making her the narrator. Describing *Zami* as "really fiction" that "has the elements of biography and the history of myth," Lorde consciously constructs a narrative self, purposefully evading the naive referentiality behind the idea of objectively chronicling a life.[31] Her hybrid genre, biomythography, fuses the opposing discursive categories of "myth" and "biography" signaling *Zami*'s thematic project of creating an embodied identity that transgresses all boundaries. The prologue describes the work's fundamental concern with bridging dichotomous, narrowly restricting classifications of self.

> I have always wanted to be both man and woman, to incorporate the strongest and richest parts of my mother and father within/into me—to share valleys and mountains upon my body the way the earth does in hills and peaks. (*Zami* 7)

Zami thus begins with the premise that Audre's lived and felt experience is at odds with normative categories of identity. She speaks of herself as "grow[ing] up fat, Black, nearly blind, and ambidextrous in a West Indian household" (*Zami* 240). Although this description thwarts valued self-representations, Lorde defiantly claims it nevertheless. From the pages of *Ebony,* to the "wasting" expression of whites, to the favoring of light skin in her family, to the special classroom for children "with various serious deficiencies of sight," Audre learns from early on that her body is not only different but wrong (*Zami* 5, 24). *Zami*'s mission is to reconstruct the narrative of deviance carried by *fat, blind, lesbian,* and *Black* to create a discursive self that incorporates the bodily traits and experiences upon which these terms are based yet infuses the words with value, power, and fresh meaning.

For Lorde, rigid oppositional categories such as man/woman, self/other, normal/abnormal, and superior/inferior straitjacket her lived, physical experience. *Zami* vigorously resists such imposed definitions of the self, refusing to capitulate to self-erasure as Pecola Breedlove does in Morrison's *The Bluest Eye.* The autobiographical form eliminates the dynamics of sympathy and the potential for objectification that often emerge when a narrator mediates between the reader and a marginalized character like Audre. By establishing a subjective perspective centered on lesbian sexuality and cultivating outsiderness, *Zami* denaturalizes the dominant viewpoint and protests its ascendancy. Both invoking and retooling autobiographical form and content, *Zami* shapes a multifaceted cultural and corporeal otherness into a coherent subjectivity, grounding her narrative of self in the kind of third designation discussed at the beginning of this essay (*Zami* 15). To do this, Lorde intensifies her subject's differences from the dominant norm rather than muting them and highlights those differences in the text. Hence, what we might term *the intensely other* becomes the self in Audre's narrative, challenging the cultural norms that would shunt her to the margins.

Explicitly representing lesbian sexuality in a cultural context where heterosexuality is the norm becomes a method for contesting normalcy itself.

Zami extends Petry's and Morrison's explorations of new forms of black female identity by founding its definition of self on the extraordinary rather than the ordinary, on the exception rather than the rule. If her physical difference is the source of her social alienation, she also makes it the source of her poetic and erotic affirmation. Such self-authorization, Lorde insists, is a political and personal act of survival, a "transformation of silence into language and action" that achieves significant cultural work.[32] Thus *Zami* illustrates that identity for these extraordinary women follows the postmodern impulse of repudiating the dominant order's master narratives, conjoining subjectivity with embodied differences.

Audre/Zami draws on the conventional forms of the *Bildungsroman, Kunstlerroman,* picaresque, and autobiography to build a positive self-representation as a black, lesbian poet. Her development progresses through a series of relationships with women, beginning with her foremothers and culminating with Afrekete, the black love-goddess figure with whom Audre affirms herself as Carriacouan, woman-loving poet. By representing these relationships with women, including her mother, as both erotic and constitutive of herself as poet, Lorde connects word and body.[33] The biomythography is a surprisingly linear, teleological, picaresque, selected account of relationships with women that together form a response to the work's initial, structuring questions: "To whom do I owe the power behind my voice, what strength I have become?" and "To whom do I owe the symbols of my survival?" (*Zami* 3). *Zami*'s closing statement reveals that Audre's composite self includes aspects of herself recognized in other women. The biomythography fashions these encounters into a patchwork identity drawn from lived experience and open to alteration by subsequent relationships.[34]

> Every woman I have ever loved has left her print upon me, where I loved some invaluable piece of myself apart from me—so different that I had to stretch and grow in order to recognize her. And in that growing, we came to separation, that place where work begins. Another meeting. (*Zami* 255)

Lorde imagines this self-creation as a renaming—what Claudine Raynaud has aptly called a "fiercely active denomination."[35] She begins the transformation from Audrey to Zami with her insistence, at age four, on severing the *y* from her given name, Audrey, and completes it by invoking the biological fact that the body regenerates itself every seven years. This renaming is cast as a somatic reshaping: letters are amputated, and lovers leave imprints on Audre. The body that shifts from Audrey to Zami has supple boundaries; it transfigures and is transfigured by its history in a dialectic between body and experience that recalls Morrison's disabled women, whose bodies literally are their histories.

Moreover, Lorde's narrative departs from the master narrative of the self-determining, autonomous individual. Audre's self, produced by affiliation with a series of women, contrasts starkly with the cultural self articulated in Emerson's "Self-Reliance" or Thoreau's *Walden,* for example, which repudiates all fore-fathers, seeking to develop identity through differentiation. Audre's profound physical departure from the dominant type makes this affiliation both necessary and safe in a way that it might not be for someone closer to the norm. In other words, sameness with the loved ones could become an affirmation rather than the threat of undifferentiated effacement. Perhaps the almost obsessive denial of conformity in Emerson and Thoreau is a fear of being obliterated by ordinariness.

Lorde employs a structuring scheme similar to Morrison's, interweaving a mythic narrative of self with a realistic narrative of selected life events. For example, the italicized voice of the poet speaks the text's mythic account in such lyrical passages as "Snail-sped an up-hill day, but evening comes; I dream of you. This shepherd is a leper learning to make lovely things while waiting out my time of despair." This poetry intertwines with prosaic chronicles of education, work, family tension, tortured adolescence, and sexual initiation, such as "I had sixty-three dollars in my pocket. I arrived in Stamford on the New Haven local on Thursday afternoon. I went to the Black Community Center whose address I had gotten from a previous visit the week before" (*Zami* 190, 122). Audre's last and most affirming sexual encounter consciously weaves the mythic and realistic perspectives, portraying her lover alternately as the poetic "Afrekete" and the prosaic "Kitty." Kitty, "still trim and fast-lined, but with an easier looseness about her smile and a lot less make-up"—is of the real world, while Afrekete comes *"out of a dream to me"* bearing *"live things from the bush, and from her farm set out in cocoyams and cassava,"* conjuring the goddess in each of the women (*Zami* 244, 249). So from the devalued girl, Audrey, emerges the mythical *"Zami. A Carriacou name for women who work together as friends and lovers"* (*Zami* 255). Juxtaposing realism and myth blends robust social criticism with a utopian impulse, accomplishing in *Zami* precisely the same end as in Morrison's work: the mythic perspective dislodges the dominant viewpoint, opening a discursive space for imagining new ways of being.

Lorde's biomythography fully realizes Petry's tentative use of physical difference as a means to a positive-identity politics. While *The Street*'s Mrs. Hedges possesses both vision and voice, *Zami*'s viewpoint confers upon Audre a gaze and voice produced through the autobiographical form, not simply as an effect of content. Because Audre's consciousness determines the narrative per-spective, *Zami* not only generates a discursive self but also creates an entire world apprehended, spoken, and legitimized by that self. Whereas Mrs. Hedges must protect herself from the intrusive stares of others, including the reader, to whom her body seems deviant, Audre cannot become a spectacle of otherness because her voice and perspective constitute the text. Thus a narrating Audre can resist becoming a grotesque spectacle while still parading her difference as a mark of distinction, of identity: "I was fat and Black and very fine. We were without peer or category and on that day I was conscious of being very proud of it" (*Zami* 223). In *Sister Outsider,* Lorde writes movingly about the problem of exposure the risk of becoming a spectacle when one intensifies difference. Discussing self-revelation, she mentions fear of contempt or censure but asserts that "we fear the visibility without which we cannot truly live"; the "visibility which makes us most vulnerable is that which also is the source of our greatest strength."[36] Caught between rage at being negated and the self-protective impulse for concealment, Lorde uses the biomythography to discursively display the extraordinary body and to simultaneously disengage from the exploitative dynamics of spectacle. Thus, Audre/Zami's self-display exalts the extraordinary body and banishes all mediators, insisting upon a direct, intimate relation with her readers.

The Poetics of Particularity

Petry's Mrs. Hedges, Morrison's marked women pariahs, and *Zami's* Audre explore a politicized model of embodied selfhood inflected by collective and individual history. I want to suggest here that writers influenced by the black civil rights movement and the subsequent early women's movement found in the extraordinary body precisely the trope with which to express a notion of self that literally incorporated into the body the essential distinctions implied by racial and gender identity.[37] The problem of representation in a post–black power era was that if black was to be beautiful, it had to be distinguished from standardized whiteness. The figure of the marked woman offers a vehicle for representing the extraordinary body that contradicts, even insults, the privileged normative body that claims neutrality yet enjoys higher status and constitutes the cultural center. Thus, post-1960s black women writers such as Morrison and Lorde use the extraordinary body in the discourse of positive difference so integral to their fictional perspective, while Petry's much more ambivalent portrayal of Mrs. Hedges, written in 1946, was created before a positive-identity politics was commonplace. For these writers, the extraordinary body is a physical testimony to individual and collective experience. At the same time, these figures are differentiated absolutely from characters whose undistinguished bodies grant them the cover of banal, often fraudulent, normative status. In political terms, these extraordinary bodies demand accommodation, resist assimilation, and challenge the dominant norms that would efface distinctions such as racial differences and the marks of experience.

These black women writers not only appropriate marked figures for national-ist cultural work; they also rescue the extraordinary body from its modern, deviant incarnation. The disabled women are not only the racialized bodies of positive-identity politics but also nonconformity incarnate, the quality lauded in Emerson's and Thoreau's visions of an independent self. These figures regain the power subdued by equality's assumption of sameness in standardized, mass culture.

It is not surprising that the cultural work undertaken by African American women writers is reformulating the dominant model of self, particularly the female self. In her history of African American women, Paula Giddings stresses black women's uneasy relationship with dominant versions of femininity, from the ideology of True Womanhood in the nineteenth century, the New Woman image at the century's turn, the 1950s middle class housewife, to the contempo-rary mainstream feminist. Black women have always, as a group, been excluded by ideology and economics from these roles yet simultaneously judged according to them. As early as 1861, for example, Harriet Jacobs pointed to this double standard in her narrative of slave women's sexual exploitation: "the slave woman ought not to be judged by the same standards as others."[38] Similarly, the stan-dards of feminine beauty, based on Caucasian characteristics, have made black women's assigned physical inferiority seem an inherent characteristic. Cast pri-marily as slaves, sexualized prey, and domestic workers, black women's bodies have traditionally been opposed to white women's, even while they are praised or condemned by the same standards. As if in recognition of this paradoxical snare, all three writers deploy the extraordinary women figures in response to the judgment of deviance that has been imposed on the black female body.

The marked women inspire awe at the profusion of difference their bodies flaunt, challenging the supposedly superior status of normalcy by rendering it banal. These literary representations accentuate the marked body's historical context, infusing the material body with social meaning rather than metaphorical significance. By connecting physical being with individual history and culture, the extraordinary women figures define the self in terms of its uniqueness rather than its conformity to the norm.

NOTES

1. Audre Lorde, *Zami: A New Spelling of My Name* (Freedom, CA: Crossing Press, 1982), 15. All future references are to this edition and will be given parenthetically in the text. In *Writing a Woman's Life* (New York: Norton, 1988), Carolyn Heilbrun discusses the lack of language and narrative forms with which to analyze the lives of nontraditional women. Like Lorde's term, *third designation,* Heilbrun's term, *ambiguous woman,* allows

262 · The Body and Physical Difference

one to appropriate the strengths of gender identity and reject the liabilities. Both terms
attempt to affirm and amend the concept of womanhood.

2. Ann Petry, *The Street* (1946; reprint, Boston, MA: Beacon, 1974); Toni Morrison,
The Bluest Eye (New York: Washington Square Press, 1970); Toni Morrison, *Sula* (New
York: New American Library, 1973); Toni Morrison, *Song of Solomon* (New York: New
American Library, 1977); Toni Morrison, *Tar Baby* (New York: New American Library,
1981); Toni Morrison, *Beloved* (New York: New American Library, 1987). All future
references are to these editions and will be cited parenthetically as *Street, BE, Sula, SS, TB,*
and *Beloved,* respectively.

3. In her essay "When We Dead Awaken: Writing as Revision" (in *On Lies, Secrets,
and Silence* [New York: Norton, 1979]), Adrienne Rich defines "re-vision" as reading,
writing, and interpreting women's lives "with fresh eyes." More than simply cultural
history, literary criticism, or autobiographical writing, Rich's well-known feminist concept
is "an act of survival" that enables women to refute the "self-destructiveness" inherent in
conventional womanhood (35). The African American novels discussed here revise black
female identity in precisely Rich's sense. However, this study complicates the notion of
simple racial or gender identity, "re-visioning" it by highlighting the sociohistorical
category "physically disabled." Each of these novels approaches the disability category
only obliquely, unselfconsciously; none confronts the disabled identity directly. The relationships among the stigmatized identities of blackness, femaleness, and physical disability
are never explicitly enunciated.

4. Some examples of physically disabled characters in other African American
women's writing are the protagonists in Harriet Wilson, *Our Nig; or Sketches from the
Life of a Free Black* (1859; reprint, New York: Vintage Books, 1983); and Harriet Jacob,
Incidents in the Life of a Slave Girl (1861; reprint, Cambridge, MA: Harvard University
Press, 1987); Miss Thompson in Paule Marshall's *Brown Girl, Brownstones* (1959; reprint, Old Westbury, NY: Feminist Press, 1981); Uncle Willie in Maya Angelou, *I Know
Why the Caged Bird Sings* (Toronto: Bantam, 1969); the protagonist of Alice Walker,
Meridian (New York: Pocket Books, 1976); and Milkman Dead—Morrison's only
disabled male—from *Song of Solomon.* The prevalence of such figures is perhaps due more
to historical accuracy—disability occurs more frequently under conditions of poverty and
oppression—than to metaphorical intent.

5. These rhetorical figurations of disability roughly correspond to a broad historical
shift in cultural sensibility that can be briefly characterized as follows: the rhetoric of
sympathy assumes unity (expressed, for example, in millennialism), a cultural and cosmic
principle that dominated nineteenth-century American thinking but was eclipsed by the
secularized and naturalist aesthetic of the century's end. The modernist rhetoric of despair
that displaced and mourned the loss of such faith yielded the grotesque, the antihero, and
existential thinking. The postmodern rhetoric of difference no longer mourns unity, even
though it grapples with multiplicity; it is the most congenial cultural mode in which
disability is represented. The terms *modern* and *postmodern* are used here in Fredric
Jameson's sense, as "cultural dominants" that can be resisted but not transcended ("Postmodernism, or the Cultural Logic of Late Capitalism," *New Left Review* 146 [July/August
1984]: 53–92). The transition from one cultural dominant to the next would necessarily be
perceptible not only in literature but also in politics.

6. This historical shift in interpretation of disability is suggested in several studies of the history of disability legislation; see Richard K. Scotch, *From Good Will to Civil Rights: Transforming Federal Disability Policy* (Philadelphia: Temple University Press, 1984); Deborah A. Stone, *The Disabled State* (Philadelphia: Temple University Press, 1984); Claire H. Liachowitz, *Disability as a Social Construct: Legislative Roots* (Philadelphia: Pennsylvania University Press, 1988); and Joseph P. Shapiro, *No Pity: People with Disabilities Forging a New Civil Rights Movement* (New York: Times Books, 1993).

7. For example, Robert Bone in *The Negro Novel in America* (New Haven, CT: Yale University Press, 1958) sees Petry's novel as a successor to Richard Wright's *Native Son* (New York, London: Harper and Brothers, 1940). Addison Gayle Jr. analyzes *The Street* as a naturalist novel in *The Way of the New World: The Black Novel in America* (New York: Anchor/Doubleday, 1975, 192–97).

8. Definitions of True Womanhood and New Womanhood can be found in Barbara Welter, "The Cult of True Womanhood: 1820–1860" *American Quarterly* 18, 2 (1966): 151–74; and in Carroll Smith-Rosenberg, *Disorderly Conduct: Visions of Gender in Victorian America.* New York: Oxford University Press, 1985, esp. 245–96.

9. Deb and Lutie are parallel in this respect: their actions accomplish exactly the opposite of what was intended, and both women are defeated, while for Mrs. Hedges there is no disparity between intention and effect.

10. Nina Baym, *Women's Fiction: A Guide to Novels by and about Women in America, 1820–1870.* Ithaca: Cornell University Press, 1978, 11–12.

11. In Nancy F. Cott, *The Bonds of Womanhood: Women's Sphere in New England, 1780–1835* (New Haven: Yale University Press, 1977). Nancy Cott analyzes the nineteenth-century ideology of feminine "passionlessness" as a functional cultural reformulation of the belief in female carnality as weakness and moral turpitude. If passionlessness placed nineteenth-century women on a higher moral plane and increased their status and independence, it has now outlived its usefulness, tending to alienate women from their own sexuality.

12. Marjorie Pryse, in " 'Pattern against the Sky': Deism and Motherhood in Ann Petry's *The Street*," in *Conjuring: Black Women, Fiction, and Literary Tradition,* ed. Marjorie Pryse and Hortense J. Spillers (Bloomington, IN: Indiana University Press, 1985), 116–31, explores the implications of Lutie's identification with the Ben Franklin script, analyzing the novel and Mrs. Hedges in terms of deism. Pryse also suggests that Lutie's actions and attitudes are self-defeating and notes how she might have used Mrs. Hedges and others as models of survival, but Pryse does not go on to elaborate Mrs. Hedges's potential for becoming the new heroine.

13. John Berger, *Ways of Seeing* (London: British Broadcasting Corporation, 1972), 47.

14. For like-minded discussions of the grotesque, see Philip Thomson, *The Grotesque* (London: Methuen, 1972); Frances K. Barasch, "Introduction," in Thomas Wright, *A History of Caricature and Grotesque in Literature and Art* (1865; reprint, New York: Frederick Ungar, 1968); Geoffrey Galt Harpham, *On the Grotesque: Strategies of Contradiction in Art and Literature* (Princeton: Princeton University Press, 1982) (quotations at 30 and 11); Peter Stallybrass and Allon White, *The Poetics and Politics of Transgression* (Ithaca: Cornell University Press, 1986); Mikhail M. Bahktin, *The Dialogic Imagination,*

ed. Michael Holquist, trans. Caryl Emerson and Michael Holquist (Austin: University of Texas Press, 1981); and Leonard D. Cassuto, *The Inhuman Race* (New York: Columbia University Press, 1996). Like every other theorist I cite except Goffman, these theorists of the grotesque never make an explicit connection between their theories and actual disabled people. Although Harpham, for example, mentions "the various cripples and amputees" in Flannery O'Connor's fiction, he never explores the distinctions between fantastic and human grotesques. Considerations of disability as a social category are limited almost exclusively to scholarly works that announce themselves as disability studies. Also see Victor Turner, *The Forest of Symbols: Aspects of Ndembu Ritual* (Ithaca: Cornell University Press, 1967), quotation at 97.

15. I want to stress that this refiguration is different from the use of disability as a trope. These disabled figures are not metaphors; rather, their representation mediates both the life experience and the social identity of disability, potentially recasting its cultural meaning. Robert F. Murphy's ethnography of disability as liminality (*The Body Silent* [New York: Holt, 1987]) focuses primarily on loss of role and status because this was his own experience of becoming disabled. However, Michelle Fine and Adrienne Asch suggest that disabled women's rolelessness can be freeing (*Women with Disabilities: Essays in Psychology, Culture, and Politics* [Philadelphia, PA: Temple University Press, 1988], 1–31). In any case, women, particularly black women, often have less cultural capital to lose by becoming disabled than do white men such as Murphy.

16. Donna Haraway, "A Manifesto for Cyborgs: Science, Technology, and Socialist Feminism in the 1980s," *Socialist Review* 80 (1985): 67.

17. Identifications such as "powerful woman" and "disabled person," which I am calling oxymoronic here, function similarly to the dual ethnic identities, such as African American, that W. E. B. Du Bois famously notes express the "double-consciousness" of their bearers. See W. E. B. Du Bois, *The Souls of Black Folks* (1903; reprint, New York: New American Library, 1982).

18. For a discussion of prosthesis as a cultural concept, see David Wills, *Prosthesis* (Stanford, CA: Stanford University Press, 1995).

19. Haraway, "A Manifesto for Cyborgs," quotations at 65, 91, 73, and 95. Although Haraway does not develop a connection between cyborgs and disabled people, she notes in passing when discussing computers that "paraplegics and other severely handicapped people can . . . have the most intense experiences of complex hybridization with other communication devices" (97). Although she refers to prosthetic devices as "friendly selves," she does not go on to acknowledge that a wheelchair is a part of the self or that disability brings together two ostensibly mutually exclusive states.

20. Toni Morrison, quoted in Claudia Tate, ed., *Black Women Writers at Work* (New York: Continuum, 1988), 129.

21. Susan Willis's essay historicizing Morrison's first four novels cursorily discusses "lack, deformity, and self-mutilation as figures for liberation" ("Eruptions of Funk: Historicizing Toni Morrison," in *Specifying: Black Women Writing the American Experience* [Madison, WI: University of Wisconsin Press, 1987], 104). Although Willis's main argument concerns the novels' resistance to bourgeois culture, she recognizes a relation between disability and social otherness in Morrison's fiction, suggesting that self-mutilation redefines the individual as a "new and whole person, occupying a radically different social

space" (103). While my reading of disabled figures agrees with her brief explication, this study extends and focuses the analysis much further, treating disability as a socially constructed identity that complicates racial and gender categories, not simply as a physical condition.

22. Henry Louis Gates Jr., "The Blackness of Blackness: A Critique of the Sign and the Signifying Monkey," in *Black Literature and Literary Theory,* ed. Henry Louis Gates Jr. (New York: Methuen, 1984), 287.

23. Adrienne Asch and Michelle Fine, "Disabled Women: Sexism without the Pedestal," *Journal of Sociology and Social Welfare* 8, no. 2 (1981): 233–48.

24. Denver, Baby Suggs's granddaughter and Beloved's sister, also is physically disabled, having become deaf for two years in a psychological refusal to hear the truth about her sister's death. I have chosen, however, not to include her in this analysis, although she conforms fairly well to the pattern, because her disability is temporary. Sethe, Denver's mother, whom I do include because of the scar on her back, also has a temporary disability that should be noted: she stutters from the time that her mother is hanged until she first sees Halle, her husband-to-be.

25. By encompassing formal aspects such as birthmarks and functional conditions such as mobility impairments in the single category of "disability," I do not mean to propose an equivalence among all physically stigmatized conditions but to suggest instead the interrelated sociopolitical nature of these identities. I am asserting that Morrison's narratives frame femaleness, nonwhiteness, and disability not as natural, inherently limiting, biological conditions but as identities shaped by the physical, institutional, and social aspects of an unaccommodating environment.

26. Tate, *Black Women Writers at Work,* 128.

27. Erving Goffman, *Stigma: Notes on the Management of Spoiled Identity* (Englewood Cliffs, NJ: Prentice-Hall, 1963), 1; Gates Jr., "The Blackness of Blackness," 300.

28. Tate, *Black Women Writers at Work,* 129.

29. I am grateful to Mae Henderson for having pointed out this detail about Sethe's mother to me.

30. Leonard Kriegel, "The Wolf in the Pit in the Zoo," *Social Policy* (Fall 1982): 16–23; Marshall, *Brown Girl, Brownstones,* 28.

31. Tate, *Black Women Writers at Work,* 115.

32. Biddy Martin's essay, "Lesbian Identity and Autobiographical Difference[s]," in *Life/Lines: Theorizing Women's Autobiography,* ed. Bella Brodzki and Celeste Schenck (Ithaca, NY: Cornell University Press, 1988), 77–103, makes similar claims for the iconoclastic potential of the lesbian perspective in autobiography, asserting that "[l]esbian autobiographical narratives are about remembering differently, outside the contours and narrative constraints of conventional models" (85). Audre Lorde is quoted from *Sister Outsider,* Trumansburg, NY: The Crossing Press, 1984, 40.

33. This poststructuralist/feminist effort is, of course, similar to *l'Ecriture Feminine* produced by Helene Cixous (see, for example, "The Laugh of the Medusa," *Signs: Journal of Women in Culture and Society* 1 [1976]: 875–93). Lorde's attempt here, however, seems grounded more in material experience and less in linguistic theory than Cixous's writing the body. For an elaboration of Lorde's poetic theory see "Uses of the Erotic: The Erotic as Power," in Lorde, *Sister Outsider,* 53–59.

34. This articulation of self is remarkably consonant with the theories of psychologist Jean Baker Miller and her associates at Wellesley College's Stone Center, who assert that women tend to develop a sense of self through relation rather than differentiation (see Jean Baker Miller, *Towards a New Psychology of Women* [Boston, MA: Beacon Press, 1976]). For discussions see also Judith Jordan et al., *Women's Growth in Connection: Writings from the Stone Center* (New York: Guilford, 1991); and Nancy Chodorow, *The Reproduction of Mothering: Psychoanalysis and the Sociology of Gender* (Berkeley, CA: University of California Press, 1978).

35. Claudine Raynaud, "'A Nutmeg Nestled Inside Its Covering of Mace': Audre Lorde's *Zami*," in *Life/Lines: Theorizing Women's Autobiography*, ed. Bella Brodzki and Celeste Schenck (Ithaca, NY: Cornell University Press), 226.

36. Lorde, *Sister Outsider*, 42.

37. Although gender and racial essentialism are now being questioned vigorously by theorists of both subjects, the occasional emphasis on difference to ground a positive-identity politics or nationalism is important politically for both movements.

38. Harriet Jacobs, *Incidents in the Life of a Slave Girl* (1861; reprint, Cambridge, MA: Harvard University Press, 1987), 56.

Muteness and Mutilation ▶ The Aesthetics of Disability in Jane Campion's *The Piano*

Caroline Molina

When three women earned Academy Awards in 1994 for their roles in the making of Jane Campion's *The Piano* (best director, best actress, best supporting actress),[1] this unconventional "art film" had already become both an uncontested commercial success and an object of continuous media attention. But the (largely enthusiastic) discussions of this film in the media tended to focus on the traditionally appealing aspects of the genre (eroticism, narrative tension, visual pleasure) while neglecting to comment on the more "touchy" subject of the protagonist's muteness as not only a central feature of her character but, indeed, a significant force impelling the action through its various entanglements and complications. The heroine Ada's vocal "disability" reflects her deliberate rejection of conventional forms of human communication, and the film repeatedly raises the issue of the value of silence (or music) as opposed to conversation (verbal, visual, and mental) as alternative varieties of human expression. Besides marking the protagonist's body as "defective" and therefore—according to the dominant aesthetic of Hollywood cinema—as the unlikely object of erotic desire, the verbal disability represents, at various narrative levels, the universal problematic of linguistic interpretation, of speaking and understanding the "other." In tension with its counterpart, piano music, and its opposite, speech, muteness also becomes a surprisingly powerful medium of sexual seduction and a metaphor for the dialectic between art and life.

While other romantic films involving speechless heroines have been criticized for their objectification of the disabled body (e.g., Randa Haines's *Children of a Lesser God*), Campion's film endows the disabled woman with a striking eroticism that is heightened—rather than diminished—by her disability. Because this new filmic eroticization of the disabled body is inseparably linked to the role of muteness per se as a catalyst for the narrative, my discussion of *The Piano*, which is divided into six parts, has a turning point in the middle: the first half focuses on the functions of muteness as a narrative device, while the second half deals with the cinematographic and genre-specific means by which this narrative device is exploited. Part 1 defines the peculiar nature of the protagonist's muteness as a "disability," and part 2 sets this muteness in relation to the many disturbed or disrupted languages of the film, including nonverbal languages used as art. Part 3 examines the relationship between muteness and the many images of illness, woundedness, bodily impairment, or sheer physical vulnerability throughout the narrative. In part 4, the focus shifts to the function of muteness and its counterpart, music, in magnifying the visual pleasure of the film and heightening its erotic tension. Part 5 continues to explore the visual representation of the mute body, particularly the deployment of sign language and signs of bodily mutilation to establish boundaries between the (nondisabled) self and the (disabled) other—boundaries that nonetheless are continually blurred as the disabled body becomes increasingly eroticized. The final section, part 6, places *The Piano* in the context of other films with vocally impaired protagonists and identifies the melodramatic and fairy-tale components of Campion's film as investing its depiction of muteness with a distinctive aesthetic that marks *The Piano* as a singular contribution to the genre of disability film.

I

The first words of *The Piano* serve to orient the viewer with regard to the protagonist's "handicap," and this initial definition of her disability, articulated (literally) in her own words, predisposes the viewer at the outset to understand Ada's strange speechlessness from her own perspective, rather than hastening to attribute to it a freakish quality that would brand her disabled body as irredeemably "other." Ada's voice-over describes both the (medically unexplained) muteness and its musical compensation.

The voice you hear is not my speaking voice, but my mind's voice.

I have not spoken since I was six years old. No one knows why, not even me . . .

The strange thing is I don't think myself silent, that is, because of my piano.[2]

What makes this disability doubly mysterious is the fact that it is self-willed, resulting from a "dark talent" so potent as to be fatal in the event that the will should prove spontaneously life-negating rather than life-affirming.

My father says [my silence] is a dark talent and the day I take it into my head to stop breathing will be my last.[3]

Besides the striking content of these opening lines, their very form suggests the complexity of Ada's handicap as both an apparent limitation and a conspicuous, many-sided gift. For not only is the disability phrased as an uncanny *ability* ("dark talent"), but the corollary manifestations of this talent are both musical (piano playing) and lyrical (the poetic "free verse" of her "mind's voice"). Still, it is *in spite of* the handicap—and not because of any appreciation for, or even awareness of, the gift—that the Scottish Ada can be married off to a pious if somewhat insensitive New Zealand landowner whom she has never met. Stewart, her mismatched if well-intentioned husband, says Ada's muteness "does not bother him," since "God loves dumb creatures, so why not he" (9). Yet his sovereign indifference to Ada's condition gives way, after her arrival on the island, to a critical scrutiny and then a puzzled disparagement of her unusual constitution. One of Stewart's first remarks to Ada after her landing on the beach is a disapproving assessment of her physical stature: "You're small. I never thought you'd be small" (22). And only a few lines later, it becomes clear that Stewart regards his wife's fragile (yet by no means abnormal) appearance as evidence that she is "stunted" (22). Within just a few days of her arrival, Stewart has begun to perceive her muteness—and what to him is the incomprehensible behavior she displays as a result—as a sign that she may well be "brain-affected" (39). The invisible handicap thus appears to have both undesirable visible, physical repercussions (stunted growth) and negative mental consequences or causes (brain damage). To Stewart's puritanical Aunt Morag, these apparent defects make Ada somewhat less than human. When Stewart muses hopefully that "with time [Ada] will, I'm sure, become affectionate," Morag responds with a condescending naïveté that equates disability with animal primitivism (and its necessary domestication): "Certainly, there is nothing so easy to like as a pet, and *they are quite silent*" (40, original emphasis).

Being thus repeatedly confirmed as Ada's most distinguishing characteristic, her aphasia—along with its imputed physical and mental cosyndromes—becomes the major impetus for the primary plot as well as a point of narrative connection with the second story line involving the Maoris, whose language and behavior are likewise incomprehensible to the Europeans and who are similarly, unsuccessfully, "domesticated." Let us first examine the role of speechlessness as a catalyst for the primary narrative. Ada relies on two external "voices" to express herself: one resides in the piano and the other in her ten-year-old daughter, Flora, who translates aloud her mother's silent sign language. When Stewart refuses to include the piano among Ada's other belongings that are transported from the beach inland to Stewart's house, he effectively refuses to accept that crucial vehicle of her self-expression. At the couple's very first encounter, then, Stewart gives Ada every reason to reject *him*, and it is this tension between man and wife at the outset that leads Ada to try to regain possession of her piano—an attempt that involves her in the adulterous love triangle whose complications make up the film's primary plot. Because Stewart does not embrace all the ramifications of Ada's disabled condition—most significantly, her need for the piano—he unwittingly sets in motion the remaining components of the narrative.

II

If the piano is Ada's musical voice, it is also associated with her (sexual) body. Just as Flora represents, in many respects, Ada's younger mirror image in terms of mannerisms and temperament, the piano serves as a kind of surrogate female body for the speechless woman. In the screenplay (although not in the film itself), the blind piano tuner calls the instrument "my dear Miss Broadbent" (Broadbent being the brand name), and he refers to it/her as "tuned, but silent" (48). The European George Baines, who lives among the Maoris and has partially adopted their culture, understands the function of the piano as an instrument of Ada's sensuality, as the appendage by way of which he can get to Ada's body itself. When he bares his own body and nakedly caresses the piano with his shirt (49), he enacts the same erotic encounter that he will later orchestrate with Ada.

It is no wonder that Baines understands the unconventional communication that takes place when Ada plays the piano, for he himself speaks the mysterious and musical language of the Maoris (deliberately left, for the most part, untranslated in the film) and shares their unashamed celebration of the body (wearing Maori markings and practicing a discreet and tender version of their open sexuality and affectionate nature).[4] But he also comprehends the "dominant" language of the film, which is the language of commerce—that is to say, the language of negotiation and, sometimes, that of lying. To lead Ada to the point of successful seduction, Baines needs to follow a progressive plan of approach involving a continuous process of bargaining. After making a deal with Stewart to get possession of the piano in exchange for eighty acres of land, Baines proceeds to make an "arrangement" (76) with Ada by which he will enjoy increasingly obliging sexual favors from her in exchange for an agreed-on number of keys from the piano keyboard, until the entire instrument belongs to Ada again. As the most dialectical form of communication, negotiation represents the polar opposite of speechlessness. Yet it is precisely through the constant back-and-forth that bargaining entails that we become aware of how fragile human communication always is—how "defective" every speech act (and, by extension, every speaker). In this film fraught with negotiations—between colonialist and Maoris over land, between mother and daughter over permissible behavior, between husband and wife over regulating marital fidelity, and between the two lovers over the degree of their mutual possession—muteness becomes the background against which all language reveals itself as both disturbed and disruptive. It is only fitting, then, that the willfully speechless Ada should harbor the "strong" and "unholy" opinion that "most people speak rubbish and it's not worth the listen" (57).

In this film riddled with contradictions, however, it is precisely "worth the listen" to pay careful attention to what is said and then denied, for the very speechlessness that initially impels the plot is exactly what is denied in the end when Ada "chooses" to speak. We are prepared for such reversals throughout the film, since repeatedly the characters make assertions only to retract them or later to act in a way that belies what they have said. For example, Flora announces at the beginning that she is "not going to call [Stewart] Papa" and, in fact, is "not even going to look at HIM" (17, original emphasis).[5] Yet in keeping with the shifting alliances of the four central characters in the film, Flora later goes back on her word in order to side with Stewart as her "Papa" (87), feeling, like him, neglected and betrayed by Ada. In an apparently less motivated reversal, Baines agrees to take Ada and Flora back to the beach (and the abandoned piano) even though he originally claims that he doesn't "have the time" to do so (33). Stewart likewise says what he doesn't mean, but his "lying" stems from his puritanical politeness—as, for example, when he pretends that he "wants [the piano] to come" with Ada's other belongings and is indeed "very pleased" (23)—all the while arranging to leave the piano behind—or when he insists that "the girls are very excited" about Baines's piano lessons, although it is evident that they dread the prospect (46). But the most outrageous, if "innocent," lying occurs through Flora's made-up stories about her mother's past and, specifically, about the origin of Ada's muteness.

One day when my mother and father were singing together in the forest, a great storm blew up out of nowhere. But so passionate was their singing that they did not notice, nor did they stop as the rain began to fall, and when their voices rose for the final bars of the duet a great bolt of lightning came out of the sky and struck my father so that he lit up like a torch . . . And at the same moment my father was struck dead my mother was struck dumb! She — never — spoke — another — word. (31–32)

Situated as this story is immediately after a similar fairy tale of Flora's invention—one which Flora admits, however, is "a lie" (31)—this fantasy narrative of erotic union culminating in death and muteness parallels the "real" narrative of Ada and Stewart's "wedding ceremony," which takes place in the form of a staged photograph taken under similarly stormy conditions. Yet both the fairy tale and the "real" marriage are equally constructed as lies, as artifice. If the cartoonish drawing of a puppetlike figure going up in flames intrudes on the screen during Flora's tale to call attention to the workings of her childish imagination, the parallel scene of the wedding photograph, complete with fake costumes and a painted backdrop, is no less contrived. Thus the film draws attention not only to the interchangeability of fantasy and "reality" but to the ultimate pervasiveness of fictionality in all representation: to art as the ultimate lie.

Yet let us remember that the fairy tale is not just about death and dumbness but about consummate art combined with passion: the most intimate and refined communication culminating in its opposite—silence and separation. If the film's primary narrative moves toward silence (the stillness of the piano in its watery grave) and separation (the severing of Ada's umbilical connection to the rope of the piano), it also constantly reminds us of multiple modes of artistic communication and expression. Nonverbal art is a vital ingredient of life in this film—from the spontaneous dancing of the child on the beach to the giant sea horse designed out of shells in the sand; from Stewart's fetishization of Ada's photograph to the ironic playfulness of the Maoris' mimicry; from the all-important piano playing to Ada's articulate "pantomimes" of stories: art has the power to captivate and unnerve. Nowhere is this more apparent than in the scenes that purposefully cast art at odds with life and expose the lure of theatrical illusion in the "play within the film," the shadow drama of Bluebeard. The film audience is well prepared for the rudimentary if gory performance, since we have been warned in advance that bleeding heads and amputated hands will contribute to the "dramatic" effect of the scene (39). Yet the Maoris witnessing the play are drawn in by its murderous plot, their warrior reflexes mobilized to avenge the crime behind the curtain. This comical if temporarily unsettling "misreading" of the play by the natives unmasks yet again the fragility of human communication, since even without a language barrier, the Maoris fail to understand the theatrical signs, even as so many other verbal and visual signs are gravely misunderstood in the film.

The drama performance enacts on a large scale the same deficiency of language that permeates the entire film in countless minute and subtle ways. At one point or another, virtually every character fails to communicate or to comprehend something in some way. Stewart understands neither the Maoris' speech nor Ada's finger language; Baines cannot read Ada's written messages; Flora is puzzled by her mother's mixed signals; and even Baines's dog Flynn becomes confused by Flora's contradictions. Yet what the Bluebeard drama also makes clear—albeit only later in the film—is that we the film audience have also failed to understand: have failed to read the play as a foreshadowing of Stewart's brutal "crippling" of Ada, failed to comprehend the full import of the performance's disruptive messages. For there is a way in which we want to react as the Maoris do, protecting and avenging, when we see the real-life drama of Stewart threatening Ada with the ax.[6] In response to his question: "Is it [Baines] you love?" (97), Ada accepts all the painful consequences of refusing to speak (and refusing to lie). The punishment for her silence—the withholding of an answer Stewart understands all too well—is amputation. The counterstroke to muteness is mutilation.

III

Aunt Morag: I can't imagine a fate worse than being dumb . . .
Nessie: To be deaf?
Aunt Morag: Oh yes, deaf too—*terrible! Awful!* (56, original emphasis)

What Aunt Morag, characteristically, fails to understand when she utters these lines is that at one point or another, everyone is deaf, dumb, or otherwise disabled. That, at least, is a message *The Piano* drives home repeatedly, not just in the obvious stage descriptions, as when, for example, Stewart is "struck dumb with pride" (30) at the sight of Ada in a wedding dress, or when he turns a deaf ear to her requests for the piano. Physical disorders become manifest both concretely and symbolically, and sickness and vulnerability become the standard conditions, not the exceptions. We see this time and again with Flora, who vomits on the beach, gets nauseated from twirling around with Ada in the bedroom, and tries to vomit again from the boat on its return. We see it more figuratively in Baines's "lovesickness" for Ada, which nevertheless has diagnosable symptoms: loss of appetite and insomnia (77). We don't see it in the Maori characters in the film, but the script tells us that "many of the Maoris have coughs, running noses and sores" since "they have no immunity to European diseases" (128). And a similar vulnerability afflicts Stewart, who is "unmanned" and "helpless" when confronted with Ada's erotic curiosity and aloofness (92). One scene in the script (deleted from the film) has the blind piano tuner describe his wife, who has stopped singing out of sadness (49), and even the piano—like its human counterpart, Ada—seems "wounded" from the start: strips of cloth wrap its legs like bandages, it suffers under Stewart's ax, and it even loses a "limb" when Ada willfully cuts out a key to send to Baines as a token of love. Just as Ada is rejected by Stewart when he sees what he perceives as her multiple handicaps, so does Ada finally reject her piano as "spoiled" (120), even though it is presumably as functional as before (Baines has saved the severed key). It would seem that in the final movement of the film toward restoration and renewal—with the promise of a happy future for the reunited "family" of Baines, Ada, and Flora—all signs of damage would have to be erased, and all handicaps removed. This, at least, is the first impression we get when Ada begins to "speak" at the end of the film, and we see that her amputated fingertip has been "repaired" by Baines. But in keeping with the contradictory voices of this film, another message resounds in the final scene: that Ada has chosen a kind of blindness in exchange for a speaking voice (she speaks only "when . . . it is dark" and therefore covers her eyes [122]) and that her apparently restored finger on the piano keys is both a visible and an audible reminder of her lasting deformity. With her metal fingertip, she is "quite the town freak" (122)—that is, more different than ever—but her abnormality "satisfies" (122). Her disability has become a distinction.

IV

What does it mean for a physically disabled woman to be the central focus of a highly erotic film? Dramatic literature has depicted mute heroines before: for example, Kattrin in Brecht's *Mother Courage and Her Children* (1941) shares both Ada's speechlessness and a scar from a visible wound, but she is more saintly than sexy, being explicitly de-eroticized by her role of martyr in the play. Contemporary filmmakers have also experimented with silent protagonists: Werner Herzog's film *Every Man for Himself and God against All, or The Enigma of Kaspar Hauser* (1974) enacts the story of the speechless (male) outsider who personifies loneliness and isolation. Yet the combination of vocal disability and eroticized female sensuality is an unlikely choice for a cinematic character. How does *The Piano* manage this unusual role?

To begin with, film is a medium that traditionally privileges "visual pleasure."[7] The screen is the space where beautiful bodies are displayed, larger and infinitely more perfect than in real life, and the naked female body is the quintessentially eroticized form, arousing the viewers' voyeuristic delight, if not their desire. Moreover, because the visual component dominates in narrative cinema, dialogue can be foreshortened or replaced with other diegetic as well as nondiegetic sounds—that is, sounds within or outside the narrative frame. (Silent film, of course, relies only on external music and the *visual* representation of dialogue.) The introduction of the protagonist's muteness limits the opportunities for spoken dialogue in *The Piano,* but it also sharpens the focus on the visual and, specifically, on the visual representation of language.

The very opening shot, a blurry dark image accompanied by the voice-over of Ada's "mind's voice," introduces the theme of *looking,* as the spectator assumes the perspective of Ada peering through her fingers before viewing the woman from the camera's viewpoint as a filmed object. Throughout the film, the camera will take us to places normally hidden from view—the inside of the piano crate, the inside of Stewart's pocket, the underside of the piano itself. Whereas it is common for film to display what is usually unseen (sex scenes are the most obvious example of the camera's intrusiveness into private space), *The Piano* repeatedly thematizes the act of voyeurism by positioning the looking audience in the perspective of another, *visible* voyeur. This occurs not only in the lovemaking scenes, which we witness as Flora and Stewart do, by peeping through holes and cracks in Baines's hut, it also occurs when we watch Stewart step behind the camera before the wedding photograph, since he assumes the same angle of vision that we the audience will later share. In a film that highlights the act of viewing as both irresistible and forbidden, it is not surprising that we should hear the characters themselves both asking to be seen and asking to be hidden. Thus Flora, dancing on the beach to her mother's piano playing, revels in her mother's gaze: "*Look,* Mama! Mama, *look*!" (original emphasis), but the same Flora will not be allowed to watch during Baines's music lessons. Her pledge not to "look at him" (55), which echoes her earlier remark about Stewart, proves ineffectual as a means of keeping her "in the picture" (one recalls that she is also left out of the crucial wedding photograph). In another play of showing and hiding, looking and being looked at, Aunt Morag peers at the school hall audience through one of the many peepholes in the stage curtain for the Bluebeard play (65). It is also Aunt Morag who will later insist on being hidden by a cape when she relieves herself in the forest (92; the perspective of the film audience, ironically, is not obstructed by the cape). Aside from playing off the Victorian notions of propriety and modesty, the frequent illustrations of glances stolen or blocked create a running subtext of commentary on the experience of film viewing itself.[8] The stage descriptions make this all but explicit when, backstage in the school hall, "there seem to be more peep-holes than curtains as eyes press themselves to the little flap" (65). To magnify and multiply the layers of vision, *The Piano* makes abundant use of the traditional filmic props of viewing: mirrors (55, 87), windows (32, 79), and even a photograph doubling as a mirror (19) reappear as the privileged sites of both the gaze and the display.

It would seem, then, that muteness functions in the service of visual pleasure in this film—taking our attention away from the dialogue to focus it on the image. But that is not to say that the muteness creates a kind of sensual void to be filled up with pictures. For what fills the silence, more often than not, is its necessary counterpart, music. As much as the mirrors, windows, and photographs, the piano becomes the instrument by which to magnify visual pleasure, since it is through the medium of music that the film prolongs our gaze, lingering over a minimum of images until the music has run its course. We have to consider it somewhat of a lie, then, when Baines claims of his piano lessons that he "just wants to listen" (50), since music in this film is not only the consummate nonverbal art form, but it also becomes—for Baines, at least—the medium through which to gain access to other sensual, sexual experience, allowing him not only to prolong his gaze but ultimately to explore Ada's eroticism through the other senses as well (smelling her clothes, touching her body). It is only when the music stops, however, that a complete erotic union takes place between the lovers, and it is significantly also then that Ada first begins to whisper. Thus silence, music, and speech constitute a continuum of communicative possibilities and the media for varying degrees of erotic encounter.

I mentioned earlier that the piano serves as a kind of inanimate double to Ada's sexual body, making possible her musical voice but also echoing her silence (when she abandons the instrument for Baines's body or finally leaves it to lie mute on the ocean bed). In a sense, then, the piano functions as a kind of character in the film—the titular character, complete with human attributes (48, 96) and an existence that ends in a "grave" (122). The many scenes in which piano playing predominates for up to sixty or ninety seconds of film time (see, e.g., 129, 130)—an extraordinary duration for an average feature film— underscore the centrality of music as the ongoing complement to muteness in the narrative. The fact that Michael Nyman's sound track enjoyed a commercial success parallel to but independent from the box office popularity of the film testifies to the music's status as a complete artwork despite its complementary narrative function.

V

So far, I have discussed the muteness in its relation to the visual and musical components of the film. But part of the aesthetics of silence in *The Piano* is to highlight the *verbal*, often through visual means. This occurs through the elaborate sign language that Ada "speaks" with her face and hands. Most of the time, her language is translated by Flora, but sometimes it is rendered instead through subtitles, so that two layers of visual signs (finger language and written text) represent Ada's part of the dialogue. In a written narrative such as a novel, Ada's "speech" would presumably be rendered through descriptions of her movements along with verbal translations in direct or indirect quotations. Both of these, however, would obviously be *written* equivalents of the mute character's language. In a stage performance, Ada's sign language would either stand alone or be translated by another speaker—visual and aural signs complementing one another. But the subtitled film uniquely allows for a third possibility: two layers of visual signs at once, some written and some enacted. Moreover, even without subtitles, the film integrates written language into its dialogue when Ada uses her writing pad (and at one point, the piano key) to communicate via a written text. Here, too, the genre of film is unique in its capacity to incorporate such a multiplicity of visual signs into the narrative and to make muteness so visually eloquent.

But there are other aspects to Ada's sign language that add narrative depth to the film. The fact that Flora is the only character who can translate Ada's signs into spoken words emphasizes the symbiotic relationship between mother and daughter that prevails in the first part of the film. Yet in contrast to the other paired women, Morag and Nessie, who often speak in unison since the younger woman parrots what the older woman says, Ada and Flora are not always of one voice (or of one mind). This makes their relationship dynamic and, toward the end of the film, often strained. But the fact that they alone share the sign language indicates the special strength of this mother-daughter dyad. Only when music, sexuality, "telepathic" speech, and, finally, spoken words progressively replace Ada's sign language does the mother-daughter bond begin naturally to loosen, like the rope kicked off Ada's foot when she "chooses life."

In another respect, however, Ada's various "languages" mark her as distinctly other, somewhat like the Maori natives on this island of English-speaking colonialists. Like Ada's, the Maoris' speech is sometimes subtitled, marking it visually (and not just audibly) as alien, even while the written text renders their spoken dialogue comprehensible. As with the Maoris, whose culture Stewart not only misunderstands but also violates, Stewart approaches Ada's strangeness with similar suspicion, his initial good will yielding to antagonism and lasting mistrust. Her otherness holds him long in abeyance, then finally repulses him. Yet if Ada's difference renders her, too often, frightening to Stewart, it also arouses Baines's fascination. What makes her unattractive to her husband renders her sexually intriguing to her lover. Ada herself implicitly describes that quality of mystery and eroticism that derives from her muteness—the "dark talent" that makes her captivating and terrifying—when she explains the effect she once had on Flora's father: she "could lay thoughts in his mind like they were a sheet," but "he became frightened and . . . stopped listening" (51). Her uncanny telepathic ability is borne out later in the film when Stewart claims to have heard her voice "in his head" (114), telling him to send her away. The muteness, time and again, gives rise to strange messages—sometimes misunderstood, sometimes painfully clear—that signal communion or rejection.

What, then, of Ada's other handicap—the wound inflicted on her hand, that part of her body that makes both music and visual language? How does this mutilation define her identity within the film? How does the amputation affect her eroticism? Although we never actually see her wound, the missing finger represents a visible counterpart to the missing voice. But if the lack of a voice oddly empowers Ada vis-à-vis Stewart by making her foreign and untouchable to him, the lack of a finger strangely eroticizes her as his wife, for it is only after Stewart has symbolically castrated Ada—has "clipped her wing," as he calls it (112)—that he dares to approach her sexually in bed (although this attempt, like the attempted rape in the woods, abruptly fails). Ada's truncated hand, like her language, which seems incomplete without a translation, also marks her as having something in common with the Maoris, since they, too, wear visible scars (and, in the script, have sores on their bodies). Like the Maoris, Ada loses her "immunity" in the course of the colonialist enterprise: she becomes susceptible to the lure of the encounter with the other—in this case, the discovery of her sensuality with the Maori-like Baines—and to the punishments that that transgression entails.

In one sense, however, the ending of *The Piano* blurs the boundaries between self and other that are so strictly upheld by the Victorian ideology that pervades most of the film. While it would seem that the conclusion points toward a restoration of the self (the regained voice, the regained piano, the reconstructed finger, the restored family) at the exclusion of the foreign other (the Maori landscape and culture are exchanged for the urban, Europeanized setting of Nelson), the purity of each realm has been contaminated by the colonial process. Take Baines, for example: marked by his Maori scars and lacking literacy, he cannot return to the dominant European culture without being somewhat of a "town freak." Or consider Stewart: having forfeited part of his arsenal of guns to the Maoris for their land, he becomes ever more vulnerable to their impending aggression (retribution); having lost not part of his hand but his "right-hand man" and translator, Baines, Stewart threatens to become "unmanned" again by the warrior spirit of the Maoris, who already consider their pale-faced oppressor an impotent "old dry balls" (26). By the end of the film, all of the main characters have been marked not only as partially "disabled" but potentially or conspicuously other as well. The only exception here is Flora, who, once more turning playful cartwheels in her white petticoat, seems still untouched by the unsettling proximity of stability and disruption, of integrity and dissolution.

Ada's position at the end of the film remains characteristically unstable. On the one hand, she moves in the direction of (bourgeois) conformity, finally conceding to speak in the dominant language. On the other hand, she celebrates her status as other, satisfied at being the "town freak." The closing underwater image of the silent piano with the specter of Ada floating above it, accompanied by the voice-over of her "mind's voice" with its girlish ring, marks a regression to the realm of muteness in which the film's narrative began. Quoting the sonnet "Silence" by Thomas Hood (123), and speaking of the underwater stillness as a "lullaby" (122), the voice-over connects the lyrical image of the "cold [ocean] grave" (123) with the visual image of the womblike ocean embracing Ada, the piano, and the umbilical rope that binds them. For all its visual, verbal, and musical eloquence, the film's final message is startlingly plain: that muteness is not something to be overcome but something to return to.

VI

If one tries to place *The Piano* within the historical context of disability film, one soon recognizes two striking characteristics of this genre: first, its seeming ubiquity, with portrayals of the disabled abounding in feature films since the early twentieth century and, more recently, in television series and made-for-TV movies;[9] and second, the relative scarcity of elective muteness as a central narrative device in these popular films. Almost uniformly, muteness is depicted as a "cosyndrome"—most often paired with deafness but sometimes shown as a side effect of a specific brain-damaging accident.[10] In keeping with the long-standing tradition of film adaptations of the Helen Keller story, which focus on the heroism of the teacher as much as on the successful mainstreaming of the disabled character, more recent filmic portrayals of mute heroines tend to emphasize the role of the (male) lover as a catalyst or teacher instrumental in the process of getting the heroine to speak. Robert Markowitz's *Voices* (1979) and Randa Haines's *Children of a Lesser God* (1986), both centering on deaf-mute heroines, follow this narrative pattern. Michael Apted's 1994 film *Nell*, whose title character is speech impaired as a result of her extremely sheltered upbringing, similarly highlights the healing power of male affection and, finally, familial love. These films share with *The Piano* a respect for the heroine's linguistic otherness while maintaining a story line aimed at her "assimilation" or "normalization." Unlike *The Piano*, however, none of these films shows the heroine's muteness as a willful, medically unexplained disability (although, to be sure, the deaf heroine of *Children of a Lesser God* deliberately *chooses* not to speak). By contrast, Robert Siodmak's 1946 film *The Spiral Staircase* and its 1975 remake by Peter Collinson depict a woman who is electively mute as a result of a psychological trauma sustained in childhood, until a comparable psychological shock in her adult life renders her suddenly able to speak.[11]

For all their partial similarities with *The Piano,* all of these films lack a complex narrative structure that interweaves the discourses surrounding muteness (sign language, subtitles, telepathic or translated speech, written messages) with other aural and visual discourses—in particular, music and pantomime. In this regard, *The Piano* represents not so much a typical example of disability film as a combination of two other, partially related genres—namely, the melodrama and the fairy tale. Peter Brooks, a leading theorist of the melodrama, has singled out that genre as privileging disability in general and muteness in particular. According to Brooks, the "use of extreme physical conditions" corresponds to the "extreme moral and emotional conditions" that characterize melodramatic plots, and muteness has "a special place" in those plots because melodrama is primarily concerned with (hyperbolic) "expression."[12] Any survey of the history of melodrama, going back specifically to its heyday in the mid-nineteenth century, shows that music and "dumb shows" constituted defining elements of the genre, which so often took recourse in mute gesture, as Brooks explains, "to express its most extreme meanings" and to "make the terms of the moral dilemma *visible*" (original emphasis).[13] One can thus easily recognize that *The Piano,* set as it is in the mid-nineteenth century, makes use of that era's melodramatic forms not only in its primary plot but also, even more obviously, in the "play within the film," the Bluebeard pantomime. This populist tradition of vividly expressive, even graphic "dumb shows" is precisely what Morag invokes when she describes the school house play as "dramatic" (39)—a tradition that links the European-style folk theater to the playful costuming and role playing of the Maoris, despite their misunderstanding of the actual performance. In this sense, the deployment of muteness and gestural language in *The Piano* corresponds to melodrama's original intent "to recover something like the mythical primal language, a language of presence, purity, immediacy" and to reintroduce, by way of speechless gesture, the "primal spiritual meanings which the language code . . . has obscured, alienated, lost."[14]

This definition of pantomime as a "mythical primal language" suited to hyperbolic expression aligns this aspect of melodrama with its related genre, the fairy tale. As it does with elements of melodrama, *The Piano* shares characteristics of the fairy tale both in its primary and in its secondary plots. The heroine's journey away from home, her entanglements in a foreign world,[15] her sufferings and eventual overcoming of her afflictions through a marital union all point to the fairy-tale structure of the main narrative.[16] Within this larger story, the fairy tales told by Flora bring together the themes of muteness, music, and the supernatural to explain not only the origin of Ada's disability but also, by extension, her mysterious participation in a "primal language" with "spiritual meanings." For it is our association of Ada with the fantastic events of the fairy tale, as well as her own acts of pantomimic fairy tale narration and other storytelling (17, 51), that renders plausible her uncanny ability to "lay thoughts out in [one's] mind like they were a sheet" (51). The research on the connections between disability and folklore shows that fairy stories are conventional narrative modes of justifying physical disabilities as well as explaining supernatural or extraordinary abilities.[17] According to this research, one remarkable ability typically associated with physical or mental impairment is musical skill[18]—a gift that, in Ada's case, represents (along with her "unbelievable" finger signing,[19] telepathic speech, and the self-willed muteness itself) just one of her many "dark talents." It is no coincidence that Ada's pantomimic storytelling, depicted in two separate scenes in the film, combines elements of both the fairy tale (the narrative content) and the melodrama (the form of a "shadow play" [17, 51]). The narrative language of muteness in *The Piano* thus takes us beyond the generic conventions of disability film and explores, repeatedly and explicitly, other popular genres that, through their long-standing traditions of graphic and fantastic expression, multiply this film's evocative and expressive power.

While *The Piano* reinforces some enduring stereotypes of disability (the association of muteness with mental illness and physical deformity, the voiceless woman's "cure" by assimilation into the verbal culture of the male), it also shatters several other stereotypical images. The emphasis on the woman's will as the cause of both her muteness and her speech, the depiction of her transgressive sexual morality as deliberate and autonomous, the element of mystery surrounding the origin and the persistence of her silence, and finally the "explanations" offered from the heroine's perspective both at the beginning and at the end of the film—all these aspects serve to challenge conventional representations of disability. While the film resists glorifying images of the disabled figure—it dwells on her internal struggles, her punishments, and her suffering more than on her "heroic" deliverance—it also aestheticizes and eroticizes the disabled woman in unprecedented ways. If *The Piano* does little to further our practical understanding of disability as encountered in the real world, it nevertheless offers new ways of conceptualizing muteness through a variety of visual and aural languages that converge in a complex narrative combining the expressivity of melodrama with the haunting mystery of a fairy tale.

NOTES

1. Jane Campion won Best Director, Holly Hunter (Ada) Best Actress, and Anna Paquin (Flora) Best Supporting Actress.

2. Jane Campion, *The Piano* (New York: Hyperion [Miramax Books], 1993), 9. All further references will be to this edition, with page numbers indicated parenthetically. It should be noted that the published script differs from the film version in several respects. In instances in which the film version is cited, the corresponding page number of the script will be given.

3. The reference to Ada's father may suggest to some viewers that a paternal authority, not Ada herself, has determined the nature and the cause of her muteness. But other passages in the dialogue—spoken by Ada's voice-over or attributed to her—confirm that Ada's silence is indeed a product of her will; note the references to her will as being "strange and strong" (115) as well as unpredictable and uncontrollable (115, 121).

4. This connection between Baines and Ada based on their shared mystery, musicality, and sensuality is unwittingly reinforced by Stewart when he refers to Baines's "hidden talents" (41), echoing Ada's "dark talent."

5. In the film version, the spoken emphasis is on the word "look," which accords well with the work's pervasive theme of voyeurism.

6. This, at least, has been a response experienced by one film critic (Lizzie Francke, "The Piano," review of *The Piano, Sight and Sound* 3, no. 11 [1993]: 50) and thematized by another (Carol Jacobs, "Playing Jane Campion's *Piano*: Politically," *Modern Language Notes* 109 [1994]: 764).

7. For a discussion of "visual pleasure," a concept that in feminist and psychoanalytic terms defines the male viewer as the bearer of a desiring gaze focused on the eroticized female object, see Laura Mulvey's widely anthologized and influential article "Visual Pleasure and Narrative Cinema" (1973), along with her "Afterthoughts on 'Visual Pleasure and Narrative Cinema' inspired by King Vidor's *Duel in the Sun* (1946)" (1981), both reprinted in Laura Mulvey, *Visual and Other Pleasures* (Bloomington, IN: Indiana University Press, 1989): 14–26 and 29–38, respectively.

8. For more on the film's (self-referential) treatment of the theme of viewing, see Jacobs, "Playing Jane Campion's *Piano*," 763–70.

9. See Martin F. Norden, *The Cinema of Isolation: A History of Physical Disability in the Movies* (New Brunswick, NJ: Rutgers University Press, 1994); Lauri E. Klobas, *Disability Drama in Television and Film* (Jefferson, NC: McFarland, 1988); Paul K. Longmore, "Screening Stereotypes: Images of Disabled People in Television and Motion Pictures," *Images of the Disabled, Disabling Images,* ed. Alan Gartner and Tom Joe (New York: Praeger, 1987) 65–78; and E. Keith Byrd and Randolph B. Pipes, "Feature Films and Disability," *Journal of Rehabilitation* 47, no. 1 (1981): 51–53, 80.

10. On deafness in film, see John S. Schuchman, *Hollywood Speaks: Deafness and the Film Entertainment Industry* (Urbana, IL: University of Illinois Press, 1988); on the filmic portrayal of muteness or "aphasia" as a result of brain damage, see Klobas, *Disability Drama,* 369–435 passim.

11. For a brief discussion of Siodmak's film and its remake, see Klobas, *Disability Drama,* 370f., 376f. For a discussion of a rare television drama that, in the manner of these

films, integrates elective mutism into a romantic plot, see Klobas, *Disability Drama,* 395f. (on "Hotel").

12. Peter Brooks, "The Text of Muteness," *New Literary History* 5, no. 3 (1974): 549.

13. Ibid., 552.

14. Ibid., 555, 559.

15. The deliberate representation of the New Zealand bush as exotic intensifies the fairy-tale quality of the setting, underscored cinematographically by the preponderance of blue-greenish hues and "tentacled," "anarchical" landscapes that purposefully replicate a "prehistoric," "underwater" world (140–42). The imitation of archaic, "autochrome" photography also lends the images an antique quality that, together with the exoticism of the setting, positions the narrative as both spatially and temporally far removed from the present (141).

16. A random sampling of audience responses to the film at a recent Women's Studies conference at the University of Wisconsin-Madison (26–28 October 1995) revealed that several feminist spectators shared the view that *The Piano* is "a fairy tale"—a response that, unless further qualified, tends to minimize the disturbing (melodramatic) aspects of the film, including its violence against women.

17. See Susan Schoon Eberly, "Fairies and the Folklore of Disability: Changelings, Hybrids, and the Solitary Fairy," *The Good People: New Fairylore Essays,* ed. Peter Narváez (New York: Garland, 1991), 227f.

18. Ibid., 238.

19. Stewart intimates that he finds Ada's sign language rather uncanny when he tells Baines in the script (not in the film): "you can't believe what [Ada and Flora] say with just their hands" (46).

"Making up the Stories as We Go Along" ▶ Men, Women, and Narratives of Disability

Madonne Miner

> This is the important point about the stories we tell
> ourselves about our lives. We make them up as we go
> along . . . We can't select every event and detail, of course.
> We can't decide, for instance, whether or not someone gets
> MS. MS just *happens*. But—and this is the exciting part—
> we can choose how we will respond to that happening,
> what kind of role we will give it in the story we're making
> up as we go along.
>
> —Nancy Mairs, "Good Enough Gifts"

> The less evident social aspect of stories is that people do
> not make up their stories by themselves. The shape of the
> telling is molded by all the rhetorical expectations that the
> storyteller has been internalizing ever since he first heard
> some relative describe an illness, or she saw her first
> commercial for a non-prescription remedy, or he was
> instructed to "tell the doctor what hurts" and had to figure
> out *what* counted as the story the doctor wanted to hear.
>
> —Arthur Frank, *The Wounded Storyteller*

Arthur Frank's observation—"people do not make up their stories by themselves"—complicates but does not contradict Nancy Mairs's claim that "we make up our stories as we go along." Mairs's "we," surely, is no simple, essential self. Rather, this we includes a range of voices speaking through any individual storyteller; we are shaped from and by relatives' stories, commercial narratives, medical interpellations, and countless other tales in which we find ourselves. Striving to create ourselves in stories, we simultaneously are created by stories; this curious tension speaks to and of the postmodern human condition—and reminds us of the importance of attending to stories.[1]

This importance has not been lost on scholars working in the relatively new area of disability studies.[2] Early on, disability critics asked: "where are we to find stories that speak of disability?" In the mid-1980s, scholars Leonard Kriegel, Deborah Kent, and Paul K. Longmore each published essays describing representations of disability in fiction, drama, television, or film.[3] Each expressed dismay over the stories he or she found: stories that yoke disability to criminality and social isolation, that highlight dependency and suicidal tendencies, that speak, most often, from the perspective of the nondisabled. Both Kriegel and Kent concluded their essays with pleas for stories by men and women who are themselves disabled.

Not long after Kent's essay appeared in print, two collections of writing by women with disabilities were published. Those collections represent the next phase in disability studies: that is, the publication of works by disabled authors.[4] As I write this essay, I can call upon recently published disability narratives by Nancy Mairs, Andre Dubus, John Hockenberry, Cheri Register, May Sarton, Molly Haskell, Anne Finger, Reynolds Price, Irving Zola, William Styron, Oliver Sacks, and others.[5] Following in the wake of these stories are critical questions similar to those that readers of other minority literatures have been asking in recent years: what unique point of view does this new literature express? does the experience of disability result in particular types of narratives? how does this experience "write" those who undergo it? how might the disabled writer rewrite this experience? how might readers identify a "disabled writer?" how might this writer identify him- or herself? The contemporary critical reader of disability narratives soon becomes entangled in postmodern/poststructural discussions of nature and narrative, biology and culture, bodies and books.

A particularly insightful contributor to these more recent discussions is Arthur Frank, sociologist, heart attack and cancer patient, and author of *The Wounded Storyteller: Body, Illness, and Ethics*.[6] In *The Wounded Storyteller*, Frank approaches stories of illness and disability as opportunities for patients to resolve moral problems of postmodern identity. He suggests that patients may *become* themselves in the stories they tell: "Those who have been objects of others' reports are now telling their own stories. As they do so, they define the ethic of our times: an ethic of voice, affording each a right to speak her own truth, in her own words."[7] While we might question Frank's seemingly uncritical acceptance of the possibility of speaking one's "own truth" in one's "own words," his claim that the "ethic of voice" is the ethic of our times seems beyond question. As divided and troubled as this voice may be, its existence is apparent in an outpouring of stories from subjects previously muted or voiceless. Frank listens to the stories of numerous patients, discerns typical narrative patterns, and challenges readers to see how many of the stories require their tellers to shape themselves anew. Frank's analysis of illness and disability stories is remarkably insightful; his careful employment of nonsexist prose is admirable. But Frank does not go far enough in pursuing the implications of his own insights, especially with respect to the ways in which rhetorical expectations, and hence, possible "self-stories" written out of disability or illness, vary depending upon a subject's history of embodiment within discourses of gender, race, and sexual orientation. Frank argues, for example, that "[s]elf-change seems remarkably unrelated to gender"[8] and cites stories from Audre Lorde and Robert Murphy—both of whom call upon metaphors from ancient cultures to represent their new selves—to substantiate his claim. Postmastectomy Lorde identifies herself with Amazons; Murphy, paralyzed in a chair, compares himself to the stationary myth-telling shamans of Peru. Murphy's metaphor wouldn't work for Lorde, just as hers wouldn't work for Murphy, not simply because of the differing nature of their losses but also because of the differing discourses and rhetorical expectations that have shaped and continue to shape this white man and black woman. Frank repeatedly alludes to the "culturally elaborated" nature of bodies and selves,[9] but he does not pursue the implications of different cultural elaborations of women's and men's bodies, bodies of color and white bodies, as these cultural elaborations intersect in narratives of illness and disability.

In the pages that follow, I look closely at two disability narratives, highlighting ways each narrative's representation of disability takes place within a gendered discursive field. These discourses color narrated experiences of the texts' subjects both *before* and *during* disability. In focusing on gender, I neglect other, equally important features affecting narrational possibilities/identity possibilities, but I also avoid the temptation (to which I think Frank falls prey) of ascribing all representational choices to a subject's experience of illness or disability alone.[10] Sidonie Smith observes that the autobiographical subject, "coming out of a complex experientially based history . . . speaks not from one overdetermined position within the webs of discourse . . . [but rather becomes] 'multiply designated,' severally situated within diverse, sometimes congruous, often competing, even contradictory discursive fields."[11] In this essay, I analyze intersections between two discourses—gender and disability—as these discourses contribute to the construction of the narrative projects of Andre Dubus and Nancy Mairs.

To preview my argument: in telling stories of their losses (Dubus, of his legs to an accident; Mairs, of her stability and partial mobility to multiple sclerosis [MS]), Dubus and Mairs initially seem to employ traditionally gendered narrative paradigms. Where Dubus repeatedly returns to stereotypically masculinized questions of agency, responsibility, and guilt, Mairs concerns herself with more stereotypically femininized issues of being, speaking, and shame. When Dubus tells his story of throwing a woman out of the path of an oncoming car, he focuses upon his decision to act and upon guilt and anger consequent to that act. In contrast, when Mairs tells her story of living with MS, she focuses upon being a woman, being a cripple, and how this being implicates her in a system of shame. Narrating their tales, each gives voice to stereotypical expectations; each articulates the culture's discourse with respect to male and female bodies.

But as we look more carefully at these disability narratives, it becomes clear that the stories actually move in different ways. Dubus's narrative repeatedly returns to the site of loss, because for Dubus, this site simultaneously represents presence. Although the accident robs Dubus of the use of his legs (and, by implication, of an independence and mobility conventionally associated with "manhood"), Dubus's activity during the accident speaks of his male presence as agent and actor; that is, recitation of this tale reaffirms Dubus's manliness and heroism. Overtly, Dubus's narrative never challenges gender roles; instead, its narrator returns time and time again to a story that allows him to position himself as "a man among men, and among women."

In contrast, Nancy Mairs's story of loss attendant upon disability actually becomes a story of gain. Prior to the onset of MS, Mairs suffers discontinuities between her self and cultural expectations for female selves. She is uncomfortable and uneasy as a midcentury white American woman, a woman who wants to write, a woman who wants to establish a public voice. As MS pushes Mairs further away from model womanhood, she happily chucks such models and begins to delight in the liberatory possibilities of stepping out of bounds, of pushing the envelope. Rather than mourning losses, Mairs glories in new opportunities. Rather than looking backward, she looks forward. Ironically, Mairs's disability stories suggest that her disease frees her from a subordinate gender position; in contrast, Dubus's stories betray the keen loss felt by a man accustomed to privileges of a superordinate position, a man who deems himself no longer qualified to hold this position but who remains emotionally and psychologically caught within the confines of a traditional gender system.

In substantiating my thesis, I take cues from Mairs and Dubus with respect to semantics. Both writers elect to identify themselves as *cripples,* and I shall do the same. Mairs declares her preference for this term ("a clean word, straightforward and precise") in her essay "On Being a Cripple,"[12] where she also notes that the word tends to make people wince—and she wants them to do so. Unlike Mairs, Dubus does not explain his choice, but he repeatedly enacts it. Throughout the essays in *Broken Vessels* he elects to describe himself as crippled, a man wounded and injured, a man whose body is a "living sculpture of certain truths."[13]

Readers of Dubus's essay collection, *Broken Vessels,* come to the first full account of Dubus's crippling in a short piece entitled "Lights of the Long Night."[14] Here, and then in later essays, Dubus provides details of an accident that occurred on the morning of 23 July 1986. Driving north on Route 93 from Boston Dubus notices a car stopped in the lane ahead of him. To check on the situation of the driver, he pulls to the left of the car; he observes Luz Santiago, with forehead bleeding, near the driver's side door. When he stops to help her, she says, "There's a motorcycle under my car" ("Lights," 129). Fearing that Luz has run over a cyclist but also fearing that she is in danger of shock, Dubus walks Luz and her brother Luis, a passenger in Luz's car, to the left side of the highway. As the three get to the side of the road, another car's lights appear on the highway, headed north. Dubus waves to the car, hoping to get more help. Apparently this motorist doesn't see him; coming upon the stopped cars, the driver of the oncoming car swerves toward Dubus, Luis, and Luz. Dubus notes that the driver turns toward them: "Then I was lying on the car's trunk and asking someone: *What happened?*" ("Lights," 130).

Although Dubus cannot remember in detail what happens between the time he realizes the car is going to hit them and when it does so, he meticulously pieces together what must have happened: he must have pushed Luz Santiago away from the car, sacrificing himself in order to save her. Filling in the gap, we have the evidence of Dubus's wounds and the testimony of Luz. But more important to Dubus is a personal sensation, a conviction: "I knew, from the first moments in the stationary ambulance, that a car struck me because I was standing where I should have been; and, some time later, in the hospital, I knew I had chosen to stand there, rather than leap toward the guard rail" ("Lights," 130). "I knew I had chosen"—with these words Dubus revises what might have been an account of an accident into an account of choice; we move from horror story to heroic story. Certainly, Dubus is victimized by the oncoming car; but he also asserts himself as agent in confronting this car.

Reiteration of choice assumes a central position in Dubus's narrative of the accident. In the concluding paragraph of "Lights," Dubus tells us several times that Dr. Wayne Sharaf, the doctor who worked on him and on Luz after the accident, confides that Luz told him Dubus had pushed her away from the car. Dubus thanks Sharaf: "I said: *Now I can never be angry at myself for stopping that night. He said: Don't ever be. You saved that woman's life*" ("Lights," 131). Why this repetition? In one of the epigraphs with which this essay begins, Nancy Mairs suggests that we "make up" the stories of our lives as we go along. Dubus's stories of his crippling reveal a tremendous desire to envision himself as *acting,* as *doing* something. Within Dubus's narratives, to be a man is to be an actor; this action may result in the loss of limb, perhaps even of life, but such losses are minor in comparison to the loss of manhood associated with agency's alternative: passivity.

It is perhaps not surprising then, that when the postaccident Dubus finds himself in decidedly passive positions (when his body is being worked on by his physical therapist, for example), his thoughts turn toward cultural models of agency—specifically, toward the military forces. He conjures up "memories of myself after my training at Quantico, those times in my life when I had instinctively moved toward action, to stop fights, to help the injured or stricken, and I saw myself on the highway that night, and I said: *Yes. It makes sense. It started as a Marine, when I was eighteen; and it ended on a highway when I was almost fifty years old.*"[15] Marines learn they must move: "*Don't just stand there, Lieutenant . . . Do something, even if it's wrong*" ("Broken," 173). Dubus *does* do something, and then, having lost most of the use of his legs as a result of this doing, constructs narratives that foreground the doing instead of the loss. In other words, while the result of his act may have been an "unmanning," the act itself positions him as man beyond question. Focusing on that act and on the antecedents to that act, Dubus encourages us to recognize (misrecognize) him according to ideology's interpellation of him as an autonomous male agent.[16]

What about a second desire repeatedly articulated in Dubus's narratives: the desire to avoid feeling angry with himself? Most obviously, it is Dubus's choice to stop at the scene, to throw Luz out of the way, that leads to his crippling and to potential feelings of anger with himself. In conversations with Doctor Sharaf, Dubus uses Sharaf's reassurances to reassure himself; her life was worth the sacrifice of his legs. But this explanation of Dubus's desire to ward off self-destructive anger doesn't go far enough in accounting for the essays' repetitions of Dubus's fear of anger and guilt.

If we look again at Dubus's story of the accident in "Lights of the Long Night," we find that although Dubus acts with absolutely the best intentions, his actions contribute to a combination of factors that make the accident possible. Quite probably, there wasn't a right way to do things that night on Route 93; and Dubus did the most important "right thing" by pulling over in the first place. But curiously, as Dubus narrates what happens after he pulls over, he leaves open the possibility of his own contributory negligence. For example, rather than pulling into the breakdown lane when he sees Luz Santiago's stalled car, Dubus pulls ahead and to the left, into the speed lane. Having parked, partially blocking the lane, he approaches Luz, who asks for his help. She says there's a motorcycle under her car, but Dubus imagines a dead cyclist and so also imagines that Luz is in danger of shock: "I had to get Luz off the highway and lie [sic] her down" ("Lights," 129). This series of mistakes, of misapprehensions, precipitates Dubus into the position of military leader: "We walked in a column: I was in front, Luz was behind me, and Luis was in the rear" ("Lights," 129–30). When an oncoming car swerves to avoid Luz's car, and then toward the blinking lights of Dubus's Subaru, Dubus, Luz, and Luis are sitting ducks.

Dubus is not culpable. But Dubus's essays suggest that he isn't fully convinced of his innocence. Assuming the position of "the man," of the leader, Dubus assumes responsibility for bad decisions as well as good ones; both his account of the accident and his insistence upon shoring up a case for the defense suggest that numerous bad decisions were made. Arthur Frank notes that disability stories often involve repetition and recollection so as to "set right what was done wrong or incompletely."[17] Dubus never consciously talks about what was done wrong, never suggests that marine imperatives might be incomplete, but the stories he tells undermine such imperatives, revealing their gaps and inconsistencies.

Essays in *Broken Vessels*, with their repetitions, elisions, and apparent meanderings, describe to us the high costs of being a man. In these essays, we see that a man must act, but in doing so, he runs the risk of harming others and thereby harming himself. He has the opportunity of writing himself into a hero's role; but this role, as evidenced by Dubus, is an increasingly problematic one. If a hero's acts result in his own death, the narrative works; but when the hero remains alive, he may very well find himself crippled by doubts and angers that follow upon making a choice about where to stand, about what to do.[18] Ironically, Dubus's tales work against the overt value system of their teller; where Dubus clings to the values of traditional manhood, his essays call these values into question.

Throughout essays in *Broken Vessels*, Dubus describes a man *becoming* a cripple. The essays of Nancy Mairs, in contrast, more often describe a woman *being* a cripple. Arthur Frank points out that during illness or when confronted with disability, "people who have always *been* bodies have distinctive problems *continuing* to be bodies."[19] Dubus and Mairs invoke different strategies for responding to these problems: the former emphasizes the decisiveness of his preaccident body; the latter represents her body as it is now—in its almost laughable unreliability, social unconformability, and outspoken volubility.[20] We can get a sense of Mairs's approach by examining her essay "Carnal Acts," included in the anthology *Carnal Acts* and written in response to a student's request that Mairs talk about disability and writing.[21] Where Dubus casts his story as one in which he initiates action, Mairs positions herself quite differently; something happens to her and she reacts, adjusts. Actually, Mairs puzzles over the nature of this presumed "happening," wondering whether an external agent is at work or if this something *is* her. In the account of her MS, Mairs initially figures the disease as a ghost who haunts the house of her body, an alien invader who trips her up and weighs down her body with weariness. Then she retracts these figures: "But of course it's not [an alien invader]. It's your own body. That is, it's you" ("Carnal," 84). No exorcism, no ghostbusting: "it's you."

Early on, Mairs does struggle against the ramming of her *self* "straight back into the body I had been trained to believe it could, through high-minded acts and aspirations, rise above" ("Carnal," 84). Very quickly, however, she recognizes that to reject this body as herself is to concede to a Western European convention that subordinates body, treats it as "other," and marks it as that for which we must feel shame. She also realizes that the very idea of "rising above" one's body, of presenting the body as other, runs parallel to this convention's conception of men rising above women and of male "culture" asserting superiority over female "nature."[22] Meditating on, in, and from her bodied self leads Mairs away from the struggle to transcend body and toward the struggle to accept body. Throughout her essays, she presents herself/her "self" *as* body—a body to be attended to, not denied: "What I am saying is that I must now *attend* to my body—both in the sense of 'fix the mind upon' and 'watch over the working of' it—in ways that I never dreamed of and that you may still find foreign."[23]

To be a female, crippled self: in late-twentieth-century America, such a self conventionally will be tutored in shame. Not surprisingly, the subject of shame (rather than of anger) occupies much of Mairs's essay "Carnal Acts." As Mairs explains, American culture gives her many reasons to feel this emotion. First, she fails to live up to the ideals for a woman of her generation. She observes: "I was never a beautiful woman, and for that reason I've spent most of my life (together with probably at least 95 percent of the female population of the United States) suffering from the shame of falling short of an unattainable standard" ("Carnal," 87). With dark hair, flat chest, and narrow hips, Mairs doesn't come close to the Marilyn Monroe ideal of 1950s femininity. When the symptoms of MS become worse, Mairs's failure is exacerbated: "The real blow to my self-image came when I had to get a brace . . . it meant the end of high heels. And it's ugly" ("Carnal," 88). So shamed is she by this lightweight piece of plastic molded to her foot and leg that Mairs for many years wears trousers. She comments: "The idea of going around with my bare brace hanging out seemed almost as indecent as exposing my breasts" ("Carnal," 88). Respectable women protect onlookers from any sight of difference, whether that difference be a braced leg or a flat chest.

But despite losses associated with MS, Mairs continues to "expose" herself in public venues. As fatigue takes more of a toll on her, Mairs comes to rely upon yet another "shameful" aid: an Amigo, a three-wheeled electric scooter. She characterizes her reaction to this aid as one of ambivalence. The Amigo lessens her fatigue and widens her range but "also shouts out to the world, 'Here is a woman who can't stand on her own two feet'" ("Carnal," 89). We might compare Mairs's experience of her Amigo to Dubus's experience of his wheelchair. While both machines telegraph to the world, "this person cannot stand on his or her own two feet"—somehow this message conveys different things about a man (and to a man) than it does about and to a woman. Mairs sees her electric cart as signifying failure (according to conventional gender stereotypes), while Dubus can position his chair to signify success. Her Amigo says she is not a beautiful woman, while his chair says he is (and has been) a powerful, active man. I certainly do not intend to suggest that Dubus feels unambivalently positive about his chair, but his remarks in *Broken Vessels* imply that there are discourses available to him that do not associate wheelchairs with shame. For Dubus, the chair functions first as a signifier of his willingness to lose his legs by acting on someone else's behalf; second, it functions as a machine over which he exerts control.

We can better understand how these machines suggest different things about men and women if we look at a passage from Dubus's essay, "A Woman in April," which suggests that men in wheelchairs retain a conventional social standing unavailable to women similarly situated.[24] Crossing Lincoln Center plaza, Dubus notes an especially lovely woman about forty feet away. He says to the friend pushing his chair, "'Skipper . . . Accidently push me into *her*'" ("Woman," 142). She turns, smiles, and says with a softness in her voice: "'I heard that'" ("Woman," 142). Dubus senses that although her first response may have been "instinctive anger or pride," when she sees him in a wheelchair, she feels "not pity but lighthearted compassion" ("Woman," 143). And while we too feel positive about what Dubus terms "the infinite possibilities of the human heart" ("Woman," 144), his essay, quite unintentionally, speaks to Mairs's predicament: she will never be the woman striding across the plaza of Lincoln Center, attracting the appreciative attention of men like Dubus. Note how Dubus describes this woman: "She wore a dark brown miniskirt . . . she strode with purpose but not hurry, only grace" ("Woman," 142). While grace is out of the reach of both Dubus and Mairs, only the latter will feel shame upon not being able to achieve it; culturally, only the latter is held and holds herself responsible for such an achievement.

We might parallel Dubus's portrait of the woman in the miniskirt to a self-portrait provided by Mairs in the middle of "Carnal Acts." There, Mairs writes in excruciating detail about giving a reading at the University of Arizona. Having smashed three teeth in a fall on her concrete porch, she wears temporary crowns; at a dinner prior to the scheduled reading, the crowns fly off, and Mairs must read in public with her smashed teeth: "So, looking like Hansel and Gretel's witch, and lisping worse than the Wife of Bath, I got up on stage and read" ("Carnal," 90).[25] Despite the shame she's been tutored in, despite the lessons she's received about hiding her female body weakened and misshapen by disease, Mairs eventually defies all such strictures; she strides *and* holds up her head in the very act of telling stories about herself as crippled. Foregrounding the way her body differs from conventional expectations for women's bodies, Mairs refuses shame. As a whole, Mairs's narrative, speaking as forthrightly as it does about misshapen female bodies, challenges conventional gender expectations (she will not "suffer and be still") while that of Dubus continues to enact them.

Telling the story of her lost teeth and found voice provides Mairs with a transition into the second part of "Carnal Acts." Having discussed her "disability," which encompasses "shame" as well as MS, Mairs shifts the focus of her attention to a discussion of voice. As Mairs observes, the two topics are intimately intertwined; she copes best with her disability by "speaking about it, and about the whole experience of being a body, specifically a female body, out loud, in a clear, level tone that drowns out the frantic whispers of my mother, my grandmothers, all the other trainers of wayward childish tongues: 'Sssh! Sssh! Nice girls don't talk like that'" ("Carnal," 91).

To avoid shame, one must abandon the "nice girl" routine, and utter the "hidden, dark secret[s]" of one's life. Mairs does so. She tells us about her early, maudlin prose voice, a voice "that had shucked off its own body" and is so vaporous that Mairs abandons all prose writing for nearly twenty years. She tells us how she comes to her new voice when she returns to prose after a suicide attempt, writing about this particular bodily event in an essay that does not gloss over her matted hair, gray and swollen face, nightgown streaked with blood and urine. Knowing the rules of "polite discourse," she knows she should keep quiet; but her voice wins out, and she produces at least two accounts of this failed suicide attempt. These accounts exemplify what Mairs now sets as her task: "to scrutinize the details of my own experience and to report what I see, and what I think about what I see, as lucidly and accurately as possible" ("Carnal," 94). Given her identity as a crippled woman, her experience cannot avoid the body; Mairs states emphatically that her voice "is the creature of the body that produces it . . . No body, no voice; no voice, no body" ("Carnal," 96). This last set of parallels sums up the argument of "Carnal Acts," as it not only reiterates the claim that if one is bodiless, one can have no voice but also introduces the claim that if one doesn't use her voice, then one doesn't exist.

Before bringing "Carnal Acts" to a close, Mairs observes that "[p]aradoxically, losing one sort of nerve has given me another. No one is going to take my breath away. No one is going to leave me speechless" ("Carnal," 96). Yes: MS is a loss, but in Mairs's stories about her self, this loss results in a gain of another sort. Mairs's disease, which demands that she attend to her body, gives her an understanding of her own embodiment as a woman, as a cripple. When, many years earlier, Mairs learned that she had MS, she started a poem with the line, " 'My body is going away,' " imagining her body fading "to the transparency of amber."[26] She was wrong. As she says, this body "has, on the contrary, grown thicker and more opaque over time. It looms in my consciousness now as it never did when all my gestures were as thoughtless as yours perhaps still are."[27] Mairs comes to be her body not only because MS demands this of her but also because of her history of female embodiment; Mairs's experience of the intersection of gender and disability pushes her to insist on her own opacity—over and against any cultural claims of feminine transparency.

Arthur Frank suggests that one "rises to the occasion" of being ill or disabled "by telling not just any story, but a good story."[28] The narratives of both Dubus and Mairs are remarkably good disability stories, but they are radically different stories. I've argued in the preceding that an important causative factor of these differences is the differing gender histories Dubus and Mairs bring to their experience of disability. Prior to his accident, Dubus need not think much about his male body. He does, of course, think some about this body; he writes about being scrawny as a young man, about being bullied, about joining the marines— "destined by my body and my feelings about it"[29]—but in none of Broken Vessels' essays does he reveal anywhere near the bodily preoccupation that Mairs documents as a facet of American womanhood in Plaintext, Carnal Acts, Remembering the Bone House, and Voice Lessons. Female bodies, like bodies of color, homosexual bodies, *and* disabled bodies, are positioned culturally so as not to forget their embodiment. We might say that Mairs has had more practice than Dubus in shaping a story from her body; it really should come as no surprise then, that her "self-story" throws off convention more readily than his and that it looks with faith toward the future, while his invests more belief in the past. Mairs emphasizes what she has become; Dubus, what he was.

Relying on a sample of two, I can make no large claims about autobiographical narratives of disability—except to say that when negotiating this relatively unanalyzed terrain, storytellers bring their bodies—with all of these bodies' complex rhetorical and cultural histories—along with them. Arthur Frank says, "[t]he stories that ill people tell come out of their bodies."[30] It is up to disability scholars to show how varied the discourses shaping these bodies, and their stories, really are.

NOTES

1. For at least the past three decades, minority critics (feminist, black, lesbian and gay, working class) have issued similar reminders. Much of the early work of such critics was devoted to finding, publishing, and analyzing stories that spoke of the lives of women, of people of color, of lesbians, and of working class people. A second phase of this work moved away from "image analysis" to the production (and reproduction) of stories by members of these minority groups; "the authority of experience" was invoked repeatedly in support of this narrative production. More recently, critical work has addressed itself to questions about stories' roles in identity construction and identity politics and in contestations of "authority" and univocality.

2. Although, as I argue later, most scholars still do not pay *enough* attention to the plurality and power of discourses affecting who we are and the stories we tell.

3. See Leonard Kriegel, "The Cripple in Literature," in *Images of the Disabled, Disabling Images,* ed. Alan Gartner and Tom Joe (New York: Praeger, 1987), 31–47; Deborah Kent, "Disabled Women: Portraits in Fiction and Drama," in *Images of the Disabled, Disabling Images,* ed. Alan Gartner and Tom Joe (New York: Praeger, 1987), 47–63; and Paul K. Longmore, "Screening Stereotypes: Images of Disabled People," *Social Policy* 16 (1985): 31–37.

4. See Michelle Fine and Adrienne Asch, eds., *Women and Disabilities: Essays in Psychology, Culture, and Politics* (Philadelphia, PA: Temple University Press, 1988); Susan Brown, Debra Connors, and Nanci Stern, eds., *With the Power of Each Breath: A Disabled Women's Anthology* (Pittsburgh, PA: Cleis Press, 1985); Marsha Saxton and Florence Howe, eds., *With Wings: An Anthology of Literature by and about Women with Disabilities* (New York: Feminist Press, 1987).

5. I am grateful for Nancy Mairs's essay "The Literature of Personal Disaster" in *Voice Lessons* (Boston, MA: Beacon, 1994), 123–35, which provided me with an initial bibliography; and for Arthur Frank, *The Wounded Storyteller: Body, Illness and Ethics* (Chicago, IL: University of Chicago Press, 1995), which offered a marvelous supplement.

6. Arthur Frank, *The Wounded Storyteller* (Chicago, IL: University of Chicago Press, 1995).

7. Ibid., xiii.

8. Ibid., 130.

9. Ibid. See 75, 163, 170.

10. I do not want to leave the impression that Frank consistently ignores the range of discourses across which we construct ourselves. He notes, for example, that "[d]isease happens in a life that already has a story, and this story goes on, changed by illness but also affecting how the illness story is formed" (54). Later, too, he argues that "the plurality of the self that is reclaimed needs to be noted. The issue for most ill people seems to be keeping multiple selves available to themselves" (66).

11. Sidonie Smith, *Subjectivity, Identity, and the Body: Women's Autobiographical Practices in the Twentieth Century* (Bloomington, IN: University of Indiana Press, 1993), 21. Similarly, Catherine Belsey emphasizes that subjectivity "is linguistically and discursively constructed and displaced across the range of discourses in which the concrete individual participates." Catherine Belsey, *Critical Practice* (London: Methuen, 1980), 61. Belsey's articulation is problematic in itself: where is "the concrete individual?" can we locate him or her outside of the range of discourses in which he or she participates?

12. Nancy Mairs, "On Being a Cripple," in *Plaintext: Deciphering a Woman's Life* (New York: Harper & Row, 1986), 9.

13. Andre Dubus, "Broken Vessels," in *Broken Vessels* (Boston, MA: D. R. Godine, 1991), 194.

14. Andre Dubus, "Lights of the Long Night," in *Broken Vessels* (Boston, MA: D. R. Godine, 1991), 127–31. I will include all further page citations from "Lights" in parentheses within my essay.

15. Andre Dubus, "Broken Vessels," 172. I will include all further page citations from "Broken" in parentheses in my essay.

16. In clarifying ideological interpellation, Catherine Belsey observes: "people 'recognize' (misrecognize) themselves in the ways in which ideology 'interpellates' them, or in other words, addresses them as subjects, calls them by their names and in turn 'recognizes' their autonomy" (*Critical Practice*, 61).

17. Frank, *Wounded Storyteller,* 132.

18. In positioning himself as the "subject" of the accident story, Dubus becomes not only a " 'center of initiatives, author of and responsible for its actions,' but also a *subjected being* who submits to the authority of the social formation represented in ideology as the Absolute Subject (God, the king, the boss, Man, conscience)" (Belsey, *Critical Practice,* 61, original emphasis).

19. Frank, *Wounded Storyteller,* 28.

20. Granted: Dubus writes about a crippling that occurs in a moment and with which he has lived for only a few years. Mairs writes about a crippling that occurs gradually and with which she has lived for many years. As such, Dubus and Mairs actually conform to a larger pattern with regard to sex and the etiology of disability: males are far more likely than females to become disabled as the result of injuries and amputations; females tend to become disabled as the result of chronic illnesses such as arthritis and multiple sclerosis. See Susan Lonsdale, *Women and Disability* (New York: St. Martin's Press, 1990), 37.

21. Nancy Mairs, "Carnal Acts," in *Carnal Acts* (New York: HarperCollins, 1990). I will include further page citations from "Carnal" in parentheses within my essay.

22. Sidonie Smith describes this split in her discussion of Western European Enlightenment subjects: "Discourses of the universal subject assume reciprocities of self and soul, and they assign the 'tremulous private body' to marginal status at the periphery of consciousness. Such peripheralization allows the greatest possible space in which self and soul can commingle, free of biologically determined influences. But since female identity inheres in woman's embodiment as procreator and nurturer, the female subject inhabits mostly that colorful margin; or rather, a colorful marginalization of embodiment fills her self and soul" (*Subjectivity*, 11).

23. Nancy Mairs, "But First," in *Carnal Acts* (New York: HarperCollins, 1990), 5.

24. Andre Dubus, "A Woman in April," in *Broken Vessels* (Boston, MA: D. R. Godine, 1991). I will include all further page citations from "Woman" in parentheses in my essay.

25. Sidonie Smith, discussing women's contestation of conventional gender roles, notes: "To the degree that woman contests such roles and postures by pursuing her own desire and independence from men, she becomes a cultural grotesque" (*Subjectivity*, 16). In giving her speech with broken teeth, Mairs embraces the grotesque, validates it as one path to liberation.

26. Nancy Mairs, "But First," in *Carnal Acts* (New York: HarperCollins, 1990), 5.

27. Ibid., 5.

28. Frank, *Wounded Storyteller*, 62.

29. Andre Dubus, "The Judge and Other Snakes," in *Broken Vessels* (Boston, MA: D. R. Godine, 1991), 61.

30. Frank, *Wounded Storyteller*, 2.

Contributors

Lennard J. Davis is associate professor of English at Binghamton University (SUNY). He is the author of *Factual Fictions: Origins of the English Novel* (New York: Columbia University Press, 1983); and *Resisting Novels: Fiction and Ideology* (New York: Routledge, 1987); coeditor of *Left Politics and the Literary Profession* (New York: Columbia University Press, 1991); author of *Enforcing Normalcy: Disability, Deafness and the Body* (London: Verso, 1995); and editor of the *Disability Studies Reader* (New York: Routledge, 1997).

Martha L. Edwards completed her doctoral degree in ancient history at the University of Minnesota in 1995. She is now assistant professor of History at Truman State University, Kirksville, Montana.

Maria Frawley is assistant professor of English at Elizabethtown College, Elizabethtown, Pennsylvania where she teaches Victorian literature and women's literature. Her first book, *A Wider Range: Travel Writing by Women in Victorian England* (Rutherford, NH: Farleigh Dickenson University Press) was named an "Outstanding Academic Book for 1995" by *Choice Magazine*. She has also written a book on Anne Brontë for the Twayne English Authors series and is currently at work on a study of the literature written by Victorian "invalids" about their experiences with illness.

David A. Gerber is a professor in the history department at the State University of New York at Buffalo. His field is American social history. He has written on race, ethnicity, disability, and gender, variously as sources of individual identities, bases of group oppression, and organizing elements of American social pluralism.

Jan Gordon is a professor of Anglo-American literature at Tokyo University of Foreign Studies. He is a native of Tyler, Texas, and his work on nineteenth-century and fin de siècle narrative has appeared in *ELH, Genre*, the *Journal of Art and Aesthetics Criticism, Salmagundi*, and *The Nation* among other journals. His *Gossip and Subversion in Nineteenth Century British Fiction: Echo's Economies* is forthcoming from Macmillan. Three of his previously anthologized essays have been recently reprinted in the Chelsea House Series of World Literary Criticism, edited by Harold Bloom.

Elizabeth C. Hamilton is a Ph.D. candidate in German literature at the Ohio State University, Columbus, Ohio, and is currently completing her dissertation on the representation of disability in German literature since 1750. She has presented conference papers on German and U.S. media images of disability and on strategies for teaching literature in introductory German courses. Her research interests include twentieth-century German literature and German women writers.

Cindy LaCom received her degree at the University of Oregon and is currently an assistant professor in English at Slippery Rock University, Slippery Rock, Pennsylvania. She teaches and does research in Victorian studies, women's literature, and disability studies. Other publications include "Murdering Mothers: Conduct Unbecoming" in *Scholars* and the introduction to a special issue of *Nineteenth-Century Contexts*. She is currently working on two projects: an article on disabled male characters in the nineteenth-century British novel and a piece on language and the "fallen woman."

Paul K. Longmore, associate professor of history at San Francisco State University, San Francisco, California, specializes in early American history and the history of people with disabilities. His book, *The Invention of George Washington* (Berkeley, CA: University of California Press, 1988), is a study of Washington as a political actor and conscious shaper of his political image. Longmore was featured in the documentary film *George Washington: The Man Who Wouldn't Be King,* on the PBS series *The American Experience* (November 1992). He has also been interviewed regarding disability-related issues on ABC's *Nightline* and *World News Tonight,* as well as NBC's *Today Show.* Currently he is researching a cultural history of depictions of people with disabilities in motion pictures and television.

Madonne Miner is associate professor of English and adjunct faculty in women's studies at the University of Wyoming, Laramie, Wyoming. In 1984 she published *Insatiable Appetites: Twentieth Century American Women's Best-sellers* (Westport, CT: Greenwood Press, 1984). Since then, she has published essays on fiction by Marge Piercy, Toni Morrison, Kate Chopin, Tillie Olsen, and Margaret Atwood; on the film *Pretty Woman* and television show "Murphy Brown"; and on gender dynamics in women's studies classrooms.

David T. Mitchell is an assistant professor of English at Northern Michigan University. He has published essays on shared narrative strategies in the writings of contemporary women of color such as Louise Erdrich, Julia Alvarez, and Cristina Garcia. Recently, he has codirected a documentary video entitled, "VITAL SIGNS: Crip Culture Talks Back," which uses activist footage, performances, dramatic readings, and interviews by academics and artists with disabilities to discuss the evolution of a culture of disability. He is currently writing a book-length manuscript entitled, *Narrative Prosthesis: Incapacity, Idiosyncrasy and Immobility in Contemporary Art and Theory.*

Caroline Molina is assistant professor of German at Lawrence University, Appleton, Wisconsin. She holds degrees in Comparative Literature from the University of California-Riverside, the University of Wisconsin-Madison, the University of Bonn, and Harvard University. She has published on a wide range of topics, including contemporary drama, narrative theory, dramatic theory, women's writing, and film. With Reinhold Grimm, she has coedited *Gerhart*

Hauptmann's Plays: Before Daybreak, The Weavers, The Beaver Coat (New York: Continuum, 1995) and *Friedrich Nietzsche's Philosophical Writings* (New York: Continuum, 1995). Her book *Tragic Daughters: Women, Contemporary Drama, and the Tradition of Domestic Tragedy* is forthcoming.

Felicity A. Nussbaum is professor of English at the University of California, Los Angeles. She is most recently the author of *Torrid Zones: Maternity, Sexuality, and Empire in Eighteenth-Century Narratives* (Baltimore, MD: Johns Hopkins University Press, 1995) and *The Autobiographical Subject: Gender and Ideology in Eighteenth-Century England* (Baltimore, MD: Johns Hopkins University Press, 1989), corecipient of the Louis Gottschalk Prize. Her current work focuses on issues of gender and deformity in the Enlightenment period.

Martin S. Pernick is professor of History at the University of Michigan, and holds a joint appointment in the Inteflex combined BS-MD program. He has also taught medical history at Harvard University and at the Pennsylvania State University Medical Center. Pernick has written two books, *The Black Stork: Eugenics and the Death of "Defective" Babies in American Medicine and Motion Pictures since 1915* (New York: Oxford University Press, 1996) and *A Calculus of Suffering: Pain, Professionalism, and Anesthesia in Nineteenth-Century America* (New York: Columbia University Press, 1985) and is currently working on *Changing Meanings of Death, 1740–1990.* His other publications range from yellow fever in 1793 Philadelphia, motion pictures in the TB and VD campaigns of the 1910s and 20s, and the history of informed consent.

Sharon L. Snyder is adjunct assistant professor of English at Northern Michigan University. Recently, she codirected the documentary "VITAL SIGNS: Crip Culture Talks Back" (Brace Yourselves Productions, Marquette, MI, 48 min., beta sp, 1996), which was awarded the Grand Prize at the 18th annual world congress of Rehabilitation International. Her current research traces the cultural history of representations of disability.

Rosemarie Garland Thomson is assistant professor of English at Howard University in Washington, D.C. Her essays on disability in literature and culture appear in *American Literature, Feminist Studies,* and *Radical Teacher.* She has edited *Freakery: Cultural Spectacles of the Extraordinary Body* (New York: New York University Press, 1996), and is the author of a study on disability and literature entitled, *Extraordinary Bodies: Figuring Disability in American Culture and Literature* (New York: Columbia University Press, 1996).

David D. Yuan received his doctorate in English and American Literature at Stanford University, and is the author of the forthcoming article "The Celebrity Freak: Michael Jackson's 'Grotesque Glory'" in *Freakery: Cultural Spectacles of the Extraordinary Body,* edited by Rosemarie Garland Thomson (New York: New York University Press, 1996). He is completing a dissertation provisionally titled "Curious Bodies: The Body as Spectacle and the American Body Politic, 1840–1898."